BODY/EMBODIMENT

Body/Embodiment
Symbolic Interaction and the Sociology of the Body

Edited by

DENNIS WASKUL
Minnesota State University, Mankato, USA

and

PHILLIP VANNINI
Royal Roads University, Canada

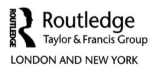

Routledge
Taylor & Francis Group

LONDON AND NEW YORK

First published 2006 by Ashgate Publishing

2 Park Square, Milton Park, Abingdon, Oxfordshire OX14 4RN
52 Vanderbilt Avenue, New York, NY 10017

Routledge is an imprint of the Taylor & Francis Group, an informa business

First issued in paperback 2020

British Library Cataloguing in Publication Data
Body/embodiment : symbolic interaction and the sociology of
    the body
    1.Body, Human - Social aspects 2.Body, Human - Symbolic
    aspects
    I.Waskul, Dennis D., 1969- II.Vannini, Phillip
    306.4'613

Library of Congress Cataloging-in-Publication Data
Body/embodiment : symbolic interaction and the sociology of the body / edited by Dennis Waskul and Phillip Vannini.
        p. cm.
    Includes index.
    ISBN 0-7546-4726-9
    1. Body, Human--Social aspects. 2. Symbolic interactionism. I. Waskul, Dennis D., 1969- II. Vannini, Phillip.

    HM636.B584 2006
    306.4--dc22

                                                                    2006009524

ISBN 13 : 978-0-7546-4726-3 (hbk)
ISBN 13 : 978-0-367-60394-6 (pbk)

Contents

List of Figures

Author Biographies

MICHAEL ATKINSON is Associate Professor of Sociology at McMaster University. His main teaching and research interests focus on body modification, violence in global sports cultures, masculine aesthetics, and figurational sociology. He has conducted ethnographic research ventures with ticket scalpers, tattoo enthusiasts, Straightedge youth, and elite-level endurance athletes. Michael is author of *Tattooed: The Sociogenesis of a Body Art* (University of Toronto Press, 2003), and co-author (with Kevin Young) of the forthcoming book, *Sport, Deviance and Social Control* (Human Kinetics). He has published in diverse academic journals including *The Canadian Review of Sociology and Anthropology*, *Sociology of Sport Journal*, *Body & Society*, *Sex Roles*, *Youth & Society* and *International Review of the Sociology of Sport*. Michael's current ethnographic projects include studies of cosmetic surgery, criminal violence in Canadian ice hockey, and cultures of ergogenic drug use among male athletes. He is Associate Editor at the journals *Deviant Behavior* and the *Sociology of Sport Journal*, and was recipient of the Social Sciences and Humanities Research Council of Canada's Aurora Award in 2004.

PAUL ATKINSON is Distinguished Research Professor in Sociology at Cardiff University, UK. He is Associate Director of the ESRC Research Centre on Social and Economic Aspects of Genomics. His publications include: *Ethnography: Principles in Practice* (with Martyn Hammersley, 2nd edition, Routledge, 1995), *The Clinical Experience* (2nd edition, Ashgate, 1997), *The Ethnographic Imagination* (Routledge, 1990), *Understanding Ethnographic Texts* (Sage, 1992), *Medical Talk and Medical Work* (Sage, 1995), *Fighting Familiarity* (with Sara Delamont, Hampton, 1995), *Making Sense of Qualitative Data* (with Amanda Coffey, Sage, 1996), *Sociological Readings and Re-Readings* (Ashgate, 1996), *The Doctoral Experience* (with Sara Delamont and Odette Parry, Routledge, 2000), *Interactionism* (with William Housley, Sage, 2003), *Risky Relations* (with Katie Featherstone, Aditya Bharadwaj and Angus Clarke, Berg, 2005). His ethnography of the Welsh National Opera Company will be published as *Everyday Arias* (AltaMira, 2006). Together with Sara Delamont he edits the journal *Qualitative Research*. He was co-editor of *The Handbook of Ethnography* (Sage, 2001).

BRONWYN BEISTLE obtained her Ph.D. in English Literature from the University of Pennsylvania in 2004. Her dissertation, titled "Honeyed Secrets" was an investigation of the meanings of Authority, Sexuality, and Flower Imagery in Women's Literature from Wollsonecraft to McGukian.

EMILY M. BOYD is a Ph.D. candidate in the Sociology Department at Florida State University. Her research interests include gender inequality, sociology of the body, identity, interaction, and mass media. She is currently examining discourse used on the television program "Extreme Makeover" to discuss bodies, body modification, and identity.

KERI BRANDT is Assistant Professor of sociology at Fort Lewis University. Her dissertation (University of Colorado, Boulder) on the human-horse communication process draws from three years (2001–2004) of in-depth interviews and participant observation and explores how the two species co-create an embodied language system to construct a world of shared meaning.

SPENCER E. CAHILL is currently Professor of Sociology at the University of South Florida. He is the immediate past editor of *Social Psychology Quarterly* and former coeditor of the *Journal of Contemporary Ethnography*. His articles and essays have appeared in such journals as *Social Problems*, *Sociological Theory*, and *Symbolic Interaction*.

KATHY CHARMAZ is Professor of Sociology and Coordinator of the Faculty Writing Program at Sonoma State University. She teaches in the areas of sociological theory, social psychology, qualitative methods, health and illness, and gerontology. As Coordinator of the Faculty Writing Program, she assists the faculty in writing for publication and leads three faculty seminars on professional writing. She has written or co-edited six books including her 2006 volume, *Constructing Grounded Theory: A Practical Guide Through Qualitative Analysis*, with Sage Publications, London and *Good Days, Bad Days: The Self in Chronic Illness and Time*, which won awards from the Pacific Sociological Association and the Society for the Study of Symbolic Interaction. She has also written a number of recent articles and chapters on grounded theory as well as on topics in medical sociology and social psychology. Charmaz serves as Vice-president of Alpha Kappa Delta, the international honorary society for sociology, and has served as the president of the Pacific Sociological Association, Vice-President of the Society for the Study of Symbolic Interaction, editor of *Symbolic Interaction*, and chair of the Medical Sociology Section of the American Sociological Association.

NICK CROSSLEY is Professor of Sociology at the University of Manchester (UK). He has published many papers on "body matters" and a book (*The Social Body: Habit, Identity and Desire*, Sage, 2001). He is currently completing a second book on the body (*Reflexive Embodiment in Late Modern Societies*, McGraw-Hill) and is conducting research on "working out," "dieting," and the martial arts. His other academic interests include social theory and the sociology of social movements.

SARA DELAMONT is Reader in Sociology at Cardiff University. She is co-editor of *The Handbook of Ethnography* (Sage, 2001) with P. Atkinson, Coffey, Lofland and Lofland, and co-editor of the journal *Qualitative Research* with Paul Atkinson. The capoeira fieldwork follows other projects in educational ethnography, and is intended both to be intrinsically interesting, and also to follow Becker's injunction to make the familiar strange, as argued in *Fighting Familiarity* (Hampton Press, 1995) written with Paul Atkinson.

CHARLES EDGLEY was lured out of retirement after a long career at Oklahoma State University. He is currently Professor and Chair of Sociology and Anthropology at the University of Arkansas at Little Rock. Charles has written, edited, or revised seven books. With the late Dennis Brissett, he authored *Life as Theater* (Aldine de Gruyter, 1990; recently re-released in a new printing by Aldine/Transaction with a new introduction by Robert A. Stebbins) and *A Nation of Meddlers* (Westview, 2000). He has published numerous works on a variety of subjects in symbolic interaction, dramaturgy, death and dying, and health and fitness.

CAROL BROOKS GARDNER is a Professor of Sociology at Indianapolis University, Indiana. A student of Erving Goffman and author of *Passing By: Gender & Public Harassment* (University of California Press, 1997), Carol has also authored articles on topics such as public place fear of crime, stalking, gaybaiting, the social lives of people with disabilities, and the sociology of pregnancy. She has published in journals including *Social Problems*, *Journal of Contemporary Ethnography*, *Sociological Inquiry*, and *Perspectives on Social Problems*; numerous articles in edited collections; encyclopaedia entries including stigma, public harassment, and street remarks.

WILLIAM P. GRONFEIN is an Associate Professor of Sociology at Indiana University, Indianapolis. He has written on topics including Goffman's analysis of mental hospitals and mental patients, the deinstitutionalization of the mentally ill, the use of subjective information in statistical models, and medical malpractice. He has published in journals such as *American Sociological Review*, *Journal of Health & Social Behavior*, *Journal of Health Politics, Policy, & Law*, *Law & Contemporary Problems*, *Perspectives on Social Problems*, and *Social Problems*. In addition, his work has appeared in several edited collections dealing with the work of Erving Goffman.

MATT HELD is a graduate student in Sociology at the University of Houston. His first experience with sociological research on athletics was to serve as an undergraduate research assistant for Dr. Joseph Kotarba's evaluation study of the "Play It Smart" Program in Houston, Texas, sponsored by the National Football Foundation. Matt is currently analyzing injury and performance among individual sports athletes.

RICHARD HUGGINS is the Assistant Dean of Social Sciences and Law, Oxford Brookes University. Richard has co-authored *Politics: An Introduction* (1997/2002, Routledge) and *New Media and Politics* (2001, Sage). He has written numerous chapters for books including *Whose Europe?* (1999, Blackwell Oxford), *Unity and Diversity in the New Europe* (2000, Peter Lang), *Vox Populi: Vox Dei* (2002, Hampton). Richard is a consultant editor for *Encyclopedia of the City* (2004, Routledge) and has authored articles published in *Innovations*, *Javnost*, *Telematics and Informatics*, *Drugs, Policy, Prevention and Education*, and *Parliamentary Brief*.

JOSEPH KOTARBA is former president of the Society for the Study of Symbolic Interaction and Professor of Sociology at the University of Houston. He is author of *Chronic Pain: Its Social Dimensions* (Sage, 1983) and editor of *Postmodern Existential Sociology* (University of Chicago Press, 1984, with Andrea Fontana) and *The Existential Self in Society* (AltaMira Press, 2002, with John Johnson). His numerous articles on music, health, and symbolic interactionist theory have appeared in such journals as *Symbolic Interaction*, *Journal of Contemporary Ethnography*, *Studies in Symbolic Interaction*, *Qualitative Health Research*, *Research in the Sociology of Health Care*, *Qualitative Inquiry* and *AIDS Education and Prevention*.

LEE F. MONAGHAN is Senior Lecturer in Sociology at the University of Limerick, Ireland. His ethnographic research draws from, and contributes to, the sociology of the body and embodied sociology. He is the author of *Bodybuilding, Drugs and Risk* (Routledge, 2001) and numerous articles on the body. He is currently working on a book titled *Masculinities and the Obesity Debate* (forthcoming, Routledge).

DON MYNATT is currently working on his Master's Degree at the University of Memphis in the Department of Sociology. He is also exploring his options for a doctorate. His areas of interest include epistemology, poverty, social justice, politics, and social policy.

SARA RENÉE PRESLEY is a graduate student in Sociology at the University of Memphis. She is currently conducting research on the discourses female exotic dancers use when constructing the identities of their clientele. Sara's other research interests include sociology of the body, human sexuality, and sexual deviance. Upon completing her Masters Degree, Sara plans to go on for a Ph.D. in Sociology.

ERICA OWENS is an Assistant Professor in the Division of Sociology and Anthropology at West Virginia University. Her main areas of interest are romantic partnership and identity, and her work has been published or is forthcoming in journals including *Qualitative Inquiry*, *Symbolic Interaction*, and *Family Relations*. She serves on the editorial boards of *Journal of Family Issues* and *Marriage and Family Review*.

CAROL RAMBO is an Associate Professor of Sociology at The University of Memphis. She co-edited *Everyday Sexism in the Third Millennium* with Barb Zsembik and Joe Feagin (Routledge, 1997) and has published on topics such as exotic dancing, childhood sexual abuse, and mentally retarded parenting. Carol has published in journals including *Deviant Behavior, Journal of Contemporary Ethnography, Qualitative Inquiry, Mental Retardation, Journal of Aging Studies* and *Perspectives on Social Problems.* To learn more about her latest research interests, visit her website at www.carolrambo.com.

DANA ROSENFELD is a Qualitative Medical Sociologist whose research interests centre on the intersection between health, identity, and embodiment. Her early work examining the identity work of lesbian and gay elders (specifically, how the early experience of a stigmatized homosexuality, on the one hand, and the emergence of gay liberation on the other, inform homosexual identity across the life course) produced a monograph entitled *The Changing of the Guard: Lesbian and Gay Elders, Identity, and Social Change* (Temple University Press, 2002), and grounded her current research into the interpretation, management, and regulation of the body, particularly the body in ill health, and their impact on identity and everyday life. Rosenfeld has also published on the use of the life course by medicine to produce unequal relations between patients and medical agents, and on the experiences of chronic illness, acute illness, and injury. She is the lead editor of *Medicalized Masculinities* (Temple University Press, 2006).

CLINTON R. SANDERS is a Professor in the Sociology Department at the University of Connecticut. He has served as President (2002-2003) and Vice-president (1994-1995) of the Society for the Study of Symbolic Interaction. Sanders' work focuses on cultural production, deviant behaviour, ethnographic research, and anthrozoology. He is author of *Understanding Dogs: Living and Working with Canine Companions* (Temple University Press, 1999) and co-author (with Arnold Arluke) of *Regarding Animals* (Temple University Press, 1996) both of which received the SSSI's Charles Horton Cooley Award. He is also the author of *Customizing the Body: The Art and Culture of Tattooing* (Temple University Press, 1989).

DOUGLAS SCHROCK is an Assistant Professor in the Sociology Department at Florida State University. He is interested in how emotions, identity, embodiment, and storytelling are implicated in reproducing and challenging inequality. He is currently examining micropolitical interactions in a men's anti-battering program.

NEIL STEPHENS is a Research Associate at the ESRC Centre for Economic and Social Aspects of Genomics (CESAGen), at the School of Social Sciences at Cardiff University, Wales, where he is conducting an ethnography of the UK and Spanish Stem Cell Banks. Concurrently he is also conducting ethnographic research on *Capoeira* teaching in the UK. He is also actively publishing from his Ph.D. thesis exploring the social construction of macroeconomic debate.

PHILLIP VANNINI has published theoretical and empirical works dealing with semiotics and symbolic interactionism, and the semiotics of the body in *Symbolic Interaction*, the *Journal of Popular Culture*, *CTheory*, *Cultural Studies <> Critical Methodologies*, *Studies in Symbolic Interaction*, *Life in the Wires* (edited by Arthur and MariLouise Kroker, NWP, 2004) and *net.SeXXX* (edited by Dennis D. Waskul, Peter Lang, 2004). Phillip is also currently co-editing (with Hans Bakker) *Sociology and Semiotics: From Peirce to Wiley*, and has co-edited the winter 2006 issue of *Symbolic Interaction* on popular music and everyday life. He is a Research Fellow in the School of Communication and Culture at Royal Roads University in Victoria, Canada.

DENNIS D. WASKUL is an Assistant Professor of Sociology at Minnesota State University, Mankato. He is author of *Self-Games and Body-Play: Personhood in Online Chat and Cybersex* (Peter Lang, 2003) and editor of *net.SeXXX: Readings on Sex, Pornography, and the Internet* (Peter Lang, 2004). His published empirical works have explored a variety of topics including Internet sex, fantasy role-playing, and chronic illness.

RACHEL WESTFALL is a *Michael Smith Foundation for Health Research* and *Canadian Institutes of Health Research* Postdoctoral Fellow in the Sociology department at the University of Victoria. Her current research utilizes mixed qualitative and quantitative methods to consider how social factors impact women's health and well-being after childbirth. She has published articles on women's experiences with prolonged pregnancy (in *Social Science and Medicine*), herbal medicine use in pregnancy and postpartum (in *Complementary Therapies in Nursing and Midwifery*, *Canadian Journal of Midwifery Research and Practice*, *Journal of Herbal Pharmacotherapy*, and *Advances in Therapy*), and historical and contemporary issues regarding midwifery care. Her research interests include the subjective experience of childbearing, human agency, alternative health movements, and the practical and symbolic uses of plants in human interactions.

Chapter 1

Introduction:
The Body in Symbolic Interaction

Dennis D. Waskul and Phillip Vannini

The body social is many things: the prime symbol of the self, but also of the society; it is something we have, yet also what we are; it is both subject and object at the same time; it is individual and personal, as unique as a fingerprint or odourplume, yet it is also common to all humanity.... The body is both an individual creation, physically and phenomenologically, and a cultural product; it is personal, and also state property.

Anthony Synnott, *The Body Social* (1993)

The body and experiences of embodiment have always been prominent in sociology. As Synnott (1993:4) suggests, we can "usefully reconsider the body at the heart of sociology, rather than peripheral to the discipline, and more importantly at the heart of our social lives and our sense of self." From this standpoint, even a cursory review reveals the body and embodiment as fundamental to numerous esteemed sociological interests including gender, race and ethnicity, sexuality, health and medicine, disability, sport, aging, death and dying. Sociologists have long articulated strong and provocative statements about the body and experiences of embodiment. Nevertheless, as Shilling (2003:17) rightly suggests, "the body has historically been something of an 'absent presence' in sociology" – an object and subject of analysis that is both "at the very heart of the sociological imagination" and "absent in the sense that sociology has rarely focused in a sustained manner on the embodied human as an object of importance in its own right."

However, since the early 1990s the body has come to bear a veritable bonanza of contemporary sociological interest. On the heels of significant social, cultural, political, and technological change, the body and experiences of embodiment appear substantially more visible than ever before – conditions that have stimulated sociological interests in a manner that is decidedly more direct, focused, and sustained compared to previous and legacy sociology. From the diffusion of plastic surgery to the mainstreaming of tattooing, from fashion to fitness, from shifting health practices to profound changes in the experience and treatment of illness, from continued preoccupations with youthfulness to the changing definitions of the aging body, from sexual to athletic performance, contemporary scholarly literatures reveal a steady flow of provocative new sociological investigations, speculations, and research inquiries on the body and experiences of embodiment.

The sheer volume and diversity of contemporary scholarly work that now characterize "the sociology of the body" is itself impressive. Simply considering a relatively small sample of published books, it is apparent that bodies are socially constructed (Crossley 2001; Featherstone, Hepworth, and Turner 1991; Shilling 2003; Synnott 1993; Turner 1984), gendered (Backett-Milburn and McKie 2001), sexed and sexualized (Fausto-Sterling 2000; Grosz, Probyn, and Grosz 1995; Laqueur 1992), customized (Demello 2000; Featherstone 2000; Gay and Whittington 2002; Hewitt 1997; Mifflin 2001; Pitts 2003; Sanders 1989) as well as fashioned (Calefato 2004; Entwistle 2000; Guy, Green, and Banim 2003; Virgili and Hodkinson 2002), electrified and digitized (Springer 1996), posthuman (Halberstam and Livingston 1995), objectified (Foster 1995; Tebbel 2003), overtaken by panic (Kroker and Kroker 1987), ascended to the heights of the mystical and sacred (Moore 1998; Newell 2002) as well as descended to the depths of the stigmatized and the freakish (Covino 2004; Elson 2004; Goffman 1963; Lebesco 2004; Thomson 1996), commodified (Falk 1994; Scheper-Hughes and Wacquant 2003), subject to the discipline of fitness, training, and diet (Moore 1997; Pronger 2002), fetishized (Stratton 2001) and, of course, subject to the politics of gender and sexual orientation (Atkins 1998; Birke 1999; Bordo 2000; Brook 1999; Burt 1995; Weitz 2002), and race and ethnicity (Mohanram 2004). Indeed, "there are many bodies social, and they are hard to count. Equally evident, the meanings imputed to the body are various: definitions are legion and there is little consensus" (Synnott 1993:228–229).

The "sociology of the body" is increasingly living up to its implicit promise: a specialized object and subject of analysis that reflects all the diversity one would expect of sociology. Thus, the bewildering array of sociolog*ies* of the body is, in fact, an encouraging sign: just as there is not a singular sociology, neither is there a singular sociology of the body. Various sociological traditions emphasize sundry dynamics and processes, a fact that is neither surprising nor alarming. After all, just as there is not a singular sociology of the body, nor is the body itself a singular object or subject of analysis. The body and experiences of embodiment *are* layered, nuanced, complex, and multifaceted – at the level of human subjective experience, interaction, social organization, institutional arrangements, cultural processes, society, and history.

While recognizing that the sociology of the body is, essentially, a dialogue among many diverse interests and points of view, this book concisely articulates and illustrates one major approach. Drawing exclusively from symbolic interactionism – an increasingly prevalent theoretical base of contemporary sociology (see Maines 2001) – we identify major interactionist frameworks for conceiving bodies and experiences of embodiment, exemplify the utility of those insights in empirically grounded contexts, and speculate about broader issues.

The Bodies of Symbolic Interaction

Symbolic interactionists utilize a constellation of related theoretical frameworks that are loosely bound by the pragmatist tradition. Owing primarily to the works of William James, John Dewey, Charles Sanders Peirce, Charles Horton Cooley, and George Herbert Mead the core assumptions of American pragmatism represent a nucleus of ideas that generally characterize the unique contributions of symbolic interaction. Although somewhat elusive, it is possible to identity several organizing assumptions of American pragmatism. Among the most important, pragmatism emphasizes human beings as active and creative agents; a human world that both shapes the doings of people and is fashioned by the doings of people; a determined emphasis on how subjectivity, meaning, and consciousness do not exist prior to experience, but are emergent in action and interaction; a grounded examination of practical problems; an approach that situates action as a primary conceptual and analytical focus (Reynolds 2003:45–46).

Pragmatism is not "a single unified body of philosophic ideas" (Martindale 1960:297), and it is even described "as a pseudo-philosophic formulation" (Mead 1936:97). Consequently, pragmatism has often shifted its fundamental formulations, direction, and form (Reynolds 2003). Thus, it is all the more understandable that, while bound by a generally shared pragmatic foundation, there remains ample diversity in the ways interactionists envisage, employ, and articulate those core assumptions. This diversity is often associated with familiar theoretical models that are commonly allied with and collectively comprise the interactionist tradition – symbolic interaction, social semiotics, dramaturgy, phenomenology, and narrative/ life history.

For these reasons, we suggest that contemporary interactionism presents both a clear articulation of body/embodiment and a variety of approaches that uniquely emphasize particular characteristics. Thus, on one hand, we can identify a relatively coherent interactionist conceptual orientation to the body and embodiment. On the other hand, we can also identify nuances and particularities that are variously emphasized, largely in association with the assorted theoretical traditions of interactionism.

From a general interactionist perspective, the body is always more than a tangible, physical, corporeal object – infinitely more than "a mere skeleton wrapped in muscles and stuffed with organs" (Moore 1998:3) – the body is also an enormous vessel of meaning of utmost significance to both personhood and society. The body is a *social* object, which is to say that "the body as an object cannot be separated from the body as a subject; they are emergent from one another" (Waskul and van der Riet 2002:510). From this perspective, the term "embodiment" refers quite precisely to the process by which the object-body is actively experienced, produced, sustained, and/or transformed as a subject-body. As explained by Waskul and van der Riet (2002:488): "a person does not 'inhabit' a static object body but is subjectively embodied in a fluid, emergent, and negotiated process of being. In this process, body, self, and social interaction are interrelated to such an extent that distinctions between them are not only permeable and shifting but also actively manipulated and configured."

In this way, interactionists generally emphasize that "the body (noun) is embodied (verb)" (Waskul and van der Riet 2002:488) – the question is *how* and by *what means*? Various answers to these latter questions reveal the diversity of interactionism. Furthermore, the various traditions that comprise interactionism have related but slightly different orientations that emphasize related but slightly different dimensions of the body and embodiment. Thus, we can identify and detail the "bodies of symbolic interaction" with relative precision: the looking-glass body, the dramaturgical body, the phenomenological body, the socio-semiotic body, and the narrative body.

Before specifying these bodies of interactionism, it is essential that we make one point clear: while, conceptually, it may be useful to recognize the difference between various interactionist theoretical traditions, in practice interactionists rarely adhere to rigid distinctions between them. Interactionists are pragmatic and borrow freely from numerous conceptual frameworks to craft provocative analytical insights. For these reasons, the bodies of interactionism are not real in any inflexible empirical or conceptual sense. In fact, at one level there is no such thing as a "looking-glass body" or a "dramaturgical body" or any of the other bodies we shall detail. These words are abstractions – ways of thinking about, seeing, and understanding the body and experiences of embodiment. They are heuristic devices and, consequently, more or less useful depending on purposes and applications. Furthermore, there is considerable overlapping between these various bodies of interactionism and, as the chapters of this book illustrate, it is unusual for an interactionist to exclusively champion one or another. An interactionist is much more likely to borrow key ideas from many of these "bodies of interactionism" to fashion a more complete understanding. However, for our intents and purposes, it is helpful to begin by thinking about the bodies of interactionism independently.

The Looking-Glass Body: Reflexivity as Embodiment

> What we call "me," "mine," or "myself" is, then, not something separate from the general life, but the most interesting part of it, a part whose interest arises from the very fact that it is both general and individual.... To think of it as apart from society is a palpable absurdity.... There is no sense of "I" ... without its correlative sense of you, or he, or they.... A social self of this sort might be called the reflected or looking-glass self.
>
> Charles Horton Cooley, *Human Nature and Social Order* (1902)

German sociologist Georg Simmel (1921:358) once wrote that "the eye has a uniquely sociological function. The union and interaction of individuals is based upon mutual glances." Simmel describes this union as "the most direct and purest reciprocity which exists anywhere.... By the glance which reveals the other, one discloses himself. By the same act in which the observer seeks to know the observed, he surrenders himself to be understood by the observer. The eye cannot take unless at the same time it gives. The eye of a person discloses his own soul when he seeks to uncover that of another." Simmel understood that the union of a glance is no mere action, but a nuanced form of *inter*action. Or, more tersely stated, "the eye *creates* the I" (Synnott 1993:225, emphasis in original) – an insight most commonly associated with Charles Horton Cooley, an early pioneer of what would come to be symbolic interaction.

The "looking-glass body" obviously and intentionally resonates with Cooley's familiar "looking-glass self" (1902:151–152). As Cooley explains, one can only reflect and form images of one's self from the imaginary perspective of others. In this basic process, Cooley identifies "three principal elements: the imagination of our appearance to the other person; the imagination of his judgment of that appearance; and some sort of self-feeling, such as pride or mortification." For these reasons, Cooley (1902:87) argued, "the imaginations which people have of one another are the solid facts of society," self and, as we suggest, the body.

Bodies are seen and the act of seeing is reflexive in precisely the same way that Cooley identifies. When we gaze upon bodies of others we necessarily interpret what we observe. Similarly, others imagine what we may be seeing and feeling, thus completing the reflections of the looking-glass. Obviously, this looking-glass body is not a direct reflection of other's judgments – it is an *imagined* reflection built of cues gleaned from others. Reflexivity is then to be understood as a necessary condition of embodiment, and embodiment must be understood as a form of reflexivity. For Mead (1934) it is precisely this tendency towards reflexivity that characterizes embodiment as a temporal process (see Crossley 2001, and Chapter Two): "the I and the me manifest two distinct forms of temporality: the I embodies and repeats its history in the form of the habit; the me, by contrast, is constructed in the web of narrative discourse and imaginative re-presentation which the I spins in its various reflexive activities and projects" (2001:148).

It is precisely to reflexive embodiment that Nick Crossley turns to in the opening chapter of Part One. Crossley argues that symbolic interactionism's pragmatist tradition – and in particular the Cooley-Mead heritage – offers sociologists of the body a rich and nuanced understanding of embodiment; one that puts a premium on the role of social networks in constituting the meanings of the human body. Social networks and their place in the formation of the looking-glass body are also the focus of Chapter Three. In that chapter, Kathy Charmaz and Dana Rosenfeld explore how from the perspective of chronically ill and disabled people, images of self and the body in space and time become twisted, blurred, or magnified. As new, discomforting images of self arise from a changed bodily appearance, tensions between bodily feelings and views of its appearance to self and others emerge, prompting individuals to strategically manage the preservation of their self-concepts in spite of bodily decay. Finally, in Chapter Four, Douglas Schrock and Emily M. Boyd draw upon ethnographic data in order to understand how reflexivity shapes the lived experiences and instrumental strategies of transsexuals undergoing status passage. Reflexivity here is manifested in complex articulations of concealment and revelation – intrapersonal and interpersonal communication processes by way of which transsexuals retrain, reshape, and redefine their newly gendered bodies in manners that are perceived as authentic by themselves and others.

As these examples illustrate Cooley's "looking-glass" reflects unto the body in an interpretive process that is, perhaps, the most elemental form by which bodies are interactively embodied. Even so, while the looking-glass body details an important basic process, it leaves many questions open and unanswered. How, exactly, are these reflections constructed? By what means? To what extent are those reflections manipulated? How is this looking-glass body related to broader interaction-, institutional-, social-, cultural-, and moral-order? The remaining bodies of interactionism, although generally sharing this basic looking-glass insight, provide a framework for more precisely handling these latter questions.

The Dramaturgical Body: Body as Performance

Critics sometimes fault Erving Goffman (1959:253) for boldly regarding the body as a "peg" on which a person's self is "hung for a time." Critics have a valid point – the body is seldom so inert; we are mistaken when we so casually dismiss the body as a mere "peg." These criticisms, however, generally miss the point. Considering key works, especially *Stigma* (1963) and "Territories of the Self" (1971), it is apparent that Goffman was quite aware of the significance of the body to identity, social order, and emotional order – and in a manner that is personal and communal, private and political, confidential and public all at once. More than a mere "peg," Goffman and the dramaturgical tradition supply a highly sophisticated framework for understanding the body and experiences of embodiment.

Stated simply, the dramaturgical body is embedded in social practices – a basic insight that dramaturgists share with the anthropological tradition: "the human body has to be constantly and systematically produced, sustained, and presented in everyday life and therefore the body is best regarded as a potentiality which is realized and actualized through a variety of social regulated activities or practices" (Turner 1984:24). This is a significant emphasis that clearly intersects with the pragmatic tradition of symbolic interaction: people do not merely "have" a body – people actively *do* a body. The body is fashioned, crafted, negotiated, manipulated and largely in ritualized social and cultural conventions. Hijacking a few often cited words from Goffman (1959:252–253, emphasis in original) magnifies this emphasis:

> In our society the character one performs and one's self are somewhat equated and this self-as-character is usually seen as something housed within the body of its possessor.... I suggest that this view is ... a bad analysis.... While this image is entertained *concerning* the individual ... this [body] itself does not derive from its possessor, but from the whole scene of his action, being generated by that attribute of local events which renders them interpretable by witnesses. A correctly staged and preformed scene leads the audience to impute a [body] to a preformed character, but this imputation – this [body] – is a *product* of a scene that comes off, and is not a *cause* of it. The [body], then as a performed character, is not an organic thing that has a specific location, whose fundamental fate is to be born to mature, and to die; it is a dramatic effect arising diffusely from a scene that is presented, and the characteristic issue, the crucial concern, is whether it will be credited or discredited. In analyzing the [body] then we are drawn from its possessor, from the person who will profit or lose most by it, for he and his [flesh] merely provide a peg on which something of collaborative manufacture will be hung for a time. And the means for

producing and maintaining [bodies] do not reside inside the peg; in fact these means are often bolted down in social establishments.

Our commandeering of Goffman's words is somewhat unfair but, even so, it does effectively magnify the essential wisdom of dramaturgy: if the body is something that people do then it is in the doings of people – not their flesh – that the body is embod*ied*; an *active* process by which the body is literally real(ized) and made meaningful. The body is wrought of action and interaction in situated social encounters and often by means of institutionalized ritual. In communicative action the body comes to be.

The dramaturgical body posits two major analytical emphases. First, the dramaturgical body is emergent from a process by which people necessarily express themselves and unavoidably impress themselves upon others. Or, stated slightly differently, people embody the body "in the manner in which they express themselves in interaction with similarly expressive others" (Brissett and Edgley 1990:3). Although somewhat oversimplified, it is fair to suggest that this expressive and impressive emphasis is akin to the looking-glass body – it is a more precisely framed approach to how the body is established in the ongoing process of association with other people as "a behavioral, socially emergent, problematic, variable, and in fact arbitrary, concoction of human interaction" (Brissett and Edgley 1990:3). Second, dramaturgy details one framework for understanding of how social and emotional order is sustained in dramatic body-rituals that are bound by and constituents of moral order. It is in this latter emphasis that dramaturgy most strongly asserts its most powerful insight: the body and experiences of embodiment are *produced* in the doings of people by social and cultural rituals that are personal *and* communal.

The dramaturgical body reveals an equally broad range of applications. For example, in Chapter Five, Spencer E. Cahill argues that we do not have one body, but rather we have one body that is (at least) divided in two: a public body for all to see and a private body that is concealed from civic view and shared only with intimates. Cahill magnifies the essential dramaturgical point: the public body is *made* public and the private body is *kept* private, and both processes are accomplished through ritual social conventions that are deeply connected to the social-, emotional-, and moral-order. In Chapter Six, Carol Brooks Gardner and William P. Gronfein explore Erving Goffman's analysis of the bodily "territories of the self" (Goffman 1971). Gardner and Gronfein expand the eight territories that Goffman originally proposed. They consider bodies that are fragile or troublesome for owners, in particular, the bodies of some people with disabilities. Instead of viewing people with disabilities as at a continual disadvantage in public, Gardner and Gronfein emphasize the ways in which the self can selectively be armoured using Goffman's primarily spatial and verbal interactive preserves. In Chapter Seven, Paul Atkinson turns his attention to the theatre as a site of everyday life interaction, rather than as a metaphorical resource for interpreting other social domains. Atkinson examines how through the rehearsal process opera directors and performers negotiate the creation of roles and relations through the physical accomplishment of gesture, orientation, gaze, and movement within the space defined by the stage set. Finally, in Chapter Eight, Neil Stephens and Sara Delamont focus their attention on the performance of *Capoeira*, the Brazilian dance/martial art whose growing popularity throughout Europe and North America has meant that many novice bodies engage in the emulation and admiration of expert performers. It is precisely out of these dynamics of ritual and performance that the bodies as sign-vehicles emerge.

As these chapters illustrate, the dramaturgical body emphasizes human agency within a conceptual and analytical framework that fully contextualizes. The dramaturgical body is a helpful corrective to the widespread assumption that bodies "just are" – an assumption that, as Goffman (1959:252) suggests, is "a bad analysis." Although sometimes intentional and manipulated – but often times not – the body is always performed, staged, and presented: the theatre of the body are the raw materials by which the drama of our everyday embodied life are produced.

The Phenomenological Body: Body as Province of Meaning

> All of these worlds – the world of dreams, of imageries, and phantasms, especially the world of art, the world of religious experience, the world of scientific contemplation, the play world of the child, and the world of the insane – are finite provinces of meaning.
>
> Alfred Shutz, *Collected Papers I* (1973)

Edmund Husserl (1893/1917:315) identified the body as a "zero-point of orientation" – a centre for all knowledge and experience; a primordial point of reference: the body inhabits and moves – not in the abstract, but in the concrete, necessarily embodied, and privileged ontological, spatial, and temporal presence of the here and now. As Alfred Shutz (1973:232) further suggests, this world of the here and now is composed of multiple realities that represent "finite provinces of meaning." In this way, phenomenologists firmly establish a focused emphasis on embodied subjects who encounter practical problems in discrete and situated circumstances and thus accentuate an approach akin to the traditions of interactionism: embodied people mindfully resolve pragmatic problems with intention and purpose in social encounters that are situated in broader social, cultural, and institutional milieus.

Phenomenological approaches to the body and embodiment concern thick descriptions of lived experience that reveal meaning in the life-worlds of individuals and groups. Meaning is embedded in our experiences within the world; meaning is not apart from either those embodied experiences or that world – an approach evocative of classic interactionist arguments. In fact, this phenomenological approach sometimes often shares a nearly identical "looking-glass" understanding of the body and experiences of embodiment. For example, in pondering the enigma of the body, Maurice Merleau-Ponty (1974:283, 284–285) suggests:

> The enigma is that my body simultaneously sees and is seen. That which looks at all things can also look at itself and recognize, in what it sees, the "other side" of its power of looking. It sees itself seeing; it touches itself touching; it is visible and sensitive for

itself.... There is a human body when, between seeing and the seen, between touching and the touched, between one eye and the other, between hand and hand, a blending of some sort takes place – when the spark is lit between sensing and the sensible...

However, phenomenological approaches to the body and experiences of embodiment are unique. Phenomenological perspectives uniquely frame the relationship between body and world in at least two major and somewhat contradictory ways. On one hand, owing primarily to Merleau-Ponty, the phenomenological body is marked by somatic *presence*; the chief contribution and founding assumption is that self, society, and symbolic order are constituted through the work of the body (Crossley 1995). On the other hand, following Drew Leder (1990:62), the phenomenological body of the modern world is often marked by corporeal *absence*. The modern world is characterized by work and leisure activities that are organized by outcome-oriented and rational actions that immerse people in goals that are external to the body. Thus, as Shilling (2003:185) suggests, phenomenological approaches may magnify the practical, somatic, and corporeal body; they may also "suggest that the body is relatively unimportant to people's sense of self in the contemporary era." In short, from a phenomenological perspective, we have a body that serves as a fundamental corporeal anchor in the world; we also experience ourselves through numerous "bodies of meaning." These "bodies of meaning" are both literal and metaphorical: meaning is comprised *in* embodied action and the body is interpreted *by* frameworks of meaning.

The importance of phenomenology for our interactionist understanding of the body is well summarized by Lee F. Monaghan in the opening chapter to this part of the book. Monaghan's eclectic approach combines the tools of ethnography, pragmatism, and social phenomenology and effectively argues for the importance of an interpretive sociology in its inevitable corporeality. For Monaghan (2002:507) "the body's primary relationship to the world is practical" and the body of the researcher as well as those of research participants cannot but constitute the primary body of meaning-making. Along these lines in Chapter Ten, Keri Brandt examines the processes of meaning-making occurring between female horse riders – such as Brandt herself – and their equine companions. Brandt argues that the signifying system used by women and horses in interaction is a complex structure of bodily clues, movement, and touch, as well as human bodily sensations – hence making a cogent point for the constitution of intersubjectivity in embodiment and for the body's non-discursive intelligence at the level of habit and somatic sensation.

In Chapter Eleven, Joseph Kotarba and Matt Held examine how women's professional American football reflects in part traditional gender expectations on the behaviour of the female body and how in part it constitutes an alternative to those hegemonic discourses, thus providing these women with an oppositional symbolic zone for the redefinition of their bodies and selves. Through fieldwork and phenomenological interviews Kotarba and Held reflects on how gender body norms inform their behaviour on the field and skill display. The rapport between discursive constructions of the body and bodily experiences is further examined in

Chapter Twelve, in which Richard Huggins focuses on the body of the heroin addict as a discursive construction in British and American popular media and on how the discursive themes of such representations are central to the phenomenological construction of addiction and the addict. In hermeneutic fashion for Huggins representations of the body of the addict act as a conceptual horizon for the perceived social significance of drug use and addiction, while at the same time public discourses inform the production of new representations and discursive constructions, and back again, magnifying the centrality of the symbolic and representational form.

The Socio-Semiotic Body: Body as Trace of Culture

Michel Foucault (1977:154) once remarked that "knowledge is not made for understanding: it is made for cutting." Indeed, much "cutting" characterizes contemporary embodied selves: from the cutting of calories, carbohydrates, sugar, or fatty foods from our diet, to the cutting of hair in a style consistent with the latest fashion, and from the cutting of excessive cellulite or unsightly features with a surgeon's knife, to the cutting of shirt sleeves and skirt lengths. For Foucault such "cutting" is a practice by which power/knowledge leaves traces on the surface and depths of our bodies; technologies of the self, in his words, that operate on the political anatomy of the body. Herein lies the fundamental premise of a socio-semiotic understanding of the body consistent with the interactionist tradition: despite its essential biological nature, as soon as the body becomes an object of discourse it is invested with symbolic meanings and symbolic value – use-value, sign-value, exchange value, and sign-exchange value – through the functioning of a discursive and material order.

Semiological (e.g. Saussurean, structuralist, and post-structuralist) conceptualizations of the body abound in contemporary cultural studies. For most of these, however, actual lived and experienced human bodies disappear from analytical sight – wiped out by conceptual emphasis on the omnipotent forces of culture and discourse (Howson 2005). The structural-semiological body thus yields to the weight of linguistic and cultural determinism, either falling into oblivion (often by the sleight of hand of a post-human, cyborgian textual world), or existing as an experienceless mirroring representation of various dynamics of intertextuality. In contrast, a *social* semiotic and interactionist understanding of the body avoids these pitfalls. For socio-semiotic interactionism there is no body without a reflexive and agentic self and there is no self without a reflexive and agentic body. Embodied interaction is therefore an active process of practical meaning-making (semiosis) occurring in an exo-semiotic field inevitably informed by power relations.

Through the body we perform, express, and present subjectivity to others. Yet, through the same activities, others also judge our body as object by means of appearance and performance. Therefore, like in other interactionist approaches, body is both a subject and object of action. More precisely, however, a socio-semiotic interactionist approach allows us to make sense of the body as source of signification and communication, while understanding how such communication occurs through social interaction with other bodies and selves. Therefore, from a semiotic interactionist perspective bodies' meanings are constituted in relation to the positioning of the body in a system of signification, but the constitution of such meaning fully remains a product of human interaction, rather than a mere result of structural relations (see Vannini 2004).

Socio-semiotic interactionism differs sharply from structural semiology as it builds upon the pragmatist semiotics of Charles Sanders Peirce and the crypto-deconstruction of John Dewey, rather than the idealist and formalist heritage of Saussure (Vannini 2004; also see Halton 1986, 1995; Wiley 1994). From the pragmatic and socio-semiotic perspective of Peirce we can make sense of bodies from three different but *inextricably inter-related* positions. The first position is that of the body as sign-vehicle (or representamen in Peircean terminology). The body as sign-vehicle is an actual lived and experienced body whose signifying and communicating practices *represent* hierarchies of meaning and value existent in the discursive order of our society. Similar to Stone (1962), Goffman (1959), Glassner (1988, 1989) and interactionists associated with other traditions, a socio-semiotic approach magnifies the importance of managing bodily appearance and impressions through careful manipulations, and thus the body as sign vehicle bears the representational traces of culture and power. For example, in Chapter Fourteen, Erica Owens and Bronwyn Beistle critically interpret the sexual meanings of the Black body – as portrayed in some racist personal ads – as both seductive and polluting. Seduction and pollution, working as opposed semiotic frames, mutually inform the meanings of the (hyper)sexualized power of the black body.

From the second position we may view the body as object. From this view we gaze at others' bodies and objectify them through our multi-sensory interaction with them. In other words, through interaction the body-material *becomes* a symbol, but it always remains a special type of symbol, being both a subject (through its relation with a self and others) and an object (to the self and to others). Following Strauss (1993) we can therefore say that there is "action *on* the body, *toward* the body, or *with respect* to the body" (Strauss 1993:120, italics in the original). As such, bodies become intertwined in a political economy of symbolic objects (Baudrillard 1968) with some objects clearly having more value than others. Bodies reside, therefore, at the centre of a social structure built around embodied inequalities. The body, subjected to various processes of commodification, becomes a commodity itself by assuming physical capital (Bourdieu 1984; also see Featherstone 1991). Bodies with high physical capital then reflect out their power onto other bodies which then attempt to emulate the performances and appearances of the former. In part, these are the dynamics by which the construct of "body image" is constituted.

Yet, such process is not as simple as the one referred to in the psychological and social psychological literature on body image, as we argue in Chapter Thirteen. The formation of what we name "body ekstasis" is in actuality dependent on a conceptualization of the body as sense, or interpretant – the third position of a socio-semiotic analytics of the body. In Peirce's (1960) triadic model of the sign the relation between object and sign vehicle (or representamen) is mediated by an emergent interpretive process which gives rise to a unique relation between the two. A socio-semiotic interactionist approach to the body is then cognizant of the active negotiation occurring between embodied selves as objects and embodied selves as subjects. As semiotic interactionists then we see the body as the medium through which embodied selves take in and give out negotiated knowledge about their world, themselves, others, and material objects (Strauss 1993:108), a body process which "serve[s] to enhance, promote, denigrate, destroy, maintain or alter performances, appearances, or presentations" (Strauss 1993:121). And, additionally, we can see embodied interaction as a form of both signification and agentic communication occurring through the body and entailing "cooperative activity with others and [being] the basis of shared significant symbols (Mead 1934), giving meaning to what one feels, sees, hears, smells and touches" (Corbin and Strauss 1988:54). The body as sense or interpretant points to the innovative, intentional, interpretive, reflexive, existentially unique, and innovative powers of the embodied self. Along these lines in Chapter Fifteen, Carol Rambo, Sara Renée Presley and Don Mynatt examine how exotic dancers "talk back," that is, how they are engaged in symbolic resistance (also see Ronai and Cross 1998) against the discourses of social researchers who have framed stripping within the restrictive categories of deviance/exploitation/ liberation.

The Narrative Body: Body as Story

Recent literatures have gainfully synthesized classic and legacy interactionist theory within a narrative framework. From this point of view, personhood is a narrative accomplishment (Denzin 1989; Holstein and Gubrium 2000). Personhood "is more than the sum of its parts, and narrative is what allows it to *be* more" (Irvine 1999:9, emphasis in original). As Douglas Mason-Schrock (1996:176) contends, "stories are like containers that hold us together; they give us a sense of coherence and continuity. By telling what happened to us once upon a time, we make sense of who we are today." Yet, narratives "are not free-floating. Neither are they whimsical. Of course, some people *do* invent elaborate lies about themselves, but we call them confidence men or bullshit artists, or we medicate them and avoid them.... I am referring to an enduring and convincing (or at least plausible) story about who one is" (Irvine 1999:9, emphasis in original). In this way, the narratives that bestow coherence and continuity to personhood are structured by the language, grammar, and syntax of social, cultural, subcultural, and institutional discourse.

From this framework, the narrative body is situated in the stories we tell *to* ourselves and stories others tell *about* their own bodies and the bodies of others. As Holstein and Gubrium (2000) suggest narrative is a form of working subjectivity and a site of discursive struggle between narratives of the self and institutional discourses which frame our (embodied) subjectivity. The symbolic interactionist and narrative study of the body, therefore, conceptualizes the embodied self as "a particular set of sited language games whose rules discursively construct the semblance of a more or less unified subjectivity centered in experience" (Holstein and Gubrium 2000:70), or more simply as a set of stories about bodies we negotiate, struggle against, create, and of which live the consequences.

Chapters Sixteen and Seventeen open this section with two in-depth analyses of the culture of beauty. Chapter Sixteen is an effervescent commentary and critique on hegemonic discourses on health and fitness found in popular media. In that chapter, Charles Edgley scrutinizes in rich detail a vast array of narratives and discursive resources available to individuals keen on shaping up their bodies and the stories they live by, in order to better "fit" in. Michael Atkinson's focus in Chapter Seventeen is on men's narratives of their experiences with plastic surgery. These men's "before and after" stories reveal a complex set of strategies of positioning and re-positioning and of writing and re-writing the meanings of the physical appearance of their bodies in a symbolic and material universe informed by traditional and novel discourses on masculinity.

In addition to viewing the body as a site of struggle between institutional discourses and counter-narratives, symbolic interactionists conceptualize the body as a site of struggle between the realm of the symbolic (i.e. the self) and the physiological (i.e. the corporeal). Such an approach is especially typical of those symbolic interactionists interested in understanding the consequences of illness for the self-concept and identity. For Kathy Charmaz (e.g. 1991, 1995, 2002), for example, the experience of illness is not only an intrusive interruption to the rhythm of healthy life, but more significantly a threat to the organization of the embodied self over time. Selves need contend with the continuing illness of their bodies by living one day at a time – thus losing the power to story their own futures – or constructing their existence day by day in an attempt to maintain control over the present (Charmaz 1991). For this reason illness disrupts the continuity of biography, at times turning the self literally at the mercy of the body (see Frank 1991, 1995).

The intersection between the socio-linguistic (i.e. narrative) and the physiological is thus representative of symbolic interactionist emphasis on narrative practice as a way of coping with traumatic experience and also a terrain for the socio-political emancipation of those whose "abnormal" bodies have been silenced by the cultural side-effects of illness, deviance, and diversity. Stories of the body and the self in this sense are told to gain empowerment through the acceptance of self and others (Denzin 1987a, 1987b, 1987c; Irvine 1999; Ronai 1995) and in this sense become techniques of care of the self (Frank 1998). Among such stories of empowerment figure the counter-narratives examined by Rachel Westfall in Chapter Eighteen. Westfall focuses her attention on the experiences of one woman whose trials and tribulations during her pregnancy demonstrate the degree to which the institutionalization of birth and the medicalization of women's bodies leave little (but ever so meaningful) space for agentic and oppositional storytelling.

In Chapter Nineteen, Clinton R. Sanders concludes the book by first identifying a loose but useful typology in which all of the chapters of this book (as well as broader body-oriented sociological discussions) can be located and understood.

Next, Sanders insightfully highlights the central themes that are woven through the narratives and analysis of this book – identity, self, and emotion; themes central not only to this text, but to the interactionist tradition as a whole. Drawing from insights gleaned from this book as they intersect with his own published works and personal experiences, Sanders reflects on the role of the body in interaction, as a vehicle of communication, as an aesthetic object, as a site of and for social control, and concludes by observing "It is a rare issue, phenomenon, or object that relates to so many matters of central interest to symbolic interactionists as does the body." We hope readers agree and also appreciate the utility of symbolic interaction to both understanding and investigating the dynamics of the body/embodiment.

References

Atkins, Dawn. 1998. *Looking Queer: Body Image and Identity in Lesbian, Bisexual, Gay, and Transgender Communities.* Binghampton, NY: Haworth.

Backett-Milburn, Kathryn and Linda McKie. 2001. *Constructing Gendered Bodies.* New York: Palgrave.

Baudrillard, Jean. 1968. *Le Systeme des Objects.* Paris: Gallinard.

Birke, Lynda. 1999. *Feminism and the Biological Body.* Edinburgh: Edinburgh University Press.

Bordo, Susan. 2000. *The Male Body: A New Look at Men in Public and in Private.* New York: Farrar, Straus and Giroux.

Bourdieu, Pierre. 1984. *Distinction.* London: Routledge.

Brissett, Dennis and Charles Edgley. 1990. *Life as Theater: A Dramaturgical Sourcebook.* New York: Aldine.

Brook, Barbara. 1999. *Feminist Perspectives on the Body.* New York: Longman.

Burt, Ramsay. 1995. *The Male Dancer: Bodies, Spectacle, Sexualities.* New York: Routledge.

Calefato, Patrizia. 2004. *The Clothed Body.* Translated by Lisa Adams. Oxford, New York: Berg.

Charmaz, Kathy. 1991. *Good Days, Bad Days: The Self in Chronic Illness and Time.* New Brunswick, NJ: Rutgers University Press.

_____. 1995. "The Body, Identity, and Self: Adapting to Impairment." *The Sociological Quarterly*, 36:657–680.

_____. 2002. "Stories and Silences: Disclosures and Self in Chronic Illness." *Qualitative Inquiry*, 8:302–328.

Cooley, Charles H. 1902 [1983]. *Human Nature and the Social Order.* Piscataway, NJ: Transaction.

Corbin, Juliet and Anselm Strauss. 1988. *Unending Care and Work.* San Francisco: Jossey Bass.

Covino, Deborah Caslav. 2004. *Amending the Abject Body: Aesthetic Makeovers in Medicine and Culture.* Albany: SUNY Press.

Crossley, Nick. 2001. *The Social Body.* London: Sage.

_____. 1995. "Merleau-Ponty, the Elusive Body and Carnal Sociology." *Body and Society*, 1 (1):43–66.

Demello, Margo. 2000. *Bodies of Inscription: A Cultural History of the Modern Tattoo.* Duke University Press.

Denzin, Norman K. 1989a. *Treating Alcoholism: An Alcoholics Anonymous Approach.* Newbury Park, CA: Sage.

_____. 1989b. *The Recovering Alcoholic.* Newbury Park, CA: Sage.

_____. 1989c. *The Alcoholic Self.* Newbury Park, CA: Sage.

_____. 1989. *Interpretive Biography.* Thousand Oaks, CA: Sage.

Elson, Jean. 2004. *Am I Still a Woman?: Hysterectomy and Gender Identity.* Philadelphia: Temple University Press.

Entwistle, Joanne. 2000. *The Fashioned Body: Fashion, Dress and Modern Social Theory.* Cambridge: Polity.

Falk, Pasi. 1994. *The Consuming Body.* London: Sage.

Fausto-Sterling, Anne. 2000. *Sexing the Body: Gender Politics and the Construction of Sexuality.* New York: Basic Books.

Featherstone, Mike. 2000. *Body Modification.* Thousand Oaks, CA: Sage.

Featherstone, Mike, Mike Hepworth and Bryan Turner. 1991. *The Body: Social Process and Cultural Theory.* Thousand Oaks, CA: Sage.

Foster, Patricia. 1995. *Minding the Body.* New York: Anchor.

Foucault, Michel. 1977. *Language, Counter-Memory, Practice: Selected Essays and Interviews/Michel Foucault.* Edited by Donald Bouchard. Ithaca, NY: Cornell University Press.

Frank, Arthur. 1991. *At the Will of the Body: Reflections on Illness.* Boston: Houghton Mifflin.

_____. 1995. *The Wounded Storyteller: Body, Illness, and Ethics.* Chicago: University of Chicago Press.

_____. 1998. "Stories of Illness as Care of the Self: A Foucauldian Dialogue." *Health*, 2:329–348.

Gay, Kathlyn and Christine Whittington. 2002. *Body Marks: Tattooing, Piercing, and Scarification.* Brookfield, CT: Millbrook.

Glassner, Barry. 1988. *Bodies.* New York: Putnam.

_____. 1989. "Fitness and the Postmodern Self." *Journal of Health and Social Behavior*, 30:180–191.

Goffman, Erving. 1959. *The Presentation of Self in Everyday Life.* New York: Doubleday Anchor.

_____. 1963. *Stigma: Note on the Management of Spoiled Identity.* New York: Touchstone.

_____. 1971. *Relations in Public.* New York: Harper & Row.

Grosz, Elizabeth and Elspeth Probyn. 1995. *Sexy Bodies: The Strange Carnalities of Feminism.* New York: Routledge.

Guy, Ali, Eileen Green, and Maura Banim. 2003. *Through the Wardrobe: Women's Relationships with their Clothes.* Berg.

Halberstam, Judith and Ira Livingston. 1995. *Posthuman Bodies.* Bloomington: Indiana University Press.

Halton, Eugene. 1986. *Meaning and Modernity.* Chicago: University of Chicago Press.

_____. 1995. *Bereft of Reason: On the Decline of Social Thought and its Prospect for Renewal.* Chicago: University of Chicago Press.

Hewitt, Kim. 1997. *Mutilating the Body: Identity in Blood and Ink.* Bowling Green State University Popular Press.

Holstein, James and Jaber Gubrium. 2000. *The Self We Live By: Narrative Identity in a Postmodern World.* New York: Oxford University Press.

Howson, Alexandra. 2005. *Embodying Gender.* London: Routledge.

Husserl, Edmund. 1893/1917. *On the Phenomenology of the Consciousness of Internal Time.* New York: Springer.

Irvine, Leslie. 1999. *Codependent Forevermore: The Invention of Self in a Twelve Step Group.* University of Chicago Press.

Kroker, Arthur and MariLouise Kroker. 1987. *Body Invaders: Panic Sex in America.* New York: St. Martin's Press.

Laqueur, Thomas. 1992. *Making Sex: Body and Gender from the Greeks to Freud.* Harvard University Press.

Lebesco, Kathleen. 2004. *Revolting Bodies?: The Struggle to Redefine Fat Identity.* University of Massachusetts Press.

Leder, Drew. 1990. *The Absent Body.* University of Chicago Press.

Maines, David. 2001. *The Faultline of Consciousness: A View of Interactionism in Sociology.* New York: Aldine.

Martindale, Don. 1960. *The Nature and Types of Sociological Theory.* Boston: Houghton Mifflin.

Mason-Schrock, Douglas. 1996. "Transsexuals' Narrative Construction of the 'True Self'." *Social Psychology Quarterly*, 59 (3):176–192.

Mead, George H. 1934. *Mind, Self and Society.* Chicago: University of Chicago Press.

_____. 1936. *Movements of Thought in the Nineteenth Century* (edited by Charles Morris). University of Chicago Press.

Merleau-Ponty, Maurice. 1974. *Phenomenology: Language and Society* (edited by John O'Neil). Portsmouth, NH: Heinemann.

Mifflin, Margot. 2001. *Bodies of Subversion: A Secret History of Women and Tattoo.* Juno.

Mohanram, Radhika. 1999. *Black Body: Women, Colonialism, and Space.* Minneapolis: University of Minnesota Press.

Monaghan, Lee. 2002. "Embodying Gender, Work and Organization: Solidarity, Cool Loyalties and Contested Hierarchy in a Masculinist Occupation." *Gender, Work and Organization*, 9 (5):504–536.

Moore, Pamela (Ed.). 1997. *Building Bodies.* New Brunswick, NJ: Rutgers University Press.

Moore, Thomas. 1998. *The Soul of Sex: Cultivating Life as an Act of Love.* New York: Harper Collins.

Newell, Phillip. 2002. *Echo of the Soul: The Sacredness of the Human Body.* Harrisburg, PA: Morehouse.

Peirce, Charles S. 1960. *Collected Papers of Charles Sanders Peirce. Vol. 1–6.* Cambridge: Harvard University Press.

Pitts, Victoria. 2003. *In the Flesh: The Cultural Politics of Body Modification.* New York: Palgrave Macmillan.

Pronger, Brian. 2002. *Body Fascism: Salvation in the Technology of Physical Fitness.* Toronto: University of Toronto Press.

Reynolds, Larry. 2003. "Early Representatives." In Larry Reynolds and Nancy Herman-Kinney (eds). *Handbook of Symbolic Interactionism.* Alta Mira. pp. 59–81.

Ronai, Carol Rambo. 1995. "Multiple Reflections of Child Abuse." *Journal of Contemporary Ethnography*, 23:395–426.

Ronai, Carol Rambo and Rebecca Cross. 1998. "Dancing with Identity: Narrative Resistance Strategies of Male and Female Stripteasers." *Deviant Behavior*, 19:99–119.

Sanders, Clinton. 1989. *Customizing the Body: The Art and Culture of Tattooing.* Philadelphia, PA: Temple University Press.

Scheper-Hughes, Nancy and Loic Wacquant. 2003. *Commodifying Bodies.* London: Sage.

Shilling, Chris. 2003. *The Body and Social Theory* (second edition). Thousand Oaks, CA: Sage.

Shutz, Alfred. 1973. *Collected Papers I: The Problem of Social Reality.* Leiden: Martinus Nijhoff.

Simmel, Georg. 1997 [1908]. "Sociology of the Senses: Visual Interaction." In David Frisby and Mike Featherstone (eds). *Simmel on Culture.* Thousand Oaks, CA: Sage.

Springer, Claudia. 1996. *Electronic Eros: Bodies and Desire in the Postindustrial Age.* University of Texas Press.

Stone, Gregory P. 1962. "Appearance and the Self." In A. M. Rose (ed.). *Human Nature and Social Process.* Boston: Houghton Muffin Company. pp. 86–118.

Stratton, Jon. 2001. *The Desirable Body: Cultural Fetishism and the Erotics of Consumption.* University of Illinois Press.

Strauss, Anselm. 1993. *Continual Permutations of Action.* New York: Aldine de Gruyter.

Synnott, Anthony. 1993. *The Body Social: Symbolism, Self and Society.* New York: Routledge.

Tebbel, Cyndi. 2003. *The Body Snatchers: How the Media Shapes Women.* Lane Cove, Australia: Finch.

Thomson, Rosemarie Garland. 1996. *Freakery: Cultural Spectacles of the Extraordinary Body.* New York: New York University Press.

Turner, Bryan. 1984. *The Body and Social Theory.* Thousand Oaks, CA: Sage.

Vannini, Phillip. 2004. "Toward an Interpretive Analytics of the Sign: Interactionism, Power and Semiosis." *Studies in Symbolic Interaction*, 27:151–176.

Virgili, Fabrice, and Paul Hodkinson. 2002. *Goth: Identity, Style and Subculture*. Oxford: Berg.

Waskul, Dennis and Pamela van der Riet. 2002. "The Abject Embodiment of Cancer Patients: Dignity, Selfhood, and the Grotesque Body." *Symbolic Interaction*, 25 (4):487–513.

Weitz, Rose. 2002. *Politics of Women's Bodies: Sexuality, Appearance and Behavior*. Oxford University Press.

Wiley, Norbert. 1994. *The Semiotic Self*. Chicago: University of Chicago Press.

PART 1
The Looking-Glass Body:
Reflexivity as Embodiment

Chapter 2

The Networked Body and the Question of Reflexivity

Nick Crossley

Since the early 1990s, the body and experiences of embodiment have become significant subjects of sociological research and theory. In particular, the works of Anthony Giddens, Michel Foucault, and Pierre Bourdieu have offered serious theoretical frameworks that have inspired a plethora of empirical studies. However, as Nick Crossley argues in this chapter, the value of these approaches is tempered by shortcomings and Crossley contends "that the interactionist theories of Cooley and, in particular, Mead, provide a persuasive way forward." Hinging his articulation of "reflective embodiment" on three claims – each of which is directly derived from the most fundamental cornerstones of the pragmatic tradition of symbolic interaction – Crossley neatly frames the body and embodiment as embedded, and actively fashioned in reflexive looking-glasses. Tracing his conceptualization of "reflexive embodiment" to both Cooley and Mead while also connecting with contemporary interests and empirical works, Crossley offers a decidedly interactionist framework that avoids pesky shortcomings of dominant theoretical perspectives of the body and embodiment.

In this chapter I argue that an interactionist framework allows us to overcome serious deficiencies in the sociological understanding of "reflexive embodiment." Interactionism has a richer and more flexible conception of reflexivity than other perspectives and embeds reflexivity within social networks and norms, without reducing it to them. Other, more dominant perspectives either fail to situate the agent or reduce the agent to the situation. The chapter begins with a brief review of these other perspectives.

Reflexive Embodiment: An Overview

Much work in the sociology of the body has been focused upon the issue of "reflexive embodiment." Sociologists have investigated the various ways in which agents "turn back" upon their own embodiment, reflecting and acting upon it so as to modify or maintain it in a variety of ways. There have been studies of such practices as tattooing, piercing, cosmetic surgery, working out, bodybuilding, dress, beauty regimes, and diet. A number of theoretical paradigms have been used to make sense of these reflexive processes. The dominant perspectives in the literature as a whole, however, are those of Giddens (1991, 1992), Foucault (1979, 1980a,b, 1984), Foucauldian feminism (Bartky 1993, Bordo 1993, Butler 1990, Lloyd 1996, McNay 1992, Sawicki 1991), and Bourdieu (1977, 1984). The emphasis of each of these dominant perspectives is quite different.

Giddens (1991, 1992) understands reflexive embodiment as an aspect of a broader process of the reflexive reconstruction of the self. The advance of modernity has led to an erosion of traditions which once secured identities and provided templates for biographical trajectories, he argues. In the absence of these traditions individuals are increasingly required to construct their own identities and projected future trajectories. This implicates the body since embodiment is intimately related to selfhood. "Self-making" necessarily involves "body work." Identities need to be embodied in order to be projected into the social world. In addition, he notes both that new technologies have opened up more aspects of our embodiment to choice (even our sex can be changed) and that the increased flow of scientific advice on health related risks has served to problematize previously habitual bodily practices, bringing them into consciousness. Eating, in particular, has been subject to continual and repeated problematization. These changes and this knowledge flow, he continues, "condemns" us to make choices with respect to our bodies and the lifestyle practices which shape them. We may elect to ignore all advice on health and diet and we would probably find it difficult to follow it consistently, given its often contradictory nature. We may reject contemporary possibilities for body modification. However, unlike earlier generations we must choose to do this. There are no deeply engrained traditions, below the threshold of reflection, for us to follow.

In sharp contrast, Foucault and those who follow him view reflexive embodiment in terms of power. Self-mastery and awareness of the body, Foucault (1980a) argues, is achieved as a consequence of the operation of "body power." We become aware of and gain mastery over our bodies as a consequence of the disciplinary training to which we are subject in the family, school, workplace, hospital, etc. And we assume the controlling function of these institutions for ourselves, in relation to ourselves. Reflexivity amounts to self-policing, derived from an internalization of external "panoptic" mechanisms. The individual is enmeshed within a disciplinary network whose functions they take over for themselves, such that the body is imprisoned by a socially and politically constructed "soul" (Foucault 1979).

There is room for resistance here. Foucault does not explore resistance in detail, however, and where he elaborates he tends to portray resistance as hyper-conformity to the dictates of power. He notes, for example, how the imposition of health regimes on the population has led to a form of resistance in which agents now demand that their health care needs are catered for (Foucault 1980a). Some now take their health so seriously that they have started to make difficult demands upon the health services that were originally constructed and deployed to encourage them to take their health more seriously. Likewise he notes how the "invention" and imposition of sexuality, as an identity, upon European populations in the nineteenth century generated a basis for resistance, both in the form of the sexual revolution of the 1960s and the early gay rights movement. In both cases the subjects of power accepted the identity imposed upon them and mounted a form of political resistance upon that basis.

Foucault's work is insensitive to gender issues. Many feminists have taken up his work, however, as a basis to reflect upon gender issues, and have identified the particular gender skew that emerges in relation to regimes of body power (Bartky 1993, Bordo 1993, Butler 1990, Lloyd 1996, McNay 1992, Sawicki 1991). Gender is a normative category, it is observed, and women are expected to both produce and regulate their embodied selves in terms of these norms. Bartky (1993) in particular focuses upon the manner in which the self-policing of gendered embodiment and self-hood is instituted in the mundane routines of everyday life.

Bourdieu too identifies gender distinctions as a key focus in his analysis of reflexive embodiment. In contrast to the abovementioned feminist writers, however, he places a stronger emphasis upon class, both in relation to gender and independently of it. And in a theoretical move which has invited both critique and confusion (see Alexander 1995, Crossley 2001a,b), he offers an account which is more strategic in focus but which downplays "reflectiveness" and "reflexivity" in favour of pre-reflective dispositions (habitus). Middle class women make a much greater investment in their bodies than working class women, he argues, at least this is true amongst married women. In part this reflects wider class differences in the nature of the relation of agents to their bodies but it also reflects differences in strategic situations. Middle class women tend to work in occupations where appearance matters and can affect career advancement; therefore they have more incentive to work upon their appearance. Working class women, by contrast, once they have secured a man in the marriage markets, have less incentive to work upon their appearance. Reflexive embodiment, in this case, is a strategic response to a situation in which profit or advantage can be accrued. However, Bourdieu appears to suggest that this strategic adaptation is rooted in acquired pre-reflective dispositions (habitus), rather than reflective deliberation. A middle class woman would not need to reflect upon the necessity that she look good or look right and would not need to reflect upon what looking good or right involves, according to this conception, because she would, as a consequence of prior experience, "instinctively" know what was required and act accordingly. Like a tennis player whose hours of practice allow her to move instinctively into the right position and play the right shot, the embodied strategies of middle class women derive from below the threshold consciousness and seldom surface there.

Investment in the body is generally lower amongst men of all classes, compared to women, in Bourdieu's view but it is not completely absent, and where it is present it too is shaped by the history of class formation. The middle and working classes, he argues, have different concepts and modes of inhabiting the body. The hard physical labour involved in many working class occupations has resulted both in a valorization of the outward signs of strength, such as muscle, and also in a more instrumental and functional attitude towards the body. Bodybuilding, as a primarily working class preoccupation, is cited as an illustration of this. It celebrates the muscularity of the labouring body.[1] Middle class men, by contrast, are more concerned with their bodily interiors (e.g. health and fitness), whose visibility presupposes both the cultural capital that middle class men have and the aesthetic and ascetic dispositions that their jobs tend to entail.

A Critique

There is much that is perceptive in these accounts. However, there are major weaknesses in each case. I do not have the space to explore all of the problems but a brief review, demonstrating the need for an alternative approach to those on offer, is necessary.

Giddens makes an interesting case for how recent social changes have undermined the traditional supports of self and lifestyle. His account problematizes that of both Bourdieu and the Foucauldians, including the feminist Foucauldians. It suggests, contra the former, that it is difficult to avoid conscious awareness and choice regarding the body in the modern era, given the fast flow of information and innovation, and the breakdown of traditions; and contra the latter, that straightforward normative templates for appearance and lifestyle are no longer available, such that individuals are forced to choose. Bourdieu and Foucault both appear implausibly "culturally dopey" in light of Giddens' analysis. However, Giddens appears to conceptualize the reflexive agent in a disembedded manner. His agents make decisions in an anomic space. This is unrealistic. Some norms persist and inform decisions and behaviour, even if others have been undermined by recent changes. More importantly, agents are portrayed as making decisions in isolation. There is no sense of the role that personal and other networks play in informing and shaping reflexive projects, and in constraining the agent. Part of the problem here is that Giddens has failed to explore the nature of reflexivity and reflexive consciousness in any detail, considering how it emerges in a social context and is populated, even in its most individualized forms, by the perspective of both particular and generalized others.

The work of the Foucauldians is almost a mirror opposite. They conceive of the reflexive agent as deeply enmeshed in a "carceral network" (Foucault 1979). Reflexivity, for them, entails rigid adherence to social norms. It is self-policing. Clearly, as the feminist accounts draw out, there are aspects of this account which resonate with aspects of the lived experience of at least some people. Part of the attractiveness of Foucault's work to some feminists lies in its theoretical articulation of issues and criticisms which they have raised and addressed in the course of their political practice (see esp. Bartky 1993). However, the account is limited because the very fact that agents can and do address these issues in political practice suggests that there is more to reflexivity than Foucault is inclined to grant. Agents do not merely reproduce the regimes that are imposed upon them, nor is resistance restricted to

---

1   Bodybuilding does involve an aesthetic, however, which doesn't accord with Bourdieu's argument. In fact, Bourdieu's claims about these class differences are highly problematic in many instances.

the embrace of previously imposed identities. Agents have the capacity to reflect upon and debate the internalized constraints they experience, both individually and collectively, and thereby to devise alternative ways of "making out" within the normative frameworks they encounter.

Interestingly, a number of ethnographic studies of specifically female "body work" have suggested that women are aware of the feminist claim that their modifications and regimes are aspects of oppression but largely reject that claim and suggest instead that they are doing what they are doing for their self, a claim which resonates with Giddens' framework (Black 2004, Gimlin 2002, Davis 1995). In this particular case it is feminist "norms" that are experienced as externally imposed constraints, and they are rejected – which is not to say that the women involved reject either feminism or other aspects of its critique of "body power" *in toto*. Foucauldians might argue that this is precisely their point about internalization: agents want, personally, to be healthy and beautiful because political technologies have moulded them in this way. However, the fact that agents are aware of the critique of body-politics and perhaps feel as oppressed by that as by the demand that they be beautiful, healthy, etc, suggests a rather more complex picture than that painted by Foucault, which comes somewhat closer to the scenario suggested by Giddens. It is not clear, at least in all cases, what prescriptions women, or men for that matter, should follow: feminist prescriptions? Patriarchal prescriptions? Post-feminist prescriptions? This dilemma opens up a space in which, as Giddens claims, individual choices can and must be made.

Bourdieu, like Foucault, suggests a more embedded conception of agency. Agents, in this case, are embedded within class cultures. And his more strategic view of agency does avoid the excessive norm-conformity of the Foucauldian view. However, his view of reflexivity is problematic too. His emphasis upon the pre-reflective level of agency and upon our "feel for the game" is very important and interesting. As I have argued before, however, to the extent that this excludes a recognition of the role of reflexive consciousness in everyday contexts on a regular basis it is deeply problematic. Studies of a number of body modification projects suggest that a great deal of deliberation, angst and research goes into them, on the agent's behalf, suggesting that reflective choice rather than habit lies behind them (Crossley 2005, Davis 1995, Sweetman 1999). Agents know more about their contexts and actions than Bourdieu is prepared to concede and this knowledge enters into and steers their actions. I have suggested elsewhere that this gap in Bourdieu's approach might be remedied by way of a conception of habits of reflection and a "reflexive habitus." I have also suggested, however, that this conception can only be achieved by way of a dialogue between Bourdieu's work and that of G.H. Mead. If we take Mead's route, however, as I believe we should, then the tight link between class and reflexive embodiment is loosened and the Bourdieusian position further challenged.

Each of the dominant perspectives on reflexive embodiment is seriously flawed then, even if each also has something of value to offer. How can we move beyond this impasse? It is my contention that the interactionist theories of Cooley and, in particular, Mead, provide a persuasive way forward.

An Interactionist Approach

My interactionist alternative hinges upon three points. Firstly, interactionists claim that social agents are embedded in a range of networks, personal and impersonal, each embodying and enforcing specific norms. In this respect interactionism avoids the disembedded and anomic conception of Giddens. Secondly, again contra Giddens, relations with others form the very basis of human reflexivity according to interactionists. Thirdly, the relational origin of reflexivity and self-consciousness is theorized in dialogical terms by interactionists, such that we overcome the normative reductionism of the Foucauldians and the class reductionism of Bourdieu. These points must be unpacked.

Interactionism, as the name suggests, locates social agents within a context populated by others with whom they interact. The individual enjoys no primacy relative to the group from this perspective. We are born into groups. Our personal histories belong to the fabric of broader social histories and even the evolutionary history of our primate ancestors was shaped by group life (Hirst and Wooley 1982). More importantly, we live in groups and in networks of interdependency. Much of our action is interaction and/or joint action within these networks and is conditioned by the accumulated weight of past interactions; that is, history (Chang 2004). We rely upon others for resources, recognition, inspiration, ideas, information and their skills, as they rely upon us. And they constrain and enable our actions in multiple ways, as we constrain and enable theirs.

Recognition of this fact could inform our understanding of reflexive embodiment in many ways. Here I will consider two. Firstly, much reflexive embodiment occurs in "worlds" akin to Howard Becker's (1984) "art worlds;" that is, networks of interdependency manifesting a complex division of labour and diffusion of skills. Tattooing, dieting, bodybuilding, dressing and personal hygiene are not the work of a solitary agent any more than a work of art is. They presuppose collective action and a division of labour wherein tools, norms, ideas, knowledge, audiences, etc. are mobilized and diffused. Tattoos generally require tattoo artists, for example, who in turn require tattooing equipment; they require designs, which, in turn, have a history much like that of art and tend to vary across time (DeMello 2000). Everything about tattoos, from their design and location through to the very fact of having them or not is embedded in complex semiotic codes to which agents orient. To reflect upon tattooing as an individual choice and action, therefore, as Giddens' approach encourages, is to ignore most of what it involves. If this example sounds too exotic note that the same is true of washing our hands and face. Soap and flannels are made for us by others who are separated from us by retailers along a supply chain; organizations pump water into our houses; plumbers maintain the supply infrastructure; heating firms install and maintain equipment to warm the water for us, using electricity and gas supplied by other firms; the wider community generates the "civilized" moral and aesthetic norms which persuade us to wash, backed up by scientists who warn of the invisible and harmful bacteria which attach to unwashed but otherwise apparently clean hands. Whatever we may think we are not alone in the bathroom. Our morning wash engages a complex web of interdependencies.

In addition to this, agents' actions are shaped by those around them. Others are our source of knowledge and information about the possibilities of body work. Moreover, if we respect them or seek their approval, recognition or love, as Mead's neo-Hegelian conception of the "struggle for recognition" predicts (Honneth 1995, Joas 1985), then our own desires and opinions, or at least our actions, can be shaped by their desires and opinions. The desire to be desired, as Kojève's (1969) famous lectures on Hegel suggest, often leads individuals to desire and desire to become what significant others desire. If alter is impressed by muscles, for example, or ego imagines that this is so, then ego too may be impressed by them and/or may attempt to cultivate them in an effort to win alter's recognition. Alternatively, we sometimes compete with others, seeking to outdo them or distinguish ourselves from them. Either way, however, our action is interaction.

Recent work on shame, pride, embarrassment and self-feelings, which traces back to Goffman and more particularly Cooley (see Scheff 2005, Franks and Gecas 1992), echo these arguments on recognition and facilitate a deeper understanding of reflexive embodiment. They allow us to see how "face," which in this case is a metonym for the body as perceived by others, is invested by emotions which are at once embodied and intersubjective, as is the self more widely, such that strong corporeal impulses come into play where it is concerned. We have a deep seated urge to be perceived in ways that we desire.

In further cases our dependence upon others gives rise to an unfavourable power balance which allows them to direct our action. A young person living at home may not be able to have a tattoo, for example, because they would need their parent to pay for it and their parent refuses, or because they know it would upset or outrage their parent and are afraid or do not wish to cause upset. Likewise an adult might be restricted in their body projects by the demands of an employer or even a spouse. Body projects all have to be negotiated within the context of social networks wherein desires, resources and power, in addition to communicative persuasion and meaning, come into play.

At a deeper level than this, however, the basic self-consciousness and bodily awareness that reflexive embodiment presupposes derives from our relations with others. Cooley's (1902) notion of the looking glass self affords us a first approximation of this view. It reminds us that much of the information that we have about ourselves is arrived at by way of the communications of others. The self is in many respects its own blind spot. The I does not see itself any more than the eye sees itself and we are therefore reliant upon others to reflect back information about ourselves. More importantly than this, however, much of what is known or thought about the body and self in reflexive projects presupposes that we take an "external" point of view upon ourselves; that we look upon ourselves as other. Consciousness of one's own body as an aesthetic, medical, or other type of object requires self-objectification which, in turn, requires that the agent learn to occupy an imaginary external viewpoint from which to perform this operation.

Foucault's claim that agent's internalize the "panoptic gaze" goes some way to explaining how this might happen. We find a much more elaborate and sophisticated, if similar, argument in Mead's (1967) work, however. Mead's argument on the role of childhood play and games in enabling and disposing agents to assume the role of specific and generalized others in relation to their self is well known. I will not rehearse it here, except to note that the agent (qua elusive "I") becomes known to their self (qua "Me"), in this schema, by adopting the role of another towards their self. And they learn to do this, in the first instance, by quite literally playing at being other people during infancy. Two features of this account are particularly important from our perspective. Firstly, what Mead is discussing here is reflexivity, the process whereby an agent turns back upon their self to become an object of their own reflection and action. In contrast to Giddens, however, his account both explains how reflexivity is achieved, developmentally, and embeds it firmly within the social world. The agent becomes aware of their self by assuming, imaginatively, the positions of others with whom they are in contact. Putting that another way, their most intimate psychological life is inhabited by the roles of others, and their reflexivity is only possible in virtue of this. Even when we are alone, from this point of view, our thoughts and reflections are embedded in a network of virtual representations and interacts with other perspectives in this network.

The others in question may be specific others and Mead suggests that in childhood, at least, agents are inclined to assume the roles of authority figures and/or those upon whom they are dependent and who consequently exert some degree of power in relation to them (e.g. parents, teachers, older siblings). He also discusses the role of "generalized others," however; that is, the more abstract view of, for example, "the community," as embodied in formalized rules or shared narratives and rituals.

This view overlaps with that of Foucault, particularly where Mead stresses the role of power and authority. At times he appears to say, as Foucault does, that the individual polices their self in the manner of external policing agents. My second point, however, is that Mead overcomes the "culturally dopey" implications of this view by stressing the conversational nature of reflexivity and psychological life more generally. Agents do not necessarily submit to the views of others. They consider them but they may equally reply back to them, and they may bring the various views of a range of others into a simulated discussion, playing off views against one another. One need only glance at the average body modification website to get a sense of this. Typical accounts focus upon "what my dad thought ... but what my mates thought ... and why I'm not bothered what other people think anyway."

This introduces an element of indeterminism into our picture, since, as Gadamer (1989:383) notes, "No one knows in advance what will 'come out' of a conversation." Conversations are directed by their own internal dynamics. Moreover, this allows for creativity too, as the interplay of viewpoints may result in a higher synthesis or alternative which surpasses them all. It may not. One view may win out and that may be the view which serves dominant interests in power relations. There is nothing automatic about this, however. Mead believes that individuals enjoy a different vantage point to that of those in authority; indeed nobody occupies exactly the same vantage point as anybody else. And he believes that different viewpoints can be brought into play in the process of reflexivity.

Reflexive dialogues are not necessarily individual. Groups of individuals can discuss and play out the rules and recommendations of experts and authorities. They can anticipate the view of, for example, medical authorities, and construct their own replies to those authorities. In these ways, I suggest, Mead allows for a more sophisticated view of reflexivity than Foucault.

It is also worth noting, in this context, the various qualifications that Cooley (1902) makes with respect to his conception of the looking glass self (see also Franks and Gecas 1992). Although this conception tends to focus upon the manner in which an agent's sense of self is shaped by the communications of others, Cooley notes that agents both select, to a degree, who they will allow to influence them and interpret the images that others entertain of them. Moreover, he stresses that the agent may still reject those images if they contradict core values that the agent has acquired. Indeed, Cooley brings the appropriative and even aggressive aspects of the self into focus. The abovementioned corporeal impulses are one aspect of this. We desire the desire of others and are moved by this but we will kick against unfavourable appraisals in defense of ourselves. Our sense of our self is important to us and is affectively charged, such that we are disposed to defend it against what we perceive to be attacks upon it.

The interactionist approach also allows us to sophisticate Bourdieu's approach. Mead's description of the emergence of the self-process is, effectively, an account of the acquisition of specific dispositions and schemas from the social world; an account of the emergence of reflexive dispositions. As such it is wholly compatible with Bourdieu's notion of the habitus. Moreover, like Bourdieu, his theorization of the "struggle for recognition" allows for the pursuit of distinction, including the pursuit of distinction through appearance and the body:

> We may come back to manner of speech and dress ... things in which we stand out above people. We are careful, of course, not to directly plume ourselves. It would seem childish to intimate that we take satisfaction in showing that we can do something better than others. We take a great deal of pains to cover us such a situation; but actually we are vastly gratified.
>
> Mead (1967:205)

This quotation appears to describe an interpersonal level of struggle, and this is important. Mead is by no means unaware of or unsympathetic to the notion of class (or ethnicity) specific perspectives and identities, however, akin to those described by Bourdieu, nor indeed to gender distinctions and divides. Where Mead differs from Bourdieu, however, is in his insistence that we are continually encountering and absorbing the perspectives of others, such that we are continually taking others' perspectives towards ourselves and, in some cases at least, moving towards a more universal position which incorporates this new perspective. As such the disposition of the agent is never reducible to their social position for Mead. In an interesting footnote in *Outline for a Theory Practice*, intended to draw a distinction between the life of the Kabyle and that of the French, Bourdieu (1979) notes how life in modern cities unsettles the taken-for-granted feel of the world which the habitus otherwise furnishes, as agents are constantly coming into contact with others (often immigrants) who have a different lifestyle to their own. This observation sits unhappily with much of the rest of Bourdieu's work, where agents of all societies appear to live naively within their own habitual perspective, taking it for granted. It captures perfectly Mead's own sense of modern life, however, where perspectives are constantly coming into contact, affording agents a new viewpoint upon their self and generating new synthetic and hybrid cultural forms which can never achieve complete taken-for-grantedness. We are creatures of habit, for Mead, but we are equally conversational agents and our conversational tendencies, whilst rooted in habit, tend to disturb at least some of our sedimented repertoires of action, bringing them into view for us. Tradition and culture lose some of their grip upon us by virtue of our experientially-rooted awareness of their relativity.

In an interesting way then, Mead brings certain aspects of Giddens' more reflexive and agentic account back into the heart of an account which is, like that of Foucault and Bourdieu, more social. Agents are multiply socially embedded and locked in relations of authority and power, for Mead, and these relations are an integral element in their reflexivity. These elements do not subordinate the agent, however. They are "voices" in reflexive and potentially critical conversations played out at multiple levels, including the level of the individual "internal conversation."

At least some body projects and aspects of body work remain matters of contemplation and choice in this respect. Some may be deep rooted habits which lie below the level of reflection and contemplation, and some may be reinforced in relations of power which make "deviance" improbable. Many, however, are available to reflexive reflection and subject to the decision of the agent.

From Theory to Analysis

Having said all of this, it is important from an interactionist point of view that we do not seek to second guess or theoretically prescribe the nature of social reality. A theoretical framework is important but it can never supplant the need for empirical research. And in our case this means empirical research on the various forms of body modification and maintenance practiced in different societies and social contexts. We need to research, not assume, how "the body" is defined by agents in the contexts of different projects and indeed whether the body is the "object" of such practices. Is "the body" really the object and target in practices of tattooing and bodybuilding, for example, or are those projects aimed elsewhere, only co-opting the body for instrumental purposes? Sam Fussell's (1991) famous account of his bodybuilding "career," for example, suggests that he opted for bodybuilding as a means of managing his anxiety and lack of self-confidence, and was aware of this motivation, such that these psychological attributes were the key object of his project rather than his musculature as such – although his muscles were obviously implicated and arguably become more important as he followed his bodybuilding career. Muscles were a means, both physical and symbolic, to other ends, and these other ends were the true object of his body building project, at least in the first instance. Similarly, questions regarding the degree of reflexivity involved in body projects and the extent to which they are constrained by different forms of power and authority is a matter for empirical research rather than theoretical speculation. Mead's model is important because it removes certain of the more obvious limitations of the dominant perspectives in the field, but we should regard it less as an answer to key questions on "reflexive embodiment," more as a means of putting reflexive embodiment into question. Mead's views on the conversation nature of reflexive life do not preclude the possibility that certain aspects of reflexive embodiment are politically dominated, nor indeed that reflexive consciousness of the body may, in some instances, amount to self-policing on behalf of external authorities. Their utility is in breaking down the Foucauldian assumption that this is always and necessarily what happens but this then leaves a question in its wake: just when, where and how is the situation as Foucault describes? Foucault himself explicitly dodged this question. When discussing prisons and power, for example, he is clear that his focus is upon prison designs, rather than what happens to them in the "witches brew" that is actual prison life:

> ...if I had wanted to describe real life in the prisons, I wouldn't indeed have gone to Bentham.... the actual functioning of the prisons, in the inherited building where they were established and with the governers and guards who administered them, was a witches brew compared to the beautiful Benthamite machine.
>
> Foucault (1981:10)

The witches brew, by contrast, is interactionist territory. And regimes of body work are no less of a brew than prisons. They call for ethnographic analysis. Of course there have been many such enthnographic studies, some of which feature or are cited in this book. My point is that, beyond the stipulation of certain basic theoretical points, such as I have outlined in this paper, the basis for an interactionist perspective on reflexive embodiment should be empirical research.

Conclusions

In this chapter I have examined how an interactionist perspective might inform debates about reflexive embodiment. My chief argument has been that an interactionist perspective enables us to embed and locate reflexive projects within the context of social networks, norms and relations of power, thus avoiding the apparent atomism of Giddens' approach, without succumbing to the culturally dopey image of agents that we find, to an extent, in Bourdieu and the Foucauldians. Interactionist theory locates social agents in the thick of social networks and explains reflexivity and self-identity by reference to the various social relations this involves. But relations are inherently conversational for interactionists and, as such, agents have the capacity both to reflect upon their own perspective and, at least in some cases, to decide against the prescriptions fed to them by expert and authority sources. This is not an end of the matter, however, since the chief accomplishment of interactionist theory is to frame the question of reflexive embodiment in such a way that it cannot be answered by reference to theoretical diktat, as it so often is in the literature, but rather must be approached through careful and detailed research.

Acknowledgements

This chapter was completed when I was on a period of research paid for jointly by my discipline area (Sociology) at the University of Manchester (UK) and by the university's Centre for Research in Socio-Cultural Change (CRESC). Thank you to both for the support.

References

Alexander, Jeffrey. 1995. *Fin de Siécle Social Theory*, London, Verso.
Bartky, Sandra. 1993. *Gender and Domination*, London, Routledge.
Becker, Howard. 1984. *Art Worlds*, Berkeley, University of California Press.
Black, Paula. 2004. *The Beauty Industry*, London, Routledge.
Bordo, Susan. 1993. *Unbearable Weight*, Berkeley, University of California Press.
Bourdieu, Pierre. 1977. "Remarques provisoires sur la perception sociale du corps." *Actes de la Recherche en sciences sociales*, 14(5):1–4.
_____. 1979. *Outline of a Theory of Practice*, Cambridge, Cambridge University Press.
_____. 1984. *Distinction*, London, RKP.
Butler, Judith. 1990. *Gender Trouble*, London, Routledge.
Chang, Johannes. 2004. "Mead's Theory of Emergence as a Framework for Multilevel Sociological Inquiry." *Symbolic Interaction*, 27(3): 405–427.
Cooley, Charles Horton. 1902. *Human Nature and Social Order*, New York, Charles Scribner and Sons.
Crossley, Nick. 2001. *The Social Body*, London, Sage.
_____. 2003. "From Reproduction to Transformation: Social Movement Fields and the Radical Habitus." *Theory, Culture and Society*, 20(6): 43–68.
_____. 2004. "The Circuit Trainer's Habitus: Reflexive Body Techniques and the Sociality of the Workout." *Body and Society*, 10(1): 37–69.
_____. 2005. "In the Gym: Motives, Meanings and Moral Careers," Working Paper 6, Centre for Research on Socio-Cultural Change, University of Manchester, http://www.Cresc.ac.uk/publications/workingpapers.
Davis, Kathy. 1995. *Reshaping the Female Body*, London, Routledge.

DeMello, Margot. 2000. *Bodies of Inscription*, London, Duke.

Foucault, Michel. 1979. *Discipline and Punish*, Harmondsworth, Penguin.

_____. 1980a. "Body/Power," in *Power/Knowledge*, Brighton, Harvester, 55–62.

_____. 1980b. "The Politics of Health in the Eighteenth Century," in *Power/ Knowledge*, Brighton, Harvester, 166–82.

_____. 1981. "Questions of Method," *I&C*, 8:3–14.

_____. 1984. *The History of Sexuality Vol 1*, Harmondsworth, Penguin.

Franks, David and Viktor Gecas. 1992. "Autonomy and Conformity in Cooley's Self-Theory," *Symbolic Interaction*, 15(1):49–68.

Fussell, Sam. 1991. *Muscle: Confessions of an Unlikely Bodybuilder*, New York, Poseidon.

Gadamer, Hans-Georg. 1989. *Truth and Method*, London, Sheed and Ward.

Giddens, Anthony. 1991. *Modernity and Self-Identity*, Cambridge, Polity.

_____. 1992. *The Transformation of Intimacy*, Cambridge, Polity.

Gimlin, Debra. 2002. *Body Work*, Berkeley, University of California Press.

Hirst, Paul and Penny Wooley. 1982. *Social Relations and Human Attributes*, London, Tavistock.

Honneth, Axel. 1995. *The Struggle for Recognition*, Cambridge, Polity.

Joas, Hans. 1985. *G. H. Mead*, Cambridge, Polity.

Kojève, Alexandre. 1969. *Introduction to the Reading of Hegel*, Ithaca, Cornell University Press.

Lloyd, Moya. 1996. "Feminism, Aerobics and the Politics of the Body." *Body and Society*, 2(2): 79–98.

McNay, Lois. 1992. *Foucault and Feminism*, Cambridge, Polity.

Mead, George Herbert. 1967. *Mind, Self and Society*, Chicago, Chicago University Press.

Sawicki, Jana. 1991. *Disciplining Foucault*, London, Routledge.

Scheff, Thomas. 2005. "Looking Glass Self." *Symbolic Interaction*, 28(2): 147–66.

Chapter 3

Reflections of the Body, Images of Self: Visibility and Invisibility in Chronic Illness and Disability

Kathy Charmaz and Dana Rosenfeld

Chronic illness and disability present circumstances in which people become conscious of their body and reflect upon them in ways that may or may not be on their own terms. Thus, as Kathy Charmaz and Dana Rosenfeld suggest, "Studying people's experiences with chronic illness and disability teaches us of the fragility of our body and its appearance, and how subject we are and have always been to contingencies that affect it." Using Cooley's looking-glass self as a tool to examine relationships between body and self, Charmaz and Rosenfeld magnify how people with illness and disability "see images of this body – and themselves – in how other people respond to them." Charmaz and Rosenfeld also unite Cooley with Goffman to investigate how illness and disability intensifies tensions between body and self, focusing here on the tension between visibility and information control. In their grounded analysis, Charmaz and Rosenfeld "take the concept of the looking glass self beyond appearances and information control about the body into the experiences of the body and to those emanating from it as they arise during illness and disability."

I just feel real self-conscious when I'm downtown and people look at me, you know, like women or something, or they notice the way I'm not walking correctly or whatever. And it really bothers me. It's almost like it brings me up short or something.... I don't know what they're thinking or anything, but I can see that they perceive something different about me because they're looking, and I get annoyed.

Charmaz Interview

I playfully asked the doctor, "When my leg heals, will I be able to walk?" The poor man, not knowing the extent of my paralysis, was a perfect foil, and gravely answered, "Yes." I could hardly contain myself, and it was only between chuckles that I could deliver the punch line: "That's wonderful. I couldn't walk before."

Beisser (1989:149)

These two statements, the first from an interview with Tina Reidel, a 44 year old woman with rheumatoid arthritis, the second from Arnold Beisser, a 63 year old man with paralysis, hint of the multiple images of self, body, and other that arise in the daily lives of people with chronic illnesses and disabilities. Tina became acutely aware of her now-altered body during the encounter, but Beisser, who had broken his leg, knew how his body appeared through long years of having a disability. Seeing that other people noticed her disability heightened Tina's consciousness of her body and forced her to reflect on it – at that moment. The incident flashed immediate images of her physical losses and difference from other people. Other women's silent recognition created an unwelcome, unanticipated intrusion and caused her discomfort and aggravation.

Beisser, in contrast, seized the moment to make the doctor's incomplete image of his body explicit. He controlled the interaction and the image of his body in it and forced the doctor's attention to it. Beisser's remarks reveal a man who learned to live with disability on his terms, but the learning was not always easy. He had contracted poliomyelitis in 1950 when people with severe disabilities remained sequestered at home or in institutions. Beisser (1989:128) realized that he navigated new ground as a sports fan, psychiatrist, and lover without "a model, someone who has suffered your loss and done the same things you want to do." For Beisser (1989:129), "Almost everything has the potential for embarrassment under new conditions. Risks are not easily taken if the consequence of failure is to feel entirely alone."

Studying people's experiences with chronic illness and disability teaches us of the fragility of our body and its appearance, and how subject we are and have always been to contingencies that affect it. Such realizations change the view we believe others hold of us and the actions we take in response to our imagined view – whether of awe and respect or of frailty or incompetence. This imagined view contains judgements of character, ranging from saintly, courageous, dependent, or slothful to morally tainted (e.g. drunk or gluttonous). Like Tina Reidel, when an event belies our taken-for granted views of ourselves as unremarkable or physically and socially competent, we likely conjure new images of ourselves during the event, whether or not these images of self last. Our self-consciousness rises, we believe that we see ourselves as more aware of others' images of us, and we select new images. As our sensitivity increases to the unexpected gaze of others, staring into the looking-glass they hold can become increasingly painful.

In this chapter, we explore Cooley's (1902) concept of the looking-glass self as a tool for looking at relationships between the body, self, and identity. For Cooley, the looking-glass self has three major characteristics: our imagined image of how we appear to another person, the judgement that we imagine he or she makes of our appearance, and our feelings about ourselves inspired by this imagined judgement, such as pride or shame. We all routinely engage in this kind of imagining, as Helen Mirren, who played Queen Elizabeth I in a recent British television production, put it when a maid offered her a mirror: "The look on your face tells the queen all she needs to know about hers" (Williams 2005). Yet a looking glass self assumes magnified meanings for many people with limited or compromised bodies because they can no longer take a competent body for granted. They see images of this body – and themselves – in how other people respond to them. The looking-glass self is, in great part, an imagined embodied self in action. Thus, we can adopt the looking glass self as a metaphor and view how the body itself becomes a looking glass reflecting images of a present self and revealing images of a future one.

People with chronic illness and disabilities confront tensions between body, self and identity that everyone faces (barring an early and sudden death); however, they experience these tensions in accelerated, intensified, and magnified form. These tensions (1) arise in such problematic concerns as maintaining a valued self, controlling information about body and self, and overruling images that others impart and (2) bring often tacit oppositions into view: visibility vs. invisibility of physical status, bodily control vs. failure, autonomy vs. dependency, victory vs. defeat, and acceptability vs. unacceptability.

We focus on visibility vs. invisibility and can only suggest how other oppositions affect relative visibility and people's lives. Thus we address how embodiment complicates self and identity for people with chronic illness and disabilities and ask the following questions: How does relative visibility or invisibility affect images of self? What strategies do people use to control these images? What are the implications of public interactions and private realizations for treating the body as a looking glass? How does scrutiny of the situations of people with chronic illnesses and disabilities inform and extend symbolic interactionist notions of the embodied self? To answer these questions, we examine how images of self and definitions of the body become problematic.

Theoretical Framework

Our analysis of the looking glass body begins with its animating concept, Cooley's looking glass self, and situates it in embodied action. The looking glass self is both social and subjective. It relies on language and meaning and typically arises in social interaction. It is a reflexive self that rests on selective interpretations, not a mechanical acceptance of imputed judgements. Like Tina Reidel, we don't know what strangers think of us, but our imagined view of their judgement can evoke strong emotions. We respond to those imagined images that we select. We may reject an imagined negative judgement by the other and or respond to it in a novel way.

Scheff (2005) emphasizes that the degree of social connectedness with others allows being attuned to the images they impart of us, and interpreting them accurately. But people with chronic illnesses and disabilities are forced to view their reflected images held by people with whom they are not attuned. They often need to make sense of reflected images of self through piecing together minimal cues imparted by strangers. Scheff (2005) shows how Erving Goffman elaborates Cooley's concept of the looking glass self in ordinary life; we point out how Goffman's ideas apply to a looking glass body. If Goffman's actor is highly self-conscious, then under certain conditions, disabled actors become even more so. They must work to overcome obstacles that undermine realizing a recognizably competent identity.[1]

---

1 This is not to say that the disability rights movement has not inspired some disabled people to embrace an easily recognizable disabled image – see e.g. Klawiter 2000.

Many of our conjured images focus on reflections others make of our surface appearances: face, form, and interactional facade. Physical limitations may either remain invisible or be intermittently visible under certain conditions, some of which people can anticipate, but many of which they cannot. Goffman's concepts allow us to examine how people with compromised bodies try to control information, minimize unwanted visibility, and manage their identities (see also Gardner and Gronfein 2005). Goffman's (see, for example, 1959) opus uncovered and documented information control and identity management. He did not explicitly engage the concept of the looking glass self however, Goffman's project and ours fundamentally assumes it: we understand that others know us through verbal and nonverbal information in interaction.

Goffman's approach focuses on immediate interaction; we can, however, reach further. We can take the concept of the looking glass self beyond appearances and information control *about* the body into the experiences *of* the body and to those emanating *from* it as they arise during illness and disability. This felt, experienced body becomes a looking-glass through which the person gains and interprets images of self. Self and body are not the same but each informs the other (Charmaz 1994). The looking-glass body in frailty and illness becomes more than a magnified image given in a moment; instead, telling images accumulate. Thus, the looking glass body forces reflexivity about self and situation through taking comparative, evaluative, normative views.

The gulf between the embodied self one wishes to present and the self one winds up presenting remains contingent, and ill and disabled people learn to imagine and try to manage this very contingency. Visibility and invisibility, then, form crucial elements in how the looking-glass self unfolds in both preparing for and conducting public action. A key question arises here: How and when do changes in bodily appearance and capacities affect images of the self on the part of ego and imagined alter?

Visibility and Information Control

People who blur or hide views of their frailty or disability employ a range of Goffmanian/dramaturgical techniques to produce a publicly and privately valued self, e.g. deference, physical grace, and props that signal healthy bodies. Those who imagine the consequences of prop failures – including the body itself – for how others see and evaluate them work to avoid these failures and/or manage their implications for self. We put ourselves together – in Goffman's words, "assemble our front" – with an eye to imagining how others will see us when we move into public view. Here, potentially discrediting visible characteristics (e.g. distorted limbs, disfigurements, and assistive devices) shape how actors manage their envisioned selves in public, prepare to enter public view, or avoid being in public (see Davis 1961; Murphy 1987). Our imagined view of how others view us relies on yet a deeper layer of images: imagined comparisons with others and imagined normative standards.

The difference between an actor's internal, private feelings and her public identity is less an obdurate reality than a constant project. We manage this difference through controlling information or bridge it in the interest of intimacy and/or authenticity. We strive to achieve as much control as possible over this information and its dissemination, but know that we cannot entirely control its content or distribution. Others may misunderstand or misrepresent its content. They can spread some or all of their reconstructed content to others. Meanwhile, we give information off through our interactions and can inadvertently let discreditable information slip.

Surface Appearances

The body is, of course, central here – information about the body, and information about the self communicated through it. The body both reflects and constitutes our biographies. Its surface can tell about our past (i.e. scars) and our current habits (i.e. through the smell of cigarettes or alcohol) and activities (i.e. perspiration signals exercise, anxiety or guilt), even our futures, as people judge us on our physical appearances.[2] Such audiences treat the body as a comparative and normative looking glass, separated from self and situation. Their taken-for-granted comparative images and normative standards result in unitary judgements imposed upon ill and disabled individuals. In one case, Charmaz interviewed a 45 year old woman with quadriplegia from multiple sclerosis who described this process. She mentioned her weight several times and recounted how other people saw it as an accountable deficit that they attributed to her inability to control her appetite. "I hardly eat anymore," she said. "You wouldn't know it by looking at me, but that's only because of being in the wheelchair and not being able to move. You can't help it even though some people think you are overeating."

How we decorate or prop up the body – the surface we place on our body's surface – reveals information and elicits evaluation. In Entwistle's (2002:133) words, dress "forms part of our epidermis – it lies on the boundary between self and other." The clothes we wear, and how we wear them and how we stand and move, shape others' image of us, and the image we hold of their image. Esther's arthritis precluded her wearing high heeled shoes, so she had to wear sneakers to a wedding even though, she explained, "that was before the sneaker age was really popular, and it wasn't as appropriate" (Rosenfeld and Faircloth 2004). To her chagrin, Clara, an elderly woman with an arthritis-related injury, had to attend her husband's funeral on crutches after her doctor gave her a cortisone shot.

Arthritis prevented these women from meeting important ceremonial demands whose adoption or rejection constituted claims about the self (Goffman 1959). These two women invoke a comparative and normative looking-glass to assess their conformity or nonconformity to standards of deference (here, rituals associated with

---

2 These appearances can be misinterpreted: not surprisingly, some individuals with neurological symptoms find that other people attribute their visible symptoms to drinking or drug use.

major life transitions) which, as Goffman (1967) has clearly shown, have direct implications for our real or imagined demeanour.[3]

Surface appearances prevail in more mundane settings as well and can transform people into objects in a distorted looking-glass. They convey an image that their audiences reflect back to them as transgressing appropriate normative standards. Nijhof (2002:191) writes about "M.," a man with Parkinson's disease, who described being stared at, even discussed, when in public because of "the stiffness of my face…. A boy, sitting opposite me in a bus, asked his mother why is it that this man looks so angry? I feel specially awkward in such a situation." The boy misinterpreted M.'s partial facial paralysis as a motivated, agentic expression of an emotion, and viewed this expression as a public display of both M.'s internal state and of his stance toward others based upon it. M.'s attributed agency makes M. feel "awkward," because whatever his actual emotional state before the encounter, being publicly misrepresented transformed him into a public spectacle.

This intrusion of the public into the private, justified by M.'s alleged intrusion of the private into the public, occurred on several dimensions. First, the incident shocked M. out of his routine civil inattention (Goffman 1963a) by a child's making him the focus of interaction when the boy should be engaging in civil inattention himself. Instead the boy converted himself and everyone within earshot into an audience, and assumed the right to speak. Second, this boy publicly declared M.'s private emotions to be a matter of public concern. Third, he called M.'s alleged emotions into account and labelled them relevant to everyone present. Moreover, the audience forced M.'s awareness of how others saw and evaluated his countenance. A stranger's unusual public announcement of his view breaches both normal relations in public and our understanding of the boundaries between our private, sacred person and the rights of others to lay claim to these relations and boundaries. M. had become, if not an open person (one to whom other people accord so little respect that he may be approached at will – Goffman 1963a:18), then someone who risked becoming one. Despite M.'s abiding by the routine rules of public transport, he is nonetheless seen (albeit by competent adults who usually appropriately refrain from public comment) as someone who did not quite belong.

To a certain degree, people can control the impact of their illness and disabilities on their surface appearances. Knowing that they wish to control their looking glass bodies reminds us of the fragility of appearance for people with physical impairment and of our own sensitivity about how others see and evaluate us. Sarah (Rosenfeld and Faircloth 2004) had severe disabilities from lupus and resultant crippling osteoarthritis, but refused to wear her prescribed neck brace in public because it caused her discomfort and constrained her movements and, moreover, because others saw her as "a walking zombie" when she wore it. Sarah imagined that self that others imagined her to be, this image derived from the affect she displayed when

---

3   Athletes with disabilities, in contrast, may startle non-disabled others because their grace and skill belie preconceived images of disability. These athletes may compare themselves and their performances with the persons they had been as well as with each other.

constrained by a device for assuaging her pain. She implied that the pain caused her self less damage than did the assumptions others made about her because she could no longer physically and thus socially engage others when in her neck brace: that she was, somehow, less than fully human, occupying a space between the living and the dead. Here, Sarah's constrained body led to constricted interactions, which in turn led to reifying unacceptable negative images of self.

These few examples show that the visibility of illness or disability affects how we imagine others view us and how our imagined images shape our experiences of and with our bodies. When everyone "knows" facts of crucial significance about us, i.e. visible disability or effects of illness, and projects images of these facts, we can seldom ignore them. Perhaps most telling and most difficult are the messages from self to self about how disability appears to self and what it means. Among these meanings are aesthetic evaluations of the body (Gadow 1982). During one interview when a woman who had lupus erythematosus was ill, but looked much healthier than she had one year before, Charmaz said, "You look pretty refreshed." She replied, "Do I? Well, you should see me on my good days then. I look totally horrible to myself today ... because my eyes hurt, my neck hurts." Surface information does not always make illness and disability visible; thus, invisibility further complicates how people think, feel, and act toward their bodies and how others view and reflect images of these bodies.

Mortification and the Contradiction of Surface Appearances

The body is a continuously signifying mechanism that provides information about the self through its movements, positioning, gestures, and the like. Just as we are never entirely certain that the verbal information we provide will jibe with the claims we wish to make about ourselves, or with claims about ourselves we have made in the past, so are we never entirely certain that the information we provide about – and through – our bodies will jibe with these claims. Hence we try to ensure that what goes on internally (e.g. our digestive processes and sexual desires) remains hidden from public view. When it does not, then observers make negative judgements about our ability to control our bodies and emotions, as Elias (1978) and those continuing his work (see e.g. Gurney 2000) have amply documented in their studies of the civilizing process. Loss of bodily control – particularly public visibility of such loss – forces reflections about our physical status, threatens personal autonomy, and prompts feeling defeated by our body and viewing self as unacceptable. A repeated image of loss of bodily control in our consciousness, if not also in others' curiosity and concern, multiplies and magnifies the meaning of this image, as though an image of one's body from a single mirror is reproduced in multiple copies and indiscriminately disseminated.

Exerting bodily control is a continuous and complex process. Ordinarily we become so adept at bodily control that we conduct it on a tacit, unconscious, or barely conscious level. Much depends on its artful and successful execution. Indeed, in the dramaturgical literature, nothing is more basic than successfully playing this information game, as it produces a morally and technically competent self and an acceptable social identity and, at least in Goffman's later work, an interactional and ritual order that constitutes society itself.

Publicly displaying information discordant with the claims we make about ourselves leads to embarrassment, shame, even mortification. In Goffman's opus, these emotions display recognition of having breached social expectations and surrendered our social standing, at least for the moment. The care we take to avoid these consequences and their relative rarity attests to their significance. When such consequences do occur, however, the results can be mortifying. Our appearance during these moments can undermine our desired self-presentation (Schneider and Conrad 1983; Goffman 1963b). In Williams and Barlow's (1998:133) study of rheumatoid arthritis, one informant described attending a cabaret while on holiday:

> When I got up to move, I couldn't move properly to start with. I had to stand there for a bit until I could get going and I know other people were looking at me and thinking that I was drunk. That's how you feel with strangers ... that they will automatically think the worst of you.

Here, the shift from competent and thus unremarkable member of the group to publicly identified "drunk" occurs rapidly. People's assumptions about themselves may shatter when observers attribute to them the "worst" qualities they can envision. The assumption that the inability to move as quickly and purposefully as others results from an unchecked appetite trumps an actor's efforts to produce herself as a competent person, and painfully lowers her standing. Note that participants imparted and received these messages with no exchange of words. The looking-glass body emerges by watching how alter watches ego. Merely having captured strangers' attention signals their having declared us unworthy of the ritual inattention due others.

Mortification can cause such an assault upon self-definition and social identification that we may sever contact with the individual who witnessed the mortifying incident. In the case of bodily failure, the "offending" person cannot forgive the self. Through losing trust in her body, the person also loses trust in her ability to continue the relationship as before. The failing body diminishes the self. The ill person feels that the relationship has fundamentally changed because the grounds on which it rested have been betrayed. Betty Rollin (1985) described her mother's relationship with her elderly admirer. Her mother suffered psychologically and emotionally from deteriorating colon cancer. The assumptions of being able to maintain *bodily control* and taking responsibility for control over appearance also figure here. This woman has lost control over both her body and appearance; therefore, from her perspective, she cannot maintain control over her identity.[4] Rollin (1985:125–126) writes:

---

4   Similarly, losing control over her appearance portends losing control over her identity. Some women who had had mastectomies regret doing so because the visible absence of their breast constantly reminded them of their difference from their past selves and other women as well as of the possible recurrence of cancer.

Her eyes were on me now, enlarged by their sorrow, like a child reporting to her mother something terrible that had happened at school that day. "I had on the pretty robe you gave me, the one with the flowers." She stopped for a moment and again pressed her lips together. Then she went on. "We were talking and he was saying all those things about wanting to see me more and not caring how I look, and then ... all of a sudden I had to go to the bathroom ... and I said excuse me and got up, and when I got there I looked at the back of my robe and it was soiled, and I looked down at the floor and I had ... left spots on the floor, and I probably smelled, too ... and I'm sure he saw. He must have seen." She wasn't crying anymore, but she looked as miserable as a person who is not crying can look.

"I am so humiliated," she said slowly, turning her head toward the window. "I'm so humiliated. I don't ever want to see him again."

In other cases, people may look well and able although they are not, or be intermittently sick and disabled. Those whose disability or illness creates a new reliance on others for mundane tasks may worry that others interpret this new reliance, and the requests for help that accompany it, as sloth. Catherine (Rosenfeld and Faircloth 2004), for example, disliked "asking people to do things that I usually do myself," and explained to the interviewer that she only does this when her arthritis is "really acting up." Catherine once misinterpreted her grandmother's requests for help as laziness, but later understood them to have been prompted by her arthritis. Catherine now worried that her husband would see her own requests for help in the same light. Although visible bodily limitations can create interactional and relational trouble and affect the looking-glass self, so can their invisibility.

I understand now why my grandmother used to always tell us, "Go bring me this and bring me that." And I used to think, "Why don't she get up and get it?" Now I understand why we were her legs, because when you sit down, and go to get up, oh, it's terrible. It feels like the bones are rubbing together.... And I find myself reaching and asking my husband, "Pass me [that]" and I guess he wonders, "Why don't you get it?" But he doesn't have arthritis, so he doesn't know.

In the absence of visible (surface) signs of illness or disability, even disclosing that one suffers from a condition can fail to make others 1) sensitive to the physical and social demands of the condition, and 2) draw positive or benign conclusions about the ill or disabled person despite that person's inability to perform certain tasks. Declarations of invisible illness and disability often elicit disbelief. Those whose claims to illness or disability are rejected view distorted images of their bodies in the looking glass given by other people who discount their symptoms or disbelieve that they have an illness. One woman told her lover of her illness but at any mention of it, he told her, "You're not sick," since her illness was not evident to him in recognizable ways. Another woman had told several acquaintances that her obvious fatigue and balance problems resulted from an episode of multiple sclerosis. In her view, they discounted her disclosure and disbelieved her account, so she became wary about seeing them. She said, "Most of the time, I think that's been probably my biggest problem is that I never looked sick ... but I always took pains not to look sick, and I always took pains never to go out when I did look sick." This woman found herself caught between social obligations to present a competent and well-organized appearance and moral obligations to be who she claimed to be (including non-verbal and embodied claims about the self).

Maintaining the difference between a private self and public identity can be an asset for those with stigma potential, when they can exercise control over discrediting information (Goffman 1963b). When this woman's acquaintances discounted her disclosure, the same difference between private self and public identity became a liability, as others used her surface appearance to gauge the authenticity of her verbal claims about self. Because this woman's surface appearance contradicted these claims, other people took her appearance as the ultimate arbiter of the validity of her claims and, thus, of her "true" identity. In their view, she did not claim her seemingly true (healthy) identity, so they negatively evaluated her self as well. She then became not only truly well rather than truly sick, but also truly inauthentic.

Thus different audiences give the gulf between inner feelings and surface appearances different weight,[5] and produce yet another disjuncture. The imagined self of a woman with severe arthritis remained strongly shaped by her glamorous appearance, in which she took pride and invested much time and energy. Yet she felt discomforted because people responded to her surface appearance without access to (or interest in) her internal experience. Her glamorous appearance was incongruent with her now fluid personal identity that she linked to her physical state:

> I may look like I'm healthy and all this stuff and I get – all these guys start making catcalls and I'm in pain and it just seems incongruous. I go, "What are they whistling at?" I usually identify with how I *feel*. Even though I go through a lot of effort to make myself look good, I still identify with how I feel. It's like being – feeling like an old person in a young person['s body]. It's like only an old person is entitled to have all this pain.
>
> Charmaz (1995:666)

This woman's body forced an immediacy upon her that negated and superseded the positive images reflected by others (Gadow 1982). Pain cracks the looking glass and refracts contradictory images. The disparity between feeling, self-definition, and projected images comes into focus when appearance belies incapacity and other people neither accept nor allow for the ill person's limitations.[6]

---

5 By the same token, the ill or disabled care more about certain people's image of them than of others. Millie (a 72 year old women with arthritis) for example, said:

> If you're in company your own age, you can joke about it....It's not so much what the public in general thinks, but I hate having the kids think that I'm such a decrepit old lady.
>
> (Taken from Rosenfeld and Faircloth 2004.)

6 This issue takes on large proportions when ill people attempt to obtain disability benefits because they can no longer work but they still look healthy.

Illness Reminders: The Self as Audience

A main audience for the self's performance is the self. Not only are ill or disabled actors aware of others' failure to recognize the reality of their physical troubles, they also become aware of their own failure to do so as well. Just as the other may give primacy to our surface appearance as a marker of our essential value and standing, so might we. Illness reminders may shock an ill person who had favoured an image of self rooted in a relatively healthy and capable past. The body becomes a looking-glass that forces comparisons between past and present. Ilza Veith (1988:69), a woman who had had a midlife stroke, writes of her:

> [P]reoccupation with my former appearance, when I appeared tall and slim, my legs appeared long and elegant in high-heeled shoes, and my face had its original lean contours. The change in my face to its present broad shape and excessively round cheeks is the consequence of several cortisone injections ... and caused the typical facial swelling which has not lessened in all the years since it first became noticeable. My absorption with my former appearance recently received another blow when I saw a new passport picture, hurriedly taken in colour, which showed that I do have some slight facial paralysis. Until then the mirror had been able to hide this disfigurement from me and I had deluded myself into believing that I had been spared this unfortunate concomitant of a stroke.

Illness reminders often fade from memory if long lapses occur between episodes. For many chronically ill as opposed to disabled people, those reminders are intermittent rather than continuous. Their appearance as ill as well as their bodily feelings of being ill may occur episodically in relatively short spaces of time between long stretches or only after many months or years. Further, the visibility of other people's symptoms may shift during the day. When people function well in the morning and become progressively less alert, agile, or capable during the day, they may hide their appearance as ill through careful scheduling and planning. When they cannot do so, a symptom such as slurred speech, imbalance, or lack of coordination could threaten the appearance they wish to project, and thus lead to intrusive questions or negative definitions of self. Those with episodic illness, like those around them, may almost forget that they have an intrusive illness. When one woman whom Charmaz interviewed became pregnant, she had a full-blown flare-up, with stiff, immobile joints, changed posture, and swollen hands with blue fingers. She wrote, "It is a reminder that I live with a chronic disease." When illness becomes invisible to self, its reappearance can shock the self. Another woman, whose red face, shortness of breath, and slowed gait marked her relapse said of it, "You forget that it is real." Later, after experiencing continued symptoms for several months, she said, "I'm on a decline, a real decline physically. And I mean, I can see it; I can feel it even on my good days." [7]

---

7   Illness reminders may come from other people who usually unwittingly, but sometimes intentionally, pronounce the person's difference. Ilza Veith's (1988:82–83) hemiplegia and wheelchair use makes her disability apparent to others. As a result of her appearance, strangers may respond with uninvited intrusive actions upon her body and self. She said:

A static disability, in contrast, provides a different looking glass with sustained images. The person may learn ways to deflect negative images and defuse physical limitation. Like Beisser, people with disabilities sometimes joke about their infirmities and use them to put other people at ease (Davis 1961). Strained encounters, however, are not equal; the person with a disability bears the interactional onus to ease the situation. Still, people with disabilities may not only become active in easing strained interactions and therefore in circumventing embarrassing situations, they may be active in meeting them head on, or like Beisser, active in forcing the other person's gaze and awareness. Thus, the body is not all of the self. Instead, the ill or disabled person presents a self which commands images of wholeness and competence extending beyond his or her impairment.

Conclusions

As recent research has theorized, when the body fails to function in expected ways, it changes from a disappearing entity (one of which we are unaware) to a *dys*appearing one, which means appearing dysfunctional to ourselves and to others (see Williams and Bendelow 1998). Just as we become excruciatingly aware of our failures when we slip up, sinking into embarrassment and perhaps even shame, so do we experience these discomforts if and when illness and disability move us from a tacit relationship with our bodies to a more conscious and reflective one. When we realize that we can no longer count on our bodies to look, behave, or move as they once did, we change the image that we imagine others have of us.

Merely *imagining* that someone might view us in negative ways can elicit similar feelings of shame as those induced by *knowing* that someone is doing so or has done so (see Scheff 2003). Our sensitivity to the evaluations of others leads us to go to great lengths to avoid being seen as incompetent or, in Douglas's (1966) words, matter out of order. Thus the time and money we spend on clothes, grooming, and the like. But making our surface appearances correspond with preferred standards of grace, tact, and timeliness becomes more difficult as we find ourselves having less control over them, or less ability to produce appearances that jibe with our own and others' expectations and with our previous appearance that comprised a legitimate claim about our selves. This legitimacy looms large at this point: we face maintaining previous claims about the self that have become technically much more difficult to sustain (and thus risk having these claims discredited by our bodies), or confront the consequences of making a new set of claims. Given the uncertain trajectory of chronic illness, making new claims is not a straightforward decision. Uncertainty

---

There are, of course, many occasions when my helplessness in dressing or seating myself becomes evident to strangers .... If, as so often happens in restaurants, a helpful soul hurries over from another table and tries to assist me in pulling on a sweater, coat, or whatever other garment, feeling I am in need of their help, they often cannot be discouraged even by a forceful rejection.

makes it difficult to plan movements, encounters, and interactions.[8] Often, the obvious solution (disclosing the reason for being unable to make the same embodied claims about the self as one did before) becomes yet another source of trouble when others view this disclosure as false, and thus the one making the disclosure as not only something she is not claiming to be, but deluded or disingenuous as well. The looking glass self, it seems, slips out of our control.

Perhaps the main issue remains: under which conditions do reflected images of body and self affect the self-concept? Charmaz's (1991, 1999) extension of Turner's (1976) argument figures here. Fleeting reflected images of the embodied self may not stick. A self-concept is relatively enduring; it has boundaries. Some attributes, characteristics, values define the "Me." Others do not. Yet repeated jarring reflections of body and self can loosen those boundaries. Tina Reidel and Arnold Beisser's stories hint of how and when reflected images matter. Tina Reidel became attuned to the images of other people; Arnold Beisser learned how to shape such images and to set the grounds *for* interaction. When earlier boundaries of the self-concept have been weakened, they become vulnerable to redefinition – whether positive or negative. To the extent that one can sustain positive images from the past and live in a world that provides positive – and meaningful – reflections in the present, then one may limit the effect of disquieting images mirrored in the looking glass body.

References

Beisser, Arnold R. 1988. *Flying without Wings: Personal Reflections on Being Disabled.* New York: Doubleday.

Charmaz, Kathy. 1991. *Good Days, Bad Days: The Self in Chronic Illness and Time.* New Brunswick, NJ: Rutgers University Press.

Charmaz, Kathy. 1994. "'Discoveries' of Self in Illness," in Mary Lou Dietz, Robert Prus, and William Shaffir (Eds), *Doing Everyday Life: Ethnography as Lived Experience.* Mississauga, Ontario: Copp Clark Longman Ltd. pp. 226–242.

Charmaz, Kathy. 1995. "The Body, Identity and Self," *The Sociological Quarterly*, 36:657–680.

Charmaz, Kathy. 1999. "From the 'Sick Role' to Stories of Self: Understanding the Self in Illness," in Richard D. Ashmore and Richard A. Contrada (Eds), *Self and Identity, Vol. 2: Interdisciplinary Explorations in Physical Health.* New York: Oxford University Press. pp. 209–239.

Charmaz, Kathy. Forthcoming, 2006, "Stories, Silences, and Self: Dilemmas in Disclosing Chronic Illness," in Dale Brashers and Daena Goldstein (Eds), *Health Communication.* New York: Lawrence Erlbaum.

---

8 This contingency is not entirely driven by the body – other contingencies such as assistive technologies, geography and architecture, and the composition of the group (strangers, intimates, fellow-sufferers, those who know of the condition or do not, and those with certain expectations over others) factor in as well.

Cooley, Charles H. 1902. *Human Nature and Social Order.* New York: Charles Scribner's Sons.

Davis, Fred. 1961. "Deviance Disavowal: The Management of Strained Interaction by the Visibly Handicapped," *Social Problems*, 9:120–132.

Douglas, Mary. 1966. *Purity and Danger: An Analysis of the Concepts of Pollution and Taboo.* London: Routledge.

Elias, Norbert. 1978. *The Civilizing Process: The History of Manners.* Oxford: Blackwell.

Entwhistle, Joanne. 2002. "The Dressed Body," in Mary Evans and Ellie Lee (Eds), *Real Bodies: A Sociological Introduction.* Basingstoke, UK: Palgrave. pp. 133–150.

Gadow, Sally. 1982. "Body and Self: A Dialectic," in Victor Kestenbaum (Ed.) *The Humanity of the Ill.* Knoxville: University of Tennessee Press. pp. 86–100.

Gardner, Carol Brooks and William P. Gronfein. "Reflections on Varieties of Shame Induction, Shame Management, and Shame Avoidance in Some Works of Erving Goffman," *Symbolic Interaction*, 28:175–183.

Goffman, Erving. 1959. *The Presentation of Self in Everyday Life.* New York: Doubleday.

Goffman, Erving. 1963a. *Behavior in Public Places: Notes on the Social Organization of Gatherings.* New York: Free Press.

Goffman, Erving. 1963b. *Stigma: Notes on the Management of Spoiled Identity.* Englewood Cliffs, NJ: Prentice-Hall.

Goffman, Erving. 1967. "The Self as Ritual Object: From 'The Nature of Deference and Demeanor,'" in Charles Lemert and Ann Branaman 2001 (Eds), *The Goffman Reader.* Oxford, UK: Blackwell Publishers. pp. 27–33.

Gurney, Craig M. 2000. "Accommodating Bodies: The Organization of Corporeal Dirt in the Embodied Home," in Linda McKie and Nick Watson (Eds), *Organizing Bodies: Policy, Institutions and Work.* New York: St. Martin's Press. pp. 55–80.

Klawiter, Maren. 2000. "Racing for the Cure, Walking Women, and Toxic Touring: Mapping Cultures of Action within the Bay Area Terrain of Breast Cancer." in Laura K. Potts (Ed.), *Ideologies of Breast Cancer: Feminist Perspectives.* New York: St. Martin's Press. pp. 63–73.

Murphy, Robert F. 1987. *The Body Silent.* New York: Henry Holt.

Nijhof, Gerhard 2002. "Parkinson's Disease as a Problem of Shame in Public Appearance," in Sarah Nettleton and Ulla Gustafsson (Eds) *The Sociology of Health and Illness Reader.* Oxford: Polity Press. pp. 188–196.

Rollin, Betty. 1985. *Last Wish.* NY, Linden Press.

Rosenfeld, Dana and Christopher Faircloth. 2004. "Embodied Fluidity and the Commitment to Movement: Constructing the Moral Self through Arthritis Narratives," *Symbolic Interaction*, 27(4):507–529.

Scheff, Thomas J. 2003. "Shame in Self and Society," *Symbolic Interaction*, 26(2):239–262.

Scheff, Thomas J. 2005. "Looking-Glass Self: Goffman as Symbolic Interactionist," *Symbolic Interaction*, 28:147–166.

Schneider, Joseph W. and Peter Conrad. 1983. *Having Epilepsy: The Experience and Control of Illness*. Philadelphia: Temple University Press.

Turner, Ralph. 1976. "The Real Self: From Institution to Impulse," *American Journal of Sociology*, 81:989–1016.

Veith, Ilza. 1988. *Can You Hear the Clapping of One Hand?* Berkeley: University of California Press.

Williams, Bethan and Julie H. Barlow. 1998. "Falling Out with my Shadow: Lay Perceptions of the Body in the Context of Arthritis," in Sarah Nettleton and Jonathan Watson (Eds) *The Body in Everyday Life*. London: Routledge. pp. 124–141.

Williams, Nigel. 2005. "Elizabeth I." Produced by Company Pictures for Channel 4. © Company Television Ltd.

Williams, Simon J. and Gillian Bendelow. 1998. *The Lived Body: Sociological Themes, Embodied Issues*. London: Routledge.

Chapter 4

Reflexive Transembodiment

Douglas Schrock and Emily M. Boyd

The status passage of transgendered people is one which arrives at the conviction that they are a gender their body contradicts, a woman in a man's body for example. In this chapter Douglas Schrock and Emily M. Boyd examine this status passage utilizing the concept of "reflexive transembodiment" that effectively highlights "the embodied nature of their transition and the central role of reflexivity." Consistent with the other chapters in this segment, Schrock and Boyd's analysis hinges on a looking-glass body in which people exercise reflexivity to resolve unique dilemmas in their transgendered status passage. Reflexive storytelling intersects with reflexive bodywork to produce a transgendered "true self." Yet the passage, in this case "coming out," is a process rife with concealment and revelation, leaking signifiers of gender, verbal and visual announcements – all of which "remind us of the importance of agency and culture in reflexive body techniques."

As Florian Znaniecki (1925:83) notes, we often use the visual cues of another's "body" to "schematize … the person into several classes [such] as male or female." At birth, medical authorities and adults define the bodies of transsexuals as indicating a sex category to which they no longer identify. As explained by Jenny, one of our interviewees, "I don't care if I have a dick, I'm a woman." Transsexuals embark on a journey to alter their bodies so as to be seen by themselves and others as announcing an identity to which they are deeply attached. Their desire to inhabit and be socially affirmed as members of the "opposite sex" is experienced so profoundly that they are willing to risk losing family, friends, and employment. Transsexuals' "status passage" (Glaser and Strauss 1971) takes considerable money, time, emotional energy, and commitment – more, perhaps, than most other forms of bodywork.

In order to highlight the embodied nature of their transition *and* the central role of reflexivity, we refer to transsexuals' status passage as "reflexive transembodiment." Reflexivity is important to transembodiment in many ways. For example, believing one is really a woman or a man requires objectifying oneself as a sexed object. Reflexivity is also central to learning, practicing, and publicly expressing the embodiment of womanhood or manhood. As Crossley (2005) points out, body maintenance and modification are by definition reflexive as they requiring viewing and treating the body as an object, and thus can be considered "reflexive body techniques." Unlike female-bodied women engaging in similar practices, male-to-female transsexuals' body projects are generally deemed deviant. As a result, transembodied people often feel compelled to carefully account for their bodywork and strategically control how they present themselves to others. The reflexive self shapes and is shaped by such accounting and controlling.

We suggest that reflexive transembodiment is also a useful concept because it emphasizes the link between transsexuals' bodywork and reflexivity, which transsexual scholarship often neglects. For example, research that suggests that the body is a tool that transsexuals use to do gender or manage stigma (Feinbloom 1976; Garfinkel 1967; Kessler and McKenna 1978) or examines the history or process of "sex reassignment" (Billings and Urban 1982; Raymond 1979) downplays the importance of reflexivity. Research that examines coming to terms with transsexuality or coming out to others (Gagné and Tewksbury 1999; Gagné, Tewksbury, and McGaughey 1997; Risman 1984) downplays the body while emphasizing the reflexive process of self-definition. Furthermore, scholarship that attempts to address the relationship between transgendered people's bodies and subjectivities often neglects the interactionist notion of reflexivity in favour of phenomenological (Rubin 2003) or postmodern (Butler 1990) concepts. The notion of "reflexive transembodiment" aims to situate transsexual scholarship more squarely within an interactionist framework on the body/subjectivity.

Although transembodiment may appear extreme, the experience reflects a common dynamic with regard to Charles Cooley's (1902) looking glass self. Most of us, at least occasionally, imagine that when certain others view us, they do not see our "true selves" through the mosaic of our bodily signs. We may envision others judging our bodies in ways that evoke feelings of shame or, if we feel particularly empowered, anger ("How dare you objectify me!"). Transsexuals, however, are usually more concerned with being judged as a *member* of their desired sex category than they are with being a particular *kind* of member. Male-to-female transsexuals usually say they feel authentic, proud, and sometimes liberated when they or others read their bodies as signifying womanhood.

In this chapter, we will examine the role of reflexivity in the experiences of nine white, middle class male-to-female transsexuals, whom the first author interviewed and observed during fourteen months of fieldwork in a transgender community (see Schrock and Reid 2006 for a more complete description of methods). We analyze how these transsexuals exercised reflexivity in their attempts to resolve several dilemmas of their status passage. More specifically, we examine how interviewees mitigate shame by adopting the transgender community as a reference group, created a sense of coherence through reflexive storytelling, and transformed their corporal and social selves via reflexive bodywork. We present in-depth analyses of previously unexplored data on how interviewees employed reflexivity in the process of coming out as women to people who had only known them as men. We show how the reflexive process shaped their coming out strategy, which involved concealing then leaking the body project, followed by verbally then visually coming out.

Taking New Perspectives

As Harold Garfinkel (1969) points out, transsexuals breach one of the key taken-for-granted assumptions of gender: that people are born into and remain in a single gender category. Contemporary gender scholars (see for example, Lorber 1994) view the maintenance of such gender boundaries as fundamental to the reproduction of inequality. While, in some ways, many transsexuals reinforce the boundaries, such as conforming to stereotypical gender norms (Gagné and Tewksbury 1998), in other ways, their challenging of the aforementioned assumption likely plays into the interactional and often institutionalized policing of their presentations. In the US, transsexuals who are "read" as men in women's clothing commonly face public harassment and sometimes violence, they are not protected from employment discrimination (on the federal level), and they are stigmatized as perverted and unnatural (Burke 1996; Namaste 2000). In contrast to those who undergo surgery to alter bodily signs of gender (such as women who have breast implants) those who undergo sex reassignment surgery must first be diagnosed with a mental illness and submit to a regimen of regulation.

Such policing can lead transsexuals to imagine a generalized other that stigmatizes them as unnatural or perverted, which, as Cooley might predict, leads to undesired emotions. Feelings of shame, fear, isolation, and powerlessness, were so intense for some of our interviewees that they planned or attempted suicide. Becoming involved in the transgender subculture, however, can change how transsexuals define and feel about themselves. For example, Taylor said that attending her first transgender support group meeting was "really good" and that "it was like I broke through a shell; an underground society that had before been out of reach.... It's almost like I had come home." As Tamotsu Shibutani (1955) might explain, transsexuals used a new reference group from which to view themselves. As interviewees interacted with other transgendered people in support groups, read community publications, and learned about or became involved in the movement for trans liberation, debilitating feelings were sometimes transformed into pride, self-efficacy, solidarity, and anger at the gender police.

Reflexive Storytelling

Newly defined transsexuals experience a disjuncture between two objects of the reflexive self: what Morris Rosenberg (1979) refers to as external features (publicly visible bodily characteristics and signifiers of social identity) and internal features (cognition and feelings). As Taylor describes, "I know up here [pointing to her head] something is not male. And yet there is absolutely no direct sensory input that confirms it. None." A key reflexive method by which interviewees reconciled the discrepancy was through what Mead (1929) discussed as the symbolic reconstruction of the past for present purposes.

One form of this reconstruction is the self-narrative, which refers to a story that selectively links biographical events so as to project a self as object (Gergen and

Gergen 1983). Interviewees' self-narratives bestowed a sense of coherency and were constructed, it appeared, to boost the chance their selves would seem credible from others' perspectives. Interviewees, for example, used childhood memories of gender non-conformity, such as failing at sports and crossdressing or desiring to do so, as evidence of transsexuality. For example, Erin said: "Even in grade school I didn't want to play with the boys. I didn't want to play football, or basketball, or baseball, or any of those things. I wanted to play jump rope with the girls." They also reframed memories of gender conformity, such as doing well at sports and not crossdressing, as evidence of being in denial about their transsexuality. Interviewees thus used gender ideology and pop psychology to overwrite cultural definitions of differently gendered bodies.

The body as sexual vessel posed a similar symbolic dilemma for interviewees. Because many, as men, had used women's clothing during masturbation rituals or in sexual encounters with women or engaged in "normal" sex with women or men, they constructed stories that distanced themselves from erotic transvestites, heterosexual men, and homosexual men (Schrock and Reid 2006). Interviewees rhetorically de-fetishized autoerotic crossdressing and refashioned transvestic sex by blaming sexual arousal while crossdressed on uncooperative penises that listened more to their male biology than their differently gendered "true selves." Interviewees straightened out gay sex and queered straight sex primarily by using gender ideology that equates submissiveness with womanhood. For example, Erin described her first sexual encounter with a man as follows:

> He treated me totally female, not male. [H]e didn't rush me into it. We sat on the couch, we talked, he put his arm around me, we hugged, we kissed, he undressed me slowly. He picked me up and carried me to the bedroom.... And we made love. Slow tender love.... When I was with him, I felt *soooo* female.... Straight people cannot understand that. They go, "He's got a dick, you've got a dick, right? That means you're gay." It was there, but the way he treated it was not like a masculine thing. It was like a feminine thing. Does that make sense? He didn't treat it like it was a, quote, penis; he treated it like it was a vagina.

Here we can see how reflexive storytelling can render insignificant one of the most potent cultural signifiers of manhood: the erect penis, or, as Jenny called it, the "hideous growth."

Reflexive Bodywork

In addition to discrediting the body's importance in signifying gender, interviewees used the reflexive process to shape and present their bodies with the hope that others would be able to imagine them as women. This involves what Morris Rosenberg (1990:3) calls "reflexive agency," which refers to the "process whereby the organism acts back on itself for the purpose of producing intended effects on itself." Transsexuals employ reflexive agency in two ways: (1) they worked backstage to change their bodies in ways that bolstered the belief that others would imagine them as women and (2) they strategically altered subjectivity in order to control front stage bodily displays to encourage others to define and affirm them as women.

Because interviewees were not pressured in childhood and adolescence to discipline their bodies to signify femaleness, they took women's perspectives in order to develop a curriculum of bodily transformation and then diligently practiced and disciplined their bodies accordingly. They retrained their physical bodies to produce feminine verbal and nonverbal gestures, redecorated their bodies with makeup and feminine accoutrements, and remade their physical bodies through dieting, electrolysis, hormone therapy, and they were saving money for genital surgery. Such reflexive body techniques (Crossley 2005) especially retraining movements and makeup application, initially increased self-monitoring and made interviewees feel inauthentic. "Applying makeup sometimes feels like I am putting on some kind of mask," said Shelly. However, similar to women who participate in self-defence classes (McCaughey 1998:290), continual repetition eventually installed the practices into "bodily memory." Kris, for example, said that she used to "really concentrate and say to myself, 'I have to always remember to make my voice go up [at the end of a sentence],' but now it's just natural." As their techniques of bodywork became more habitual, interviewees felt more authentically female. Subjectivity and bodywork are inseparable.

Whereas the relatively private work of "transgendering" (Ekins 1997) the body unintentionally shaped subjectivity, publicly embodying womanhood initially involved the intentionally shaping of subjectivity with the aim of evoking audiences' affirmation of womanhood (Schrock and Boyd 2005). If they acted anxiously when presenting themselves as women in public, interviewees feared that others would assess them more critically and notice residual signs of manhood (such as adams apples, large hands, etc.). With the aim of blending into the gendered social landscape, interviewees engaged in cognitive emotion work (Hochschild 1979) in the form of personal pep talks. For example, Kris said, "The whole key [to passing] is to get in your head that, 'I'm a woman.' So what if I do something a little bit different. As long as I don't go, 'whoops,' you know, and try to change it too quick. People notice those things." Here we can see how reflexive agency was used to evoke displays of confidence that were intended to coax audiences into reading their public bodies as signifying womanhood. While we do not know how others' actually viewed them, it does appear they avoided confrontations about discrepant signs of gender. And minimizing such confrontations enabled interviewees to imagine that others categorized them as women, which, in turn, evoked feelings of pride and authenticity.

Reflexivity and Coming Out

As transsexual women began presenting themselves as anonymous women in public settings, they continued presenting themselves as men to more familiar faces. They were in effect living a gendered variation of William James' (1892) adage: people have "many different social selves." Transsexuals' coming out process involved retiring manhood and embodying womanhood full time. Changing how others imputed gendered selves to them, however, was tricky business. Interviewees needed to control, as much as possible, the process through which they came out to friends, family, and co-workers and employers.

Interviewees believed that losing the ability to play an active part in shaping the image of themselves in others' minds could be socially devastating. Such stories were plentiful in the transgender community. For example, one interviewee explained what happened when a transsexual friend lost control over the coming out process:

> [My friend] was engaged to be married and had not told his fiancé, which is a mistake that we all make. She was over at his place when he wasn't there once and found his [women's] clothes, and decided that [the friend] was sick, sinful, and every other thing she could say about him. Called up his boss, told his boss, told his mother, his family.

Being outed in such a manner could involve not only the loss of control over one's image in others' minds, but also the loss of familial relationships as well as employment.

Although some significant others may withdraw material and emotional support regardless of how transsexuals come out, interviewees believed that the more skilfully they controlled the coming out process, the better able they were to maintain important relationships. "If you present it properly and give people enough time and information and if there's genuine love between you or a genuine friendship, then it'll work out," said Taylor. Interviewees believed that coming out "properly" required perspective taking. As Sue described it:

> It's important in everything we do to not only think of it from your perspective but from the other person's perspective and how they will react. And I guess in a way I've tried to predict how they're going to act and give them a way that they can be happy with this decision too, and not be too worried.... I think there are ways to make it easier on other people.

Making it easier on other people involved coming out to people gradually, which involved strategically concealing and leaking the body project as well as coming out verbally and visually. As others (see, for example, Cahill and Eggleston 1996; Waskul 2002) have suggested, stigmatized "others" tend to do more than their share of such emotion work. As we will show, imagining how particular others may define, judge, and treat them greatly influenced the coming out process.

Concealing the Body Project

As their transembodiment progressed, interviewees had difficulty keeping evidence of their body projects backstage. Interviewees believed that others would view them in a more accepting manner, if they did not "discover" their transsexuality.

The most basic way transsexuals concealed their projects was to limit access to the backstage. They kept friends and family out of their bedroom closets and bathrooms or temporarily stowed away the evidence when necessary. Some dramatically cut down on inviting non-transgendered friends and family members over. When asked if anyone had ever noticed something in her apartment that raised suspicion, Joyce responded, "No, I don't have a lot of people over." Such "protective strategies" helped shield the backstage from "inopportune intrusions" (Goffman 1963).

For some interviewees, however, a secure residentially-based backstage was impossible to maintain and they developed other strategies. In order to keep her transsexuality a secret from her wife and daughter, for example, Erin said, "I kept my [women's] clothes in a storage facility and I changed there or changed in the car." When Taylor was moving, she said, "My friends were going to help me pack, I was in total fear that somehow a box would break open and all this stuff would fall out. So, it was like, into the dumpster it all went." Thus when a residentially-based backstage was not secure, interviewees moved or eliminated the backstage.

Concealing the body project also involved controlling "unmeant gestures" (Goffman 1959) that could discredit masculine performances. As Sue explained, controlling feminine practices involved acute consciousness of how others may impute gendered meanings to their performances as men.

> I catch myself [gesturing like a woman] as my male side and I really have to put my hands in my pockets because I just know it's not right. [Question: Are there other things?] I touch folks. As a man, I don't mind touching a woman, but a guy freaks out over it.... Sometimes I cross my legs so that basically one leg is really high over the other as compared to the guy ninety-degree angle [cross]. I try to catch myself with that because I've heard my daughter say, "That guy is a fag. Look at the way he crosses his legs." I have to be careful also because I have taken most of the hair off my hands, so I have to be careful how much I use them and how long I let my nails grow. It's a continual editing process. Sometimes I sit down and catch myself reaching back to smooth a skirt and it isn't there.

Interviewees' continual editing of how their bodies may be signifying gender thus involved perspective taking aimed at guessing how others evaluated their gendered performances.

In terms of hiding bodily modifications, interviewees most often relied on a literal version of what Goffman (1963) called "covering." After an out-of-town friend, whom Taylor described as "homophobic," called and said he was going through a severe depression wanted to visit, Taylor wanted to be supportive but worried about him noticing her changing appearance:

> And there I was, it was the middle of summer, legs shaved, no hair on my chest, nothing. And he comes down in the middle of the summer for a visit. I spent a week with this guy wearing long sleeve T-shirts and jeans in the middle of August (mutual laughter). God, I was miserable. He kind of figured something was up, but it never really came up.

Leaking the Body Project

As interviewees' bodywork progressed, it became increasingly difficult to hide. Signs of womanhood leaked out of the backstage. Interviewees believed that gradually leaking their body projects would prime others to be more accepting of their status passage. In other words, perspective-taking led them to strategically introduce gender ambiguity into their self presentations. As Kris explained:

> I think I've done things in such a way that's made it easier for people to accept me. And I think also that if two years ago when I started having these feelings I had come out and said, "I need to live full time as a woman" … for people who had known me, it would have been a very abrupt change. But for several years now, I've been slowly changing my appearance and my actions, letting people gradually get more accustomed to how I felt and acted.

Controlled leaking sometimes targeted a specific person to whom interviewees expected to come out. For example, in hope that her current friend, Carol, would be more prepared when she came out, Joyce sometimes styled her lengthening hair in a feminine manner before getting together. She also invited Carol to accompany her when she had both ears pierced. And afterwards, Joyce reported they "haggled over which one of us were going to get to buy a particular pair of earrings. I think that's what finally got her curiosity; like, 'Okay, what's up with this?'" Carol didn't actually ask Joyce the previous question, but Joyce imagined that such leaking shaped how Carol perceived her.

For interviewees who planned on trying to transition on the job (rather than search for work after living fulltime as women), leaking the backstage was seen as a useful strategy. As Sue began experimenting with makeup, she said:

> I started wearing it to work [as a man] as part of skin protection. I would do the basic skin care package of cleansing, refresher, moisturizer, and a little base coat of makeup just to protect the skin. People had no problems. I told people at work and they'd say, "That's fine. I see you as a guy and you're just wanting to have the best skin."

Some interviewees also changed the way they dressed as men. As Sue said:

> At work I slowly faded out my male clothes – I wouldn't wear a dress or anything – but be fairly androgynous… . The clothes I was buying as a guy were very stylish, but also very much like what girls wear. So then I started substituting. "Well, gee, if I'm buying a male's vest that looks like this, I might as well buy a girl's vest." And so I started phasing out the male clothes all together in my day-to-day work.

Most interviewees similarly began expressing feminine demeanour while presenting themselves as men. Erin, for example, said:

> I found myself last fall, forgetting to walk like a boy – and having to make myself do it. But after a short time of that, I said, "Screw this, I'm not even gong to try anymore." I'm just going to walk the way I feel like walking. If people have a problem with it, the heck

with them. And so far I haven't had any overtly negative responses from people around me, like at work. I think the operative assumption among people at work is that I'm gay and just coming out of the closest. And in talking things over with the human resources person there, who I've told all about the truth, we decided that that's probably the best approach for now, just let people think that; let them wonder.

Gradually feminizing their body's décor, demeanour, and shape enabled transsexuals to imagine that friends, family members, and employers/coworkers began to view them, at minimum, as gender nonconformists. As they leaked more and more of their body project to various audiences, transsexuals thus adopted incremental looking glasses, each of which brought their differently gendered "true selves" more into focus.

Coming out Verbally

As interviewees became more comfortable embodying womanhood in public and increasingly leaked their bodywork, it became emotionally difficult to present themselves as men. As Jenny explained, "Now when I have to put on the boy face and go do the boy things again, I go, 'Oh, fuck it, I don't want to do those things anymore.'" She later added that the "social affirmation of masculinity just rubs me raw." Trying to hide their differently gendered "true selves" from others also took a toll on their relationships. Taylor said that before coming out to her family, "I'm a little more closed than normal when I'm around them." When presenting herself as a man to people to whom she had not yet come out, Joyce said, "I am inhibited in talking, period."

As their desire to embody womanhood fulltime intensified and they perceived others might be getting the wrong impression, interviewees believed that it was time to reveal their differently gendered "true selves." But coming out was carefully executed because they believed that others would see them as radically different for the rest of their lives. As Joyce said, "It's not something that you can take back either, like, 'Oops, just kidding.'" In the hope that they could minimize negative reactions, interviewees told people that they were transsexuals before they allowed these others to see them as women.

Interviewees often picked women friends to come out to first, as they believed women would be less apt than men to respond harshly and that they might also help with makeup and fashion choices. Gender-conscious perspective taking thus shaped interviewees' coming out strategy. Although such a strategy worked for some interviewees, it did not go smoothly for Joyce. Joyce was pretty sure that her friend Carol knew about her transsexuality when she came out to her. On top of the information Joyce leaked about her body project (most notably, her earrings and hair styling), Carol asked, on behalf of another friend, "if I knew where she could get size 13 shoes. Well, why would she ask me?" But when Joyce came out to her, Carol was stunned and had difficulty accepting. Erin had better luck when she came out to an out-of-town male friend over the phone:

My friend in Atlanta ... called and invited me down to go to a Johnny Winter concert – he's a blues guitarist that we both love. I said, "Don, I would love to come but there's something that you need to know about me first. I'm going to look different, I'm going to act different than the last time you saw me. The beard is gone, I've had both ears pierced and I will look to you, at best, androgynous." I then proceeded to tell him why. I explained to him I was a transsexual and gave him my best explanation of current medical interpretation of it and I realized how freaked out he was. I said, "Okay, now that you know this, you are welcome to withdraw your invitation if you wish." He says, "No, I'm interested." Then we talked for a couple of hours.

Coming out to out-of-town friends seemed less risky to interviewees, perhaps because losing remote friends would less affect their day-to-day lives than losing local friends.

Coming out to parents was especially difficult for interviewees. Not all of our interviewees had come out to their parents. One interviewee with elderly parents implied that she would not pursue sex reassignment surgery until they passed away. Interviewees' worst fear when coming out to parents was that they would be banished. As Marzie explained:

And finally while I was sitting there with my mother at breakfast and said one of the reasons that we came up here is that there is something that I wanted to talk about. And she said, "Well, what is it?" And I was just struggling. She could see that obviously there was something really emotional that I had to talk about. So she said, "Well, let's go in the other room." So we went over there, and I just started crying. Just trying to – I knew what I had to say but it was just so intense. And so she was like, "What is it? What is it? What could be this sad?" And so I started to tell her, "Well ever since I could remember I've had these feelings. I started seeing a therapist a year ago and was having these feelings about gender identity." And then she goes, "You're not going to have a sex change operation are you?" (mutual laughter) Then we talked, we talked for a couple of hours. I cried a lot. It was pretty intense, and she took it pretty well. And she was really supportive and really loving. And she was even able to make some jokes about it, which was nice. [But] she was really afraid, really afraid that I won't be accepted, that I'll be unhappy, that [my wife] would leave me, and that I'd commit suicide. She's pretty religious and she's praying a lot.... She doesn't really accept it; she's still hoping that I can change how I feel.

Marzie's experience was similar to other interviewees whose parents hoped that this was only a phase.

Colleagues and superiors within institutional settings, such as school or work, were generally the last to hear about interviewees' transsexuality. Financial concerns were paramount and transsexuals also wanted to make sure that their bodywork had progressed to the point where they would not be embarrassed by their appearance. Jenny, who humorously advised, "writing a dissertation and changing sex is guaranteed to be, like, one of the most foolish things that anybody has ever done," explained coming out to her dissertation advisor as follows:

I had to be willing to lose everything before I could tell my advisor. I had to get ready for a reaction that – well you know, actually, "That's impossible" would have been a better reaction than I got. The worst reaction I could think of was one of, "Well I understand that you have this problem but you realize that you can't stay in the field." [A]nd it turned out to be true. I had to be willing to lose, to give up something, en route to reclaim it as Jenny.

Jenny dropped her advisor and found someone more supportive of her status passage.

Sue appeared to have had better luck coming out to 225 coworkers, in part, perhaps, because transsexuality was written into the company's anti-discrimination policy. As she described it:

> Yesterday I sent a computer message to 225 people, everyone in the building and said, "Everyone, I just want you to know that I'm in the process of going through a change in my personal life that will be visible to people here at Data General. And this is a process of changing from living as a man to living as a woman and da, da, da." It was a real short little message and then finally I was like, "Up until now I have been slowly changing, living less and less as a man and with the only exception being work. Today I make the final step and beginning to live full time as a woman. Please address me as any other female employee of my company." And stuff like that. Oh, "And if you have any questions, talk to HR," because they asked me to put that in so people wouldn't come to me, they want to sort of be a buffer, I guess.... One woman I've never met before sent me a little message saying, "Welcome to the female race. I wish you luck." [E]veryone's reaction surprised me so much. I've heard so many people say, "Congratulations." It just had never occurred to me that that would be the response. But they sort of looked at it as I've made this decision and I'm making a decision that will better my life and they're all very happy for me.

As Viktor Gecas (1982) points out, there is often a difference between how others actually view us and how we imagine they see us – and this difference is often self-enhancing. While we do not know for sure, it seems likely that many of Sue's co-workers were not as accepting as those who were compelled to verbalize support. By imaging that "they're *all* very happy" for her, however, Sue bolstered her self-worth and commitment to her transembodied status passage.

Coming out Visually

After verbally coming out as transsexuals, most interviewees only then decided to let audiences see them as women. They felt that even if others offered support when they came out verbally, true acceptance only came when others literally viewed and interacted with them as embodiments of women. As one interviewee described, "It's important to let them see me and start to get used to me as Taylor." Embodying womanhood in front of these audiences helped resolve the previously discussed dilemma of the reflexive self: it gave audiences the opportunity to view them in line with interviewees' self-definitions as women.

As previously mentioned, Joyce's friend Carol was stunned when she came out to her, but they remained friends, although there was much tension. Joyce believed that if Carol saw her dressed as a woman, that things might get better. One afternoon when Carol came over to get some statistical assistance for her dissertation research, Joyce answered the door dressed in women's clothes:

> She just froze up. Basically we weren't able to start … until I went back and changed. I was looking for acceptance and maybe I shouldn't have pushed it by even being dressed that morning before she was coming over…. But I won't feel like she accepts me until she sees me dressed.

Interviewees who did not surprise others appeared to gain better reception. For example, Erin told the following story of meeting her homophobic out-of-town friend, who invited *her* to go a Johnny Winter concert:

> I showed up at his house dressed and he … said, "Welcome Erin." And we went in and talked for about an hour and decided that we were real hungry and went out for dinner… it was completely comfortable. I spent the next day in drab (dressed as a man), because he wanted to see me both ways, and then the following day I dressed as Erin again…. He said, "Thank you for spending yesterday in drab. I saw how unhappy you are. I now have a much better understanding of what it means to you." And that really meant a lot.

Fewer interviewees had visually come out to their parents at the time of their interviews. Jenny's decision to visually come out to her family during her annual Christmas visit got mixed reviews at best: "That was an odd situation, in that what made me less tense made my family more tense. There was all of that feedback." Parents of the interviewees seemed unprepared to view their sons as women.

Marzie's wife Christine was initially supportive when Marzie verbally came out and even said she desired to remain married after transembodiment was complete. But Christine started having reservations as Marzie began embodying womanhood more regularly. As explained by Marzie:

> She never had a relationship with a woman, but there had been women she felt attracted to. So she always felt it wouldn't make a difference to her whether I was male or female. But it was the person, you know, that she cared about. And so it would be okay. But I guess during the last six months as I've begun making the transition, and especially as she's started seeing me as a woman, that she's been dealing with these feelings and it's become more and more clear to her that her orientation is pretty strongly heterosexual. And she doesn't think that she can continue in the relationship.

Although Marzie's wife accepted her as a woman and had hoped to remain married, as Marzie's embodiment of womanhood progressed, she was unable to be attracted to the body of the person whom she loved.

Coming out visually led interviewees to imagine that others could never again see them as men, regardless of their masculine biographies and bodily remnants. But some were not sure if they would ever be accepted as women either. Regardless, interviewees believed that coming out visually closed down all exits off of their transembodied passage. Being a man who once thought he was a woman was perhaps too embarrassing to imagine. Taylor, who came out visually to all her friends during a weekend festival in her hometown, claimed:

> I can never be Tom-the-guy around any of these people again. And I don't know if I'll ever be Taylor-the-woman around them either. I mean, to these people I'm probably going to always be something in-between. To some of them, I hope to a large portion of them, that I'm a good person. But I'll never be able to go back to how it was. I gave up the ability to return to Tom (pause), which is great. It's like full steam ahead now.

Conclusions

As our analysis suggests, reflexivity shapes the experience, strategies, and practices of transsexuals' status passage. Interviewees used cultural notions of gender to construct biographies that essentially overwrote their masculine bodies with their differently gendered "true selves." They adopted the transgender community as an important reference group, which helped mitigate feelings of shame. How they imagined others assigned gendered meanings to their bodies shaped how they retrained, redecorated, and redesigned their corporal selves, which, over time, made womanhood feel more authentic. In terms of the coming out process, interviewees' reflexivity shaped how they chose and implemented strategies to conceal and leak their body projects as well as how they verbally and visually revealed themselves as transembodied people to those who had only known them as men.

Our analysis of reflexive transembodiment can also remind us of the importance of agency and culture in reflexive body techniques. Whereas Charles Cooley is sometimes misrepresented as positing a self that is excessively conformist, transembodied people have enough agency to transgress the cultural bodily display rules associated with the sex category to which they were ascribed at birth. Such challenges to gender ideology often simultaneously reproduce it. Interviewees reflexively employed (and thus reproduced) the cultural assumptions that women are supposed to be sexually submissive and athletically inept. Similarly, their desire to escape harassment and discrimination led interviewees to adopt stereotypical bodily displays of gender. Collectively, such transformative bodywork arguably also transforms the wider culture by making the category "transsexual" increasingly available as an identity option for people who feel deeply uncomfortable in their skin. Reflexive transembodiment is thus more than doing gender by way of bodywork, it also involves the remaking of embodied culture.

Transembodied people are not the only ones, of course, who employ reflexivity in their bodywork in ways that might reproduce or challenge the dominant themes of a society's embodied culture. Some women who adopt the perspective of feminist or lesbian communities learn to become unashamed about physical bodies that fall short of impossible-to-accomplish heterosexist media depictions. As people age and their bodies less reliably express their "true selves," they may draw on as well as challenge age-based aspects of embodied culture to create self-narratives that overwrite their material bodies. Women who see themselves through a patriarchal generalized other may view their bodies as deficient and, in the hope of changing how others evaluate them, alter their bodies through diet or cosmetic surgery. College students who have their bodies tattooed and pierced might imagine that their parents would be too shocked if they accidentally discovered their new body art and might gradually come out to them. And some professors likely imagine that wearing upper middle class costumes to campus might increase the chance that they will pass as worthy and competent intellectuals. Interactionist analyses grounded in everyday life can show how the body, subjectivity, and culture are always intertwined in ways that reproduce and/or subvert inequalities.

Acknowledgements

Thanks to Daphne Holden, Phillip Vannini and Dennis Waskul for helpful feedback.

References

Billings, Dwight, and Thomas Urban. 1982. "The Socio-Medical Construction of Transsexualism: An Interpretation and Critique." *Social Problems*, 29:266–282.

Bolin, Anne. 1988. *In Search of Eve: Transsexual Rites of Passage*. South Hadley: Bergin and Garvey.

Burke, Phyllis. 1996. *Gender Shock: Exploding the Myths of Male and Female*. New York: Doubleday.

Butler, Judith. 1990. *Gender Trouble: Feminism and the Subversion of Identity*. New York: Routledge.

Cahill, Spencer E. and Robin Eggleston. 1994. "Managing Emotions in Public: The Case of Wheelchair Users." *Social Psychology Quarterly*, 57, 4:300–312.

Cooley, Charles H. 1902. *Human Nature and Social Order*. Piscataway, NJ: Transaction.

Ekins, Richard. 1997. *Male Femaling: A Grounded Theory Approach to Cross-Dressing and Sex-Changing*. London: Routledge.

Feinbloom, Deborah Heller. 1976. *Transvestites and Transsexuals*. New York: Delta.

Gagné, Patricia and Richard Tewksbury. 1998. "Conformity Pressures and Gender Resistance Among Transgendered Individuals." *Social Problems*, 45:81–101.

Gagné, Patricia, Richard Tewksbury and Deanna McGaughey. 1997. "Coming Out and Crossing Over: Identity Formation and Proclamation in a Transgender Community." *Gender & Society*, 11:478–508.

Garfinkel, Harold. 1967. *Studies in Ethnomethodology*. Englewood Cliffs: Prentice-Hall.

Gecas, Victor. 1982. "The Self-Concept." *Annual Review of Sociology*, 8:1–33.

Gergen, Kenneth J. and Mary M. Gergen. 1983. "Narratives of the Self." in Theodore R. Sarbin and Karl E. Scheibe (Eds) *Studies in Social Identity*. New York: Praeger. pp. 254–323.

Glaser, Barney and Strauss, Anselm. 1971. *Status Passage: A Formal Theory.* Chicago: Aldine-Atherton.

Goffman, Erving. 1959. *The Presentation of Self in Everyday Life.* New York: Doubleday Anchor.

_____. 1963. *Stigma: Notes on the Management of Spoiled Identity.* New York: Touchstone.

Hochshild, Arlie R. 1979. "Emotion Work, Feeling Rules, and Social Structure." *American Journal of Sociology*, 85:551–575

James, William. 1892. *Psychology*. New York: Holt.

Kessler, Suzanne, and Wendy McKenna. 1978. *Gender: An Ethnomethodological Approach.* Chicago: University of Chicago.

Lorber, Judith. 1994. *Paradoxes of Gender*. New Haven: Yale.

Mason-Schrock. Douglas P. 1996. "Transsexuals' Narrative Construction of the 'True Self.'" *Social Psychology Quarterly*, 59:176–92.

McCaughey, Martha. 1998. "The Fighting Spirit: Women's Self-Defense Training and the Discourse of Sexed Embodiment." *Gender & Society*, 12:277–300.

Mead, George H. 1929. "The Nature of the Past." in J. Coss (Ed.) *Essays in Honor of John Dewey*. New York: Henry Holt. pp. 235–242.

_____. 1934. *Mind, Self and Society*. Chicago: University of Chicago Press.

Raymond, Janice. 1979. *The Transsexual Empire: The Making of the She-Male.* Boston: Beacon.

Risman, Barbara J. 1982. "The (Mis)acquisition of Gender Identity Among Transsexuals." *Qualitative Sociology*, 4:312–25.

Rosenberg, Morris. 1990. "Reflexivity and Emotions." *Social Psychology Quarterly*, 53:3–12.

Rubin, Henry. 2003. *Self-Made Men: Identity and Embodiment Among Transsexual Men*. Nashville, TN: Vanderbilt University Press.

Schrock, Douglas, and Emily Boyd. 2005. "Policing and Releasing Transsexual Bodies." Paper presented at the annual meetings of the Society for the Study of Symbolic Interactionism.

Schrock, Douglas, and Lori Reid. 2006. "Transsexuals' Sexual Stories." *Archives of Sexual Behavior*, 35:75–86.

Schrock, Douglas, Daphne Holden, and Lori Reid. 2004. "Creating Emotional Resonance: Interpersonal Emotion Work and Motivational Framing in a Transgender Community." *Social Problems*, 51: 61–81.

Schrock, Douglas, Lori Reid, and Emily Boyd. 2005. "Transsexuals' Embodiment of Womanhood." *Gender & Society*, 19:317–335.

Shibutani, Tamotsu. 1955. "Reference Groups as Perspectives." *American Journal of Sociology*, 60:962–965.

Waskul, Dennis D., and Pamela van der Riet. 2002. "The Abject Embodiment of Cancer Patients: Dignity, Selfhood, and the Grotesque Body." *Symbolic Interaction*, 25:487–513.

Znaniecki, Florian. 1925. *The Laws of Social Psychology*. Chicago: University of Chicago.

PART 2
The Dramaturgical Body:
Body as Performance

Chapter 5

Building Bodily Boundaries: Embodied Enactment and Experience

Spencer E. Cahill

Reflecting on both the classic work of Norbert Elias and casual observations of daily life, Spencer E. Cahill comments on conduct surrounding the fluid literal and metaphorical boundaries of the public and private body. Cahill's analysis illuminates the dramaturgical body – a body fashioned, crafted, negotiated, manipulated and largely in ritualized social and cultural conventions (see Chapter One, this volume). In this case, as Cahill illustrates, it is a body subject to the zoning ordinances of society in which, by means of cultural practice, the public body is made *"public" and the private body is* kept *"private." Cahill's reflections on public bathrooms, moments of bodily malfunction, as well as gyms and fitness centres, implicate these boundaries and practices and much more: "Whether we rigidly adhere to conventional bodily boundaries, habitually relax them, or poke meaningful holes in them, we acknowledge them" and therefore they are of much greater significance then they first appear.*

Norbert Elias's masterful *The Civilizing Process* ([1939] 1978) is often read as a history of the long social formation of contemporary Western emotionality. It is that, and more. It is also a history of the long social formation of the contemporary Western body in its complex defining relationship to self and society. As Elias ([1939] 1978: 70) documents, over the long *dureé* of Western history a "wall of affects" was built between "one human body and another, repelling and separating." First in exalted estates and then more slowly in lower ones people were repulsed by the "mere approach" of things that had been in contact with another's hands, mouth, and excretory orifices. They became embarrassed at the mere sight of another's nakedness and "bodily functions" and ashamed over the exposure of their own. What Elias ([1939] 1978) dubs "the civilizing process" enclosed the naked body and its organismic functions "in particular enclaves," keeping them "behind closed doors" and making them intimate secrets beyond the pale of public life.

Increasing mobilization of the body for publicly expressive purposes was closely related to this privatizing enclosure of the naked, organic body. With the concentration of human populations first in noble courts and then in cities, along with the corresponding growth of social interdependence, people became more observed by and observant of others. They consequently became more observant of their own bodily comportment and concerned with fashioning and controlling their bodies so as to manage others' impressions of them. That concern was first cultivated in noble courts among those of lower social stations so to avoid offending superiors. As noble courts begin to open onto streets of more socially diverse cities, those of higher social status had to concern themselves with demonstrating their own social refinement and distinction so as to justify their privilege. Finally, with the rise of the bourgeoisie and the more egalitarian ethos they championed, concealment and control of the organic body became a general qualification for participation in "decent society" (Elias [1939] 1978: 141). Much as social life was being separated into public and private spheres, so too the body was partitioned into disciplined public display and private organic secret.

By the nineteenth century, the self-declared "civilized" peoples of the West were convinced that their sartorial concealment of and highly developed control over the organic body distinguished them from the "barbaric" peoples of elsewhere (Elias [1939] 1978: 59). They were also convinced that such bodily concealment and control distinguished them from the barbarians within their midst such as children, the insane and generally untamed (Elias [1939] 1978: 141). That remains part of their legacy to us. Erving Goffman (1961: 248) once observed that "just as we fill our jails with those who transgress the legal order, so we partly fill our asylums with those who act unsuitably." Prominent among the improprieties that invite psychiatric diagnoses and custody are public exposure of the conventionally concealed body and its organismic functions. As Goffman ([1956a] 1967: 92) noted elsewhere, mental hospitals commonly decide the degree of patients' "mental illness" based on the extent to which they violate conventions of bodily comportment. Hence, the "sickest" patients relegated to so-called "back wards" are often "denudative, incontinent, and they openly masturbate; they scratch themselves violently; drooling occurs and a nose may run unchecked... " (Goffman [1956a] 1967: 80). Goffman was drawn to the study of such misconduct for what it could reveal, by way of contrast, about aspects of "good demeanor that we usually take for granted." His own brilliant analyses of the ceremonial or ritual order of social interaction are testament to the fruitfulness of that strategy. Yet, evidence of the bodily control and concealment that we expect of ourselves and is expected of us is more readily accessible than the back wards of mental hospitals.

Despite our sometimes heroic attempts at bodily self-control, the organic body is an unruly subject. It sometimes demands that we indulge its creaturely imperatives. Urine and faeces must be eliminated. Coughs, sneezes, and flatulence break through our attempted repressions, as do tears and reddened faces of anger and embarrassment. The wear and tear of everyday activities erodes our careful grooming, cosmetic decoration, and sartorial adornment of the public body. We are convinced that maintenance and repair of the body's organic functioning sometimes requires its exposure to and man-handling by virtual strangers. More recently, many of us have become convinced that a healthy and comely public body requires its extraordinary, noisy, sweaty, and revealing exercise. However inevitable and seemingly necessary such activities, they are incompatible with prevailing standards of public bodily comportment. They expose the secretive private body behind the embellished, disciplined one that we more routinely display in public.

Lest we betray our public bodies, such bodily activities must be segregated from the usual business of public life. Yet, many social settings specifically designated for the indulgence of the private body are not truly private. Public bathrooms are just that, freely accessible to anyone of the designated gender. The personnel of medical settings to whom patients reveal their most intimate bodily secrets are seldom patients' intimates. And, the many gyms and fitness centres that now dot the contemporary Western landscape are open to all willing and able to pay the requisite fee. Within such settings, the inherent tension between our publicly displayed and private organic body are particularly acute and must be delicately managed. Hence, the social conduct that routinely occurs in and around such settings may be as revealing of taken for granted aspects of publicly conventional bodily comportment as the bodily laxity often found on the back wards of mental hospitals.

This essay explores the social construction of contemporary bodily experience. Having begun with Elias's account of the historical construction of such experience, I now turn my attention to more contemporary manifestations. In what follows, I briefly review some systematic and more casual observations, including some of my own, of social conduct in public bathrooms, medical settings, gyms and fitness centres. My review of such conduct is not comprehensive but strategic. My focus is on conduct surrounding the, both literally and metaphorically, fluid boundaries between the public and private body and between different bodies. I then draw some general lessons about contemporary bodily experience from my consideration of that conduct and suggest some ways that these lessons might inform other issues of contemporary social life and experience.

Exiling the Excretory

Contemporary Western societies have virtually vanquished bodily excretion and excretions from public life. The shocked disgust that their occasional sight provokes indicates just how exceptional such sights are. It was not always so. Residents of Medieval European cities routinely emptied chamber pots out windows and onto the streets. As late as the early eighteenth century, La Salle felt compelled to instruct "civilized Christians" to "withdraw to some unfrequented place when you need to pass water" and "to perform other natural functions where you cannot be seen" (quoted in Elias [1939] 1978: 132). Even then, "almost any corner of a house, from fireplaces to cellars, might on occasion be used by ill mannered persons to relieve themselves" (Classen, Howes, and Synnott 1994: 64). Today, members of "decent society" need not be reminded to keep bodily excretion and excretions out of public sight and potential olfactory detection. Then again, it is far easier for us to do so than it was for our ancestors.

Over the years, technological innovation aided the privatization of excretory conduct. It brought running water and sewage systems to Western cities, small towns, and, eventually, even rural areas. So-called *out*houses, usually located at some remove from "living areas," were moved inside, eliminating the need for chamber pots at night and during inclement weather. Excretory conduct now had its own private enclave, often with locking doors, within private residences where its products could be spirited away upon rushing waters.

The common American English designation for such rooms – bathroom – reflected the privately unspeakable character of the excretory activities that occurred within their walls. Most other rooms in private residences are named for their characteristic activities – dining room, living room, kitchen (from the Middle English *kichene* which is from the Latin *coquina* for "to cook"), and even parlour (from the Old French *parleor* for "to speak"). In contrast, the bathroom, like bedrooms where such creaturely indulgences as sleep and sexual activity routinely occur, is named for a characteristic furnishing. Alternative designations such as "washroom" and "restroom" where visitors go "to freshen up" provide no more acknowledgement of the excretory conduct that routinely occurs in such rooms. Such conduct was not only vanquished from public life but also from public speech.[1]

Yet, so-called bathrooms in private residences were not enough to consolidate – to disseminate and constantly reproduce (Elias [1939] 1978: 140) – the new standards of excretory conduct. The social rhythms of modern public and private life and the body's excretory rhythms did not necessarily coincide. Work and other public places also needed to be equipped with bathrooms if bodily excretion and excretions were to be vanquished from public life. And, the work-a-day population of many public settings required excretory facilities that could accommodate more than one person at a time.

Public bath – or restrooms that accommodate more than a single person at a time do safely vanquish excretory conduct from the frontstage (Goffman 1959) of public places where "official" business is conducted, but they do not necessarily vanquish it from public sight. That requires additional architectural measures. In public bathrooms with multiple toilets, each usually occupies its own private inner room or is enclosed by the partial walls of so-called "stalls," often with locking doors. In men's bathrooms, long trough like receptacles for urine have been largely replaced by individual use urinals, sometimes separated by panels attached perpendicular to the wall in which the urinals are embedded. Although these panels do not completely insulate urinal users from the sight of adjacent users, such sightings take special and obvious effort. Even when they do not, they are rare.

As I have documented elsewhere (Cahill *et al.* 1985), users of public bathrooms routinely augment architectural barriers to perception with expressive ones. For example, men commonly avoid occupying adjacent urinals in public bathrooms, unless all more removed ones are occupied or inoperative (Cahill *et al.* 1985: 42; see also Oring 1975). Even when they do use adjacent urinals, they studiously avoid glancing at neighbouring urinators, fixing their eyes on the wall in front of them. Some businesses now accommodate this conventional practice by placing pages of newspapers and some marketers exploit it by placing advertisements on the wall

---

1   I thank Dennis Waskul (personal communication) for this insight.

above urinals. In any case, the obvious excretory conduct of urinal users in men's bathrooms is consequently unseen, unacknowledged, and politely, albeit somewhat fictitiously, private.

Users of public bathrooms employ related forms of "tactful blindness" (Goffman [1955] 1967: 18) when obvious evidence of flatulence and defecation emanate from toilet stalls. Excretory sounds sometimes escape the walls of such stalls despite their users heroic attempts to conceal them (Weinberg and Williams 2005:324–329) as do unmistakable odours of flatus and faeces. Yet, users of public bathrooms commonly ignore such obvious evidence of bodily excretion and excretions, although apparent efforts to do so sometimes betray their disgust. They also tend to ignore the obvious offender and whatever furtive signs of embarrassment she or he may display when emerging from the privacy of the stall. Tactfully unacknowledged, it is as if her or his creaturely private body's assault on their senses never occurred.

There are exceptions. Previously acquainted users of public bathrooms may sometimes openly acknowledge and even draw attention to sounds and smells of their own or one another's excretory conduct. Two recent observers of excretory conduct maintain that this is especially common among young men who feel empowered to flaunt social convention (Weinberg and Williams 2005:328). Yet, however powerful young men, or women or men of other ages, may feel, they are not immune to the socially dangerous powers of bodily excretion and excretions. Their scatological comments commonly remain wrapped in a circle of acquaintanceship, if not the intimacy within which the private body is typically confined. Even then, such comments are typically humorous, implying that what has just occurred is not serious or "real" (Goffman [1956b] 1967:112). Whether behind tactful blindness or friendly humour, the excretory private body is expressively veiled.

Sights as well as sounds and smells in public bathrooms also sometimes betray the secrets of our private, creaturely body. Users sometimes visually confront another's unflushed bodily excretions. Although prospective users of urine filled urinals often flush them, if mechanically possible,[2] before filling them with urine once again, those who discover unflushed faeces typically withdraw from the offending toilet stall in disgust. Yet, in such cases, the disgust does not attach itself to a culprit as it would if displayed in response to excretory smells as the obvious offender exited a toilet stall. As Weinberg and Williams (2005:323) recently document, when individuals' often repeated attempts to flush faeces out of sight fail, they commonly flee the scene in haste. Evidence of their creaturely body remains publicly exposed, but it does not betray their publicly displayed body. Those outside the bathroom's doors remain blissfully unaware of the culprit's lingering assault on bodily boundaries, however haunted she or he may be by guilty knowledge of that deed.

---

2   The recent fitting of toilets and urinals in public bathrooms with automatically triggered flushing devices may have inadvertently increased the frequency of visible excretions in public bathrooms. Although many such devices are equipped with buttons for manual flushing, many users seem unaware of them. If a urinal does not flush when stepping away or a toilet does not do so after standing up and repositioning clothing, many users simply depart seemingly unmindful.

More routinely in public bathrooms, hand washing ritually reestablishes the boundary between the publicly displayed and creaturely private body that has just been broached. Excretory conduct betrays the literal and metaphoric fluidity of that boundary. Subsequent baptism of the hands in soap and water redeems the public body from its contaminating contact with its creaturely cousin, restoring the conventional symbolic distance between the two. Although this common practice is promoted on hygienic grounds, social concerns are arguably as, if not more, influential. For example, my own earlier systematic observation suggested that users of public bathrooms are more likely to wash their hands if they think they are being witnessed by others than when they think they are not (Cahill *et al.* 1985:57, fn. 6). In addition, more than a few who do honour the post-excretion, hand washing convention ritually pass their hands under a running faucet with little apparent concern for disinfection. Bodily cleanliness would seem to be as much about preventing the spread of social disease as preventing the spread of biological disease.[3]

Although officially designed and designated for excretory conduct, public bathrooms also provide physical and interactional cover for other behaviours and activities that might broach the boundary between our publicly displayed and private body. As I have documented elsewhere, individuals whose public bodily comportment is overwhelmed by emotions often retreat to public bathrooms and behind the locked doors of their toilet stalls (Cahill *et al.* 1985:49–51). They sometimes also do so when fits of sneezing and coughing temporarily overwhelm their bodily control. More routinely, they retreat to public bathrooms to inspect and repair their publicly displayed body, combing and brushing hair, applying cosmetics, and rearranging clothing. Some may do so furtively when witnessed by others (Cahill *et al.* 1985:48), but many do so nonchalantly in full view of other bathroom users who just as nonchalantly ignore such studied management of bodily appearance. Physically and interactionally enclosed in the protective enclave of public (and private) bathrooms, the effort we devote to preparing our bodies for public display remains inconspicuous. Outside bathroom doors, our publicly displayed body and its varied adornments seem effortless and only natural. The unruly organic body lurking behind that public appearance remains safely at bay, a creature of the unspoken realm of bathrooms.

Yet, what remains unspoken and unacknowledged in everyday public life is exactly what those who study social life and experience must acknowledge and address. The boundary between our publicly displayed and secretive creaturely body is drawn within and at the doors of public bathrooms. Within those doors and underneath the prevailing tactful blindness behind them, bodily boundaries routinely dissolve and are redrawn. There the social architecture of contemporary bodily experience is

---

3   The findings of a recent observational study of hand washing in public bathrooms commissioned by the American Society of Microbiology would seem to support Weinberg and Williams' (2005:328) recent argument that men are more likely than women to flaunt excretory conventions. Based on observation of over 6,300 public bathroom users, Harris Interactive reported that while 90 percent of women washed their hands after using the "facilities," only 75 percent of the men did (Associated Press 2005).

disassembled and reassembled revealing its porous structure. And public bathrooms are not the only settings that provide such a revealing view.

Managing Malfunctions

Publicly conventional bodily comportment requires seemingly effortless bodily self-control. From early in life, we cultivate such bodily control in the young. The goal and usual consequence of such training is to transform self-conscious bodily control into an unself-conscious "second nature" (Elias [1939] 1978:167). What once took thought and effort becomes "only natural" and unthinkingly effortless. In the course of a few years, the self, with more than a little social direction, "masters the body" (Waskul and van der Reit 2002:510).

Yet, such taken-for-granted self-mastery of the body depends on its smooth organic functioning. Disruptions of its usual organic functioning can cause powerful and immediate excretory impulses that overwhelm even the most concerted efforts at self-conscious control. They may seize the body in uncontrollable spasms of coughing, sneezing, and even vomiting. Lesions and sores may erode the visible boundary between the body's public surface and private organic depths. Externally induced and internally generated organic traumas may make the body unresponsive to our usually effortless self-piloting of its movements. In these and a variety of other ways, injury and disease undermine our usual self-mastery of the body (Waskul and van der Riet 2002). Hence, maintenance of the boundary between our publicly displayed and creaturely private body requires that we keep the latter in a state of good repair and quickly and effectively fix it when in disrepair.

Today, most of us are convinced that preservation and restoration of bodily "health," which we largely equate with bodily self-mastery, requires at least occasional reliance on the expertise of medical practitioners. Yet, contemporary medical practice has little respect for the boundaries we usually draw between and upon bodies. At the same time those boundaries were being historically drawn in everyday social life, medical practitioners were erasing them in the specialized enclaves where they plied their trades (see Foucault [1963] 1975). They became increasingly convinced and increasingly convinced their patients that care and repair of the organic body required penetration below its publicly visible surface into its hidden depths. Medical practitioners visually inspected and palpated naked bodies, stared into and manually prodded inside bodily orifices, invented devices to aid them hear and see deep inside the organic body, and even surgically parted the body's surface to explore and remove pieces of what lay below. Although perhaps grudgingly, the rest of us came to accept such bodily insults as the necessary price for continued bodily self-mastery.

We did and do continue to do so, at least in part, because medical erasure of the usual boundaries between and upon bodies is often handled delicately. As Joan Emerson (1970) demonstrated some years ago with the case of gynaecological exams, the dominant medical definition of the patient's body as an object of technical interest and concern is qualified by "counter themes" of bodily privacy and self-possession. For example, "the patient's body is draped so as to expose only that part which is to receive the technical attention of the doctor" (Emerson 1970:81) in apparent acknowledgement of the intimate privacy of the naked body. Although physicians and nurses often expressively efface the patient's bodily self-possession, as when they use "the definite pronoun" *the* rather than "the pronoun adjective" *your* "in reference to body parts" (Emerson 1970:81), they sometimes briefly acknowledge the patient's bodily self-possession in order to gain the patient's cooperation as when a physician instructed a patient in a soothing voice "Now relax as much as you can" (Emerson 1970:82). In a related vein, physicians generally avoid any hint of personal intimacy while conducting bodily examinations but may make personal inquiries or otherwise acknowledge their prior acquaintanceship with a patient either before or after the examination in apparent concession to the intimacy that usually encloses contact with another's private body (Emerson 1970:85).

In these and many other respects, gynaecological exams are exemplary of medical practitioners' strategic acknowledgement of bodily self-possession and boundaries while simultaneously erasing them. For another personal example, I recently underwent radiation treatments on my left pelvic area every weekday for three weeks. Each morning, I was summoned from a waiting room by a radiation therapist who walked me to the treatment facility, engaging me in personal conversation along the way. Within two or three days, the six radiation therapists involved in my treatment knew that I was a professor at the local university, what classes I taught and research I was conducting, that I grew up near St. Louis (from where one of them had recently moved) and similar information that then provided topics for conversation on subsequent mornings. Once we arrived at the treatment facility, personal conversation ceased, and I was instructed to lie on a table. One of the therapists would then place a towel on my lap and instruct me to pull down my pants (which also implied my underwear). I did so, carefully keeping my genitals covered by the small towel. The therapists would then delicately reposition the towel, being careful to keep my genitals covered, and begin aligning my body under the radiation beam without comment to me. On many mornings, this included drawing the outline of the treatment area on my bare skin with a marking pin. One of the therapists would matter-of-factly announce "I'm going to draw on you now" and proceed to do so without further comment. The therapists would leave the room during the treatments, then return upon their completion and announce "okay, you're all done." I would pull my pants and underwear back up before getting off the table and then, as I tucked my shirt back into my pants, the therapists and I would exchange friendly farewells, wishing one another a good day or weekend and promising to "see you tomorrow" or on Monday.

These therapists' temporary suspension of conversation during my preparation for and the delivery of the treatments arguably protected my public being from possible contamination. Like occupants of public bathrooms who refrain from engaging one another in conversation while engaged in excretory conduct, these therapists disengaged from conversation the moment they initiated exposure of my creaturely private body, in apparent acknowledgement that conversation implicates a public self.[4] Holding that public self in abeyance during exposure of and technical tinkering with my organic body, it was then again evoked in conversation once my private body was safely concealed.

Medical students sometimes describe their examination of patients' private bodies as "pretty much like checking a broken toaster" or "looking under the hood" at "an automobile engine" (Smith and Kleinman 1989:61), and more veteran medical practitioners probably think of their patients' bodies similarly. Yet, as the two above examples illustrate, they routinely pay homage to the lay public's more reverential view of bodies and their boundaries. Medical practitioners often bracket their examinations and treatments of patients' private bodies with personable interaction, creating at least an illusion of the kind of intimacy that typically encloses bodily contacts. They also tend to request no more exposure of the private body than technically necessary to conduct their examinations or treatments, leaving as much of the usual boundary between the public and private body in tact as practically possible. During the actual examination and treatment of the body, they tend not to acknowledge patients' bodily self-possession any more than necessary to gain patients' cooperation, but that too may demonstrate more respect for the social structuring of self-embodiment than first appears. Some patients may feel as if medical personnel efface their very being – their bodily self-possession – but there is another possible interpretation of medical practitioners' impersonality when examining and treating patients' bodies. In a sense, they expressively levitate the boundary between a patient's public self and bodily being off the body's surface while tinkering with her or his organic body. They thereby protect the patient's public self from insult until it is safe for it to descend back onto the patient's bodily surface.

Disease and bodily injury clearly can irreparably dissolve the usual boundary between the public and private body (e.g. Waskul and van der Riet 2002). In such cases, medical practitioners can do little more than act nonchalantly when dressing open sores or cleaning oozing bodily excreta in an attempt to ease their patients' shame over their loss of bodily self-mastery and consequent privacy. Yet, when possible, medical practitioners erase no more of the boundary between the public and private body than they deem necessary and take expressive measures to insure that it can and is redrawn after their assaults upon it. We exercise similar expressive caution when we intentionally bring our private body to its public surface in the interest of enhancing our bodily self-mastery and public display.

Fashioning Fitness

Today, many of us are convinced that the maintenance or achievement of bodily health and, almost by implication, an adequately comely and controlled public body requires effortful and repeated bodily exertion. Moreover, many of us are convinced that such bodily self-mastery requires the instruction and elaborate equipment

---

4   I am again grateful to Dennis Waskul (personal communication) for this insight.

available in commercial or otherwise communal fitness centres and gyms. Ironically, our attempts to enhance the publicly displayed body in such settings expose our private bodily being to public scrutiny and potential transgression, as one social critic laments:

> In the gym people engage in the kind of biological self-regulation that usually occurs in the private realm.... Exercisers make the faces associated with pain, with orgasm, with the sort of exertion that would call others to their immediate aid. But they do not hide their faces. They groan, as if pressing their bowels. They repeat grim labors, as if mopping the floor. They huff, they shout, and they strain. They appear in tight but shapeless Lycra costumes that reveal the shape of the penis, the labia, the mashed and bandaged breasts.
>
> Greif (2004:11).

To this social critic, contemporary gyms and fitness centres signal "the liquidation of the last untouched spheres of privacy, with the result that biological life itself has become a spectacle" (Grief 2004:16).

Yet, such harsh judgments ignore that fitness centres and gyms are among those "particular enclaves" designated for indulgence and, in this case, subjugation of the private organic body, keeping it safely sequestered from the usual business of public life. The scantily clad, huffing, sweaty jogger or runner moving along city sidewalks and through public parks might fairly be accused of making a public spectacle of the private organic body, but not the exerciser within the insulating walls of the gym or fitness centre. Her or his only audience consists of those who are similarly exposed and have willingly exposed themselves to the sights, sounds, and perspired by-products of bodily exertion. As Sassatelli (1999:229) documents, gyms and fitness centres use space, light, and decoration to mark a "passage from the everyday world to the exercise world." Either before arriving at their doors or within their dressing rooms, those who frequent gyms and fitness centres shed their usual public self and don specialized exercise attire that announces a situationally specific exercising self. Even then users of gyms and fitness centres do not ignore the usual boundaries between and upon bodies but strategically shift them to accommodate the specialized activities of the setting.

Unacquainted individuals in public places commonly accord one another what Goffman (1961:84) termed "civil inattention," yet the bodily feats performed in gyms and fitness centres, and their verbal accompaniment, often make such inattention to others difficult. Users of gyms and fitness centres, especially those lifting weights or using weight training machines, sometimes emit what Goffman (1981:104–105) termed "strain grunts" at "presumed peak and consummation" of their exertion. Although these presumably spontaneous verbal ejaculations are attention attracting, they demonstrate that their emitter is fully involved in situationally appropriate activity. When such sounds or silent bodily feats attract the attention of other users, glances may repeatedly meet, making furtive diversion of the eyes less socially comfortable than some form of acknowledgement. The ubiquitous mirrors found in fitness centres and gyms further increase the likelihood of reciprocal glances, albeit reflected ones. Yet, under such circumstances, acknowledging comments tend to be limited to the bodily activity at hand. The unintentional initiator of the encounter may praise the other's performance, invidiously compare their own to it, or ask for or furnish advice about the immediate bodily activity (Sassatelli 1999:238). By carefully circumscribing these encounters, participants restrict their relation to the setting and its defining activities, limiting their interactional obligations to one another outside the setting. On the other hand, the bodily intimacy of the setting may accelerate familiarity and formation of friendships that extend beyond the setting and its defining activities (Crossley 2004:58, 61). It seems that just as interactional intimacy warrants the lowering of usual bodily boundaries, so too the lowering of those boundaries can warrant interactional intimacy. In either case, exposure of the organic body remains wrapped in a privatizing circle of intimacy.

Yet, even within the protective enclave of the gym or fitness centre and the circles of intimate familiarity sometimes found there, bodily boundaries remain. Users of gyms and fitness centres may expose their private organic bodies to public scrutiny and sometimes dramatically draw attention to them but their sweaty excretions remain repelling. Those who wet equipment or mats with their sweat often make conspicuous attempts to wipe it up with towels and may even spray the offended object with disinfectant, if available, demonstrating to anyone concerned that they honour conventional bodily boundaries (Crossley 2004:58). In a similar vein, "work-out" friends may sometimes both simultaneously acknowledge and humorously attempt to neutralize the repulsing condition of a sweaty companion with ironically delivered revulsion sound like "Eeuw" (Goffman 1981:104) or simulated facial expressions of horror (Crossley 2004:58). In either case, users of gyms and fitness centres do not allow usual boundaries between bodies to dissolve in mediated sweaty contact but expressively defend them against that threat. However much the clientele of gyms and fitness centres make the private organic body into a public spectacle, it is a carefully managed show on a clearly circumscribed stage.

Before leaving the gym or fitness centre or soon thereafter, most of its users cleanse themselves of perspiration and apply various bodily potions that promise to neutralize any lingering or subsequent creaturely odours. They thereby reopen the conventional divide between the publicly displayed and private organic body, propping it open with commercial products designed for that purpose (Classen, Howes, Synnott 1994:186). Whatever temporary erosion of bodily boundaries that occurred in the gym or fitness centres is quickly repaired. A hopefully more comely public body is put back on display with its more creaturely organic counterpart again safely secreted away.

Conclusions

At first glance, routine behaviour in public bathrooms, medical settings, gyms and fitness centres would seem to contradict my earlier characterization of socially conventional bodily boundaries in contemporary Western societies. Users of public bathrooms, gyms, and fitness centres routinely expose the organic body and its creaturely impulses and by-products to public perception. Medical practitioners routinely cross the conventional boundaries between bodies that protect the privacy of the organic body and integrity of its publicly displayed counterpart. Yet, these routine incursions across bodily boundaries are confined to "particular enclaves" and safely segregated from the usual business of public life. The very existence of such enclaves is evidence of the symbolic boundary between the publicly displayed and creaturely private body beyond their walls and doors.

Moreover, conventional bodily boundaries do not simply disappear within such enclaves. As the preceding illustrates, those who populate such settings carefully circumscribe, delicately manage, and expressively neutralize the routine incursions across bodily boundaries that occur there. They thereby attempt to limit and repair damage to bodily boundaries within these "particular enclaves" so that they can be quickly and effectively redrawn.

There are those, like the above mentioned critic of bodily exposure in gyms, who argue that the bodily conventions formed over the long *dureé* of Western civilization have declined in recent years. Some celebrate but most lament such purported relaxations of bodily boundaries. In either case, their characterizations of deteriorating bodily boundaries are not new. Elias ([1939] 1978) acknowledged in the 1930s that more open talk about organic bodily functions, new styles of dance (p. 140), bathing costumes, and sporting activities (p. 187) heralded a "certain relaxation" of social constraints on bodily comportment. Yet, he quickly added that this is a "relaxation which remains within the framework of a particular 'civilized' standard ... involving a very high degree of automatic constraint ... conditioned to become habit" (Elias [1939] 1978:187). The examples of conduct in public bathrooms, medical settings, gyms and fitness centres examined here confirm that assessment. We may playfully dance around and over bodily boundaries more today than in the not too distant past but with the implicit knowledge that they remain firm enough to withstand such cross-border traffic.

Moreover, much of what is taken as evidence of conventional bodily boundaries' recent decay may well be long-standing variations on their central theme. For example, subtle differences in bodily comportment – in the enacted firmness of the boundary between the publicly displayed and creaturely private body – have arguably long served as "signs of distinction" and social difference (Bourdieu 1989:20). Over forty years ago, Goffman (1961:205) recognized that differences in work-a-day costumes tend to be associated a more generalized "tightness" or "looseness" in bodily comportment that may convey relative social status or class standing. The everyday enactment of bodily boundaries that I have documented here is surely not played in a single key. On the contrary, there are countless variations but on a single theme of bodily integrity and self-mastery. It is only against the taken-for-granted background of that single theme that we can recognize variations as meaningful signs of difference and distinction.

Moreover, the differences and distinctions those variations convey are not limited to social status and class. Conventional standards of bodily comportment, like most standards of everyday social conduct, are enabling conventions that "make possible a meaningful set of nonadherences" (Goffman 1971:61, fn. 61). Nonaderence to conventional standards of bodily comportment perhaps most clearly conveys social distance from those members of "decent society" who most reverentially uphold those standards. For example, young people often seize upon such nonadherences to put distance between themselves and decent adult society. Young boys and men are notorious for publicly indulging the organic body by open flatulence, engagement in belching competitions, and candid talk about organic bodily functions, often with humorous intent if seldom in effect. Many young women convey similar social distance from "decent adult society" through revealing costume and ironically exaggerated cosmetic adornments. Yet again, such nonadherences are only meaningful against the background of mutually taken-for-granted standards of bodily comportment. The young can shock their elders and distance themselves from them only because they share with them taken-for-granted understandings of conventional bodily boundaries. If they did not, their intentionally shocking bodily conduct would not have the intended shocking effect.

Whether we rigidly adhere to conventional bodily boundaries, habitually relax them, or poke meaningful holes in them, we acknowledge them. That very acknowledgement serves to reproduce them both in everyday social life and experience. Our routine acknowledgement of boundaries separating bodies from one another assures us of the integrity and autonomy of our very being, of our distinct individuality. Our routine enactment of a boundary separating the publicly displayed bodily surface from its privately organic underside persuades us that our "true" being – our self – is "encapsulated 'inside'" ourselves (Elias [1939] 1978:258). Yet, the capsule that contains our seemingly private self is of our own making. It is the publicly displayed bodily surface that we keep expressively separated from others and its own organic bodily base. Perhaps in those moments of intimacy when we temporarily lower conventional bodily boundaries we may feel how nakedly open to the world our being may be. But these are fleeting feelings soon overshadowed by the bodily boundaries we expressively raise yet again. The self may not be identical to the body, as Mead ([1934] 1962:136) claims, but it may be more intimately related than he implies. The boundaries we expressively erect between and upon bodies may not only socially structure our bodily experience but our self-experience as well. Hence, routine bodily comportment in public bathrooms, medical examination rooms, gyms and fitness centres may be of far more sociological *and* psychological significance then may first appear. At least we students of social life and experience cannot afford to take such taken-for-granted conduct for granted.

References

Associated Press. 2005. "Study Confirms: Guys are Gross." *St. Petersburg* [Florida] *Times Union*, September 22:16a.

Bourdieu, Pierre. 1989. "Social Space and Symbolic Power." *Sociological Theory*, 7:14–25.

Cahill, Spencer, William Distler, Cynthia Lachowetz, Andrea Meaney, Robyn Tarallo and Teena Willard. 1985. "Meanwhile Backstage: Public Bathrooms and the Interaction Order." *Urban Life*, 14:33–58.

Classen, Constance, David Howes and Anthony Synnott. 1994. *Aroma: A Cultural History of Smell*. London: Routledge.

Crossley, Nick. 2004. "The Circuit Trainer's Habitus: Reflexive Body Techniques and the Sociality of the Workout." *Body and Society*, 10:37–69.

Elias, Norbert. [1939] 1978. *The History of Manners*. Translated by Edmund Jephcott. New York: Pantheon Books.

Emerson, Joan. 1970. "Behavior in Private Places: Sustaining Definitions of Reality in Gynecological Examinations," in Peter Dreitsel (Ed.), *Recent Sociology, Number 2*. New York: MacMillan. pp. 74–97.

Foucault, Michel. [1963] 1975. *The Birth of the Clinic: An Archaeology of Medical Perception*. Translated by A.M. Sheridan Smith. New York: Random House.

Goffman, Erving. [1955] 1967. "On Face-Work: An Analysis of Ritual Elements of Social Interaction," in Erving Goffman, *Interaction Ritual: Essays on Face-to-Face Behavior*. New York: Doubleday. pp. 5–45.

_____. [1956a] 1967. "The Nature of Deference and Demeanor," in Erving Goffman, *Interaction Ritual: Essays in Face-to-Face Behavior*. New York: Doubleday. pp. 47–95.

_____. [1956b] 1967. "Embarrassment and Social Organization," in Erving Goffman, *Interaction Ritual: Essays in Face-to-Face Behavior*. New York: Doubleday. pp. 97–112.

_____. 1959. *The Presentation of Self in Everyday Life*. New York: Doubleday.

_____. 1961. *Behavior in Public Places*. New York: Free Press.

_____. 1971. *Relations in Public*. New York: Basic Books.

_____. 1981. *Forms of Talk*. Philadelphia: University of Pennsylvania Press.

Greif, Mark. 2004. "The Fit and the Dead." *Harper's Magazine*, 309 (September):11–16.

Mead, George Herbert. [1934] 1962. *Mind, Self and Society*. Edited by Charles Morris. Chicago: University of Chicago Press.

Oring, Elliot. 1975. "From Uretics to Uremics: A Contribution toward the Ethnography of Peeing." *California Anthropologist*, 4:1–5.

Sassatelli, Roberta. 1999. "Interaction Order and Beyond: A Field Analysis of Body Culture within Fitness Gyms." *Body and Society*, 5:227–248.

Smith, Allen and Sherryl Kleinman. 1989. "Managing Emotions in Medical School: Students' Contacts with the Living and the Dead." *Social Psychology Quarterly*, 52:56–69.

Waskul, Dennis and Pamela van der Riet. 2002. "The Abject Embodiment of Cancer Patients: Dignity, Selfhood, and the Grotesque Body." *Symbolic Interaction*, 25:487–513.

Weinberg, Martin and Colin Williams. 2005. "Fecal Matters: Habitus, Embodiments, and Deviance." *Social Problems*, 52:315–336.

Chapter 6

Body Armour: Managing Disability and the Precariousness of the Territories of the Self

Carol Brooks Gardner and William P. Gronfein

Goffman's classic "Territories of the Self" is, among other things, an investigation into literal and metaphorical territories that represent defendable personal boundaries. Reminiscent of Spencer Cahill's observations (see Chapter Five, this volume), territories of the self are physical and symbolic cultural constructions that are of no small significance: trespassing in these territories risks dignity. Drawing from their studies of people with disabilities, specifically multiple sclerosis (MS), Carol Brooks Gardner and William P. Gronfein, examine how fragile and unpredictable bodies are "armoured" in public space to better defend and manage trespass. Gardner and Gronfein utilize Goffman's original typology and also add useful new ones – all of which illustrate the micropolitics of everyday life as seen through the lens of people who manage a highly variable MS body.

> All in all, I'm better off if people [in public and at work] see me as a scooter-chair than a human being.
>
> A primary care physician in his forties who has multiple sclerosis (2002)

> The armourers accomplish the knights.
>
> William Shakespeare in *Henry V*

Our general goal in this chapter is to discuss one scholarly metaphor, the territory, as applied to the body's character and actions. We begin with a discussion of Goffman's "territories of the self" as originally proposed in *Relations in Public* (1971:28–62), and apply this territorial metaphor to the study of people with disabilities, specifically multiple sclerosis (MS), in public places. Our focus here is on what might be termed the "micropolitics" of everyday life; we suggest and analyze some common ways that the people with disabilities we have observed and interviewed continue to find the body and associated public interaction difficult to predict and difficult to handle.

Our work is organized as follows. First, we summarize our method; second, we analyze Goffman's general treatment of "bodily preserves" and synopsize his proposed typology concerning these territories of the self; and finally we indicate what seem to us to be useful ways of adapting Goffman's typology to the situation of people with disabilities (multiple sclerosis specifically) in public.

Method and Sample: Procedures and Limitations

Our purpose in undertaking this research was to explore the character of some of the body-existence and body-management contingencies that can occur when one's body is not perceived by oneself or others as reliably under one's own control, as well as when a passerby or attendant holds sway over the body of another. To accomplish this, we used our own participant observations and 32 in-depth interviews of one to six hours in length (2000–2003). Our informants, about one-third men and two-thirds women, ranged in age from 18 to 73. Informants tended to be younger (20–40) and represented a variety of occupations: eight lived on disability, four were teachers, three waitstaff, one politician, six college students, six workers in the home, five workers from their home offices, and seven in the healthcare professions, among whom we included massage, occupational, and physical therapists, including one nurse who specialized in MS and two physicians. Some informants both worked and were on disability and hence can be double-counted; our total therefore is 40, not 32. All informants but one were white; MS is sometimes termed a "white disease." (Our sole nonwhite informant sometimes identified as biracial and sometimes as white.)

The data for this project was excerpted from a larger ongoing analysis about public civility with varied informants, and with IRB approval. Respondents are identified only by pseudonyms. Our fieldwork sometimes took place in areas where people with disabilities were likely to be present, including MS support groups that met in public, annual "MS runs" for a national MS charity, and in the surrounds of medical marijuana clubs. Both authors self-identified as "courtesy stigmatized" (Goffman 1963) from long experience with family members with MS; this doubtless resulted in some informant receptivity, but, contrarily in areas such as the "buyers' clubs" where medical marijuana could be purchased and where ambiguously criminal activity was involved, informants may have been more close-mouthed. In the same way, both authors were occasional but not invariable participants in public MS-related activities and for a few higher-placed individuals who recalled us from support meetings or elaborate events, less than clockwork attendance could have marked us as sunshine patriots.

Like many chronic diseases, MS manifests itself in complicated and variable ways (Strauss and Corbin 1988). First, MS can be "visible" or "invisible." Invisibility and visibility can refer to two somewhat different characteristics of the disease, one applying to differences between persons, and one referring to different manifestations of the disease in a single individual over time. Persons with "invisible" MS are those persons whose disease has not (and may not) produced visible impairment (reliable stumbling, slurred speech, difficulty walking), while persons with "visible" MS are those whose publicly available conduct such as using a cane, wheelchair or other assistive device indicates the presence of some kind of consequential infirmity.

One possibility is that the person with MS may experience an abrupt shift from being asymptomatic and hence invisible to being made visible in a deeply transgressive way.

Like persons with HIV/AIDS, the lives of persons with MS are marked by a deep uncertainty about what is possible or permissible. Upon awakening, one may feel full of vim, vigour and vitality, but feel totally drained by lunchtime; or one may experience a "flare-up" of easily perceptible public symptoms – and find that such flare-ups can last from a few hours, to several months, or to years. The person with MS truly cannot describe the effects MS has on her or him, nor could even the most qualified neurologist in the nation; an example is the situation of a woman who had worked in an office and woke up one day to find she had no use of her legs, a condition that persisted for almost a year, left her with a mildly unstable gait, but never recurred for (at least) the next 40 years of her life (a white office worker in her 70s). Another is the case of an 18-year old college student whose inability to see lasted for several months, and who experienced numbness in limbs on another occasion for several months – both to disappear for several years after these episodes, then reappear. This kind of uncertainty, when crucial areas of control are involved (such as those over ability to walk and see, as well as over bowel and bladder) makes life complicated for a person with MS in a way that cannot be fully appreciated by those whose bodies can be depended on both to (appear to) do the right thing and not to do the wrong thing.

Thus, MS can be invisible, or it can give rise to spectacularly evident conditions that can disrupt ongoing interaction or fragment the focus of an occasion entirely. Multiple sclerosis can also be reported as so mild as not to interfere very much with the person's daily life activities at all. Our examples have been gathered from among those conditions that are less predictable and likelier to have a range of others as interactants, from the familial wise to the stranger on the street; we have therefore counted the accounts as well as our opportunities for observation.

Having MS and wanting to continue one's life in public places, then, sometimes entails elaborate preparations in case the individual needs to call on passersby or to phone for help, to change clothing because of urinary or faecal incontinence, to have a mental route of pit-stops along the way, to carry a folding cane or chair/cane, to be certain a car contains a wheelchair they may need and the lift or ramp heavier wheelchairs need – thus, depending on the circumstances, needs can be many and complex.

Kicking Armour and Taking Names: Armouring Preserves for the Territory of the Self

Within the metaphor of this portion of *Relations in Public*, the self governs or inhabits or simply is subject to and active in a set of territorial preserves. We tend to think of Goffman's territories of the self in terms of the units of space that "territory" connotes (see, for example, Manning 1992:167–168); in fact, it is more accurate to say that any one type of territory is not so much a space as it is a convergence of the effects or potential effects of a physical body. Preserves are the accumulation of the body's abilities to assert itself – whether by motion (including speech), movement, products, even images of the body, or material artifacts associated with a body – on a point that is given a social connotation.

The types of preserve that Goffman describes can be spoken of serially but are meant to be understood to be capable of coexistence. In addition to the preserve of *personal space*, actually a layer of sensibility or toughness that varies according to social category and setting and that we as a society take great care to manipulate by kinesic body-movement and by the fur and feathers of apparel, Goffman mentions seven other types of territorial preserve. The next mentioned is the *stall,* space bounded by equipment that is likely to be fixed, such as a photo or restaurant booth or a theatre or airplane seat, which the body can claim as temporary territory for a performance or activity but to which one is not felt to be permanently attached or in need of; the stall can also be suddenly created by individuals (later to be razed), as when numbers of bodies on a lawn, a beach, or an overnight queue for tickets lay down towels, sleeping bags, or jackets for the specific use of resting or waiting. The use of the preserve we term the *shell* – the publicly permanent container for the body we later name as a preserve – can be as much a weapon as a shield, as when a middle-aged man who occasionally works at a homeless shelter claimed his scooter wheelchair was effective in keeping him safe from the ambulating "human crush," as well as enabling him to "run over the foot of anyone who threatens me, of which there are some number at the shelter. An older office worker said she had, for decades, used her cane to formulate an "invisible cube" so that people would allow her room to walk or sit on sidewalks or buses. Then it can be another sort of armour "in a fancy store like Macy's on Union Square," where he could enter "no matter how [I'm] dressed" and have the chair frame him as an "armour of shame," where I get a wide berth that doesn't feel like people are repulsed by me, they just feel – they can't, they're so worried about discomfiting me." In the last armour, the scooter afforded Cameron a form of respect that seemed to him very different (as another informant, Thelma Manning, user of an electric wheelchair, noted) from "being repulsed – they're afraid they'll offend me, which I use if I can."

Next is *use space,* the amount of space that the body needs to engage in and complete a task, whether the task is one to which we give little weight or definition such as simply walking down the street without bumping into another body, or whether it is more regularly articulated such as the space required to use a laptop in a coffee shop or accomplish the standing "commuter fold" of the newspaper on a bus or subway. Although it is clear in his excursus that Goffman occasionally does see private and public space as to be spoken of with the same vocabulary, there is no sense that he intended the stall or use space to prevail, much less to be considered a "life-sentence, such as a iron-lung, or a motorized wheelchair," as one informant (the healthcare worker Eileen Entwhistle) said, or a homemade vehicle where the individual can only go into public places in an oxygen tent and push-chair. (Some of these possibilities we attempt to deal with later when we speak of the "shell.") The *turn*, Goffman's next suggested preserve, is "the order in which a claimant receives a good of some kind" (35), with variable rules involving such considerations as time of arrival, possible contributions, and social category; in the last case, general rules – such as special consideration to be given to women, children, and people with visible or presumed disabilities – vary with patterns more idiosyncratic to a situation, such as giving away the individual's turn in line at the grocery store or ATM to someone who appears to be in a hurry, likely to consume far less time, or potentially dangerous and therefore to be allowed no excuse to remain behind one or observing one. The *sheath* is both the "purest" and "least" of bodily territories, consisting of the skin and apparel that cover the body (38). As is the case for personal space, the character of different parts of the sheath varies with regard to intrusions and symbolism.

The possessional territory of the body consists of the set of objects or articles that can be identified with the body and whose disposition is felt to be that of the body's owner, such as purses, cigars and cigarettes, and, for Goffman, "a claimant's co-present dependents" (38). In our society, the possessional territory of some (such as the too-general category "men") is believed to be less on certain occasions than the customary possessional territory of contrastive categories (such as "women," who are still cartoonishly portrayed with huge purses that contain armamentaria for every self-presentational occasion.

Preserves and Vulnerability: The Case of People with Disabilities

The general parallel between body and territory can be useful in explicating at least some circumstances concerning bodies that are considered disabled and some of the singular arrangements made between people who are disabled and those who interact with them, either formally and in paid positions (as attendants) or informally and spontaneously (as family, friends, and strangers).

As noted earlier, several of the preserves analyzed by Goffman (the stall and use space in particular), figure in the accounts given by our informants of their everyday encounters in the public realm. For people with disabilities, selves reinforce preserves as access baffles or barriers to the threatened bodily preserve. The threat may be one that seems mild or innocuous to the nondisabled; for the person with MS, a penetrated preserve such as an intrusion on personal space can result in an injurious fall as well as an affront to composure. The person with MS who knows she has two "good hours" – with energy enough to be out and about – may seek to forestall elaborately entrance into preserves involving draining attention and physical or verbal interaction, for fear of violations. In turn, the young woman college student can come to understand and report that she has (and, by our observation, uses) a series of "path-clearers" as she walks with her cane to lessen the time, trouble, and animate and inanimate obstacles, including saying in a mock-menacing tone, "Person with a disability coming through! Watch out, all! Get out of my way or I'll sue you under the A.D.A.!"

Goffman's more general concern emphasizes worries that might concern anyone, such as any citizen's concern about preventing theft of an everyday possession like a handbag or the usurpation of a space such as a "good" seat at the theatre or in a restaurant. We argue that our understanding of the typology of bodily territories can be expanded by exploring the experiences of people with one type of disability, MS; that the potential for violations reported by this group of people with disabilities can be very much broader and less under their control than would be the case had MS not modified the relationship between competent self and incompetent bodily territory; and that people with MS can report their sense of territory violated more broadly than had they not the divisional symptoms of MS to come between self and body, so that they have good reason to invent and utilize available and manufactured armour.

Now that citizens with disabilities are more perceptible in public and the post-Americans with Disabilities Act (ADA) legal stance is to attend to their needs, the same citizens regularly find themselves wrestling with the more everyday trials and tribulations of conscious or unconscious strategizing and managing their own bodies in public.

Territories of the Self: Some Suggestions from the Experience of People with Disabilities

While some of the categories used by Goffman in his typology can be appropriately applied to people with disabilities, such people also use strategies more specifically adapted to their disabilities. We present some examples in what follows.

We are more concerned than Goffman with public bodily vulnerability and with individuals who have special reasons to be more concerned with the armours constructed to foil vulnerability, as some people with disabilities (and in some other social categories) do. Armours are those arrangements, physical or social, which serve to protect the individual with a putative disability from those disruptive contingencies (which, again, can be physical or social) associated with her or his disability that pose a threat to interaction in public. While our focus here is on people whose public performances are vulnerable because of features associated with their bodies, we note that other types of persons, celebrities famous and infamous among them, often feel the need to protect themselves from the public gaze, and use various kinds of armour to do so. The arm upraised so as to conceal a famous actor's face as she is walking out of a nightclub, or the hat placed in front of the face of one subject to the ignominy of a forced "perp walk" constitute armour in just the sense we mean by the term.

1. *The huddle.* For the person with a disability, we propose "the huddle" as a shelter different from the stall. *The huddle* is a momentary and sometimes manufactured retreat from pain and also an armour that hides the vulnerable body accomplishing invulnerability for the body by "hollowing myself into a wedged corner of a big building till it passes or I can walk again," as a woman who works as an editor said,

or "I hide in a bookstore because you don't have to move much there, I just sink to the floor. If they bother me, I tell them I'm sick, I'll be OK in a second," in the words of a man who was formerly a postal worker. The armour – claimed space, claimed legitimate reason (disability) – worked well, both these informants said; and both also mentioned the drawbacks of the huddle, namely, that the suddenly or opportunistically chosen huddle might have to be chosen without regard for comfort so much as the mere possibility of stopping and remaining still. A teacher also mentioned that she constantly thought about places where she might have to execute the sudden self-removal from human traffic that commonly constitutes the huddle, so that a part of her time in public "on bad days" was indeed to plan – if she were walking down a sidewalk or negotiating a store – where she could "collapse without seeming to collapse and without getting too many offers of help"; her very success at this, she noted, came from using the "little bit of remaining strength I have to tell people to" leave her alone and she would "be fine in a moment."

2. *Allowable Breaches.* There has long been a formal stranger etiquette for interacting with people with disabilities in general, and it has continued from decades preceding disabilities awareness and activism into the current time, always given to certain groups like women and "the elderly," people with disabilities are to be given extra measures of help in public places by strangers. The newer etiquette has expanded to the point where written etiquette explicitly suggests that there is a self within a body; though the body is seemingly in trouble, the competence of a "real" self must not be confused with apparent bodily incompetence. One is informed by this new etiquette, then, how to "help" by handling the blind person (firm grasp of the elbow) or to act as a human crutch for the person who has trouble walking or offer juice to a diabetic, but not how to deal with the larger concerns of the self inside the body or even attempt to distinguish the person with slurring speech as not drunk, but experiencing a stroke's aftereffects. Often now the self within the body is consulted – in keeping with the new emphasis on the phrase of reference "person with a disability" – by being told to ask the person with a disability if she or he needs or wants help rather than simply beginning that action her – or himself. Note that these changed or (if one likes) "evolved" etiquette rules function as armour just as certainly as do huddles and other applications of armour we mention. Note also that these etiquette rules furnish the person with a disability with an armour for defending oneself against unwanted incursions.

3. *The shell.* As we suggested earlier, some fragile bodies or bodies unable to navigate in the manner expected use physical arrangements that can be said not only to demarcate a body's boundaries, but to create a movable shield around and transport for the person's body; examples are conveyances like wheelchairs or scooters and baby-carriages or strollers. It should be emphasized that these effective means for transport are different from other sorts of shells into which a body may be placed or may conceal itself, such as the sometimes elaborate creations used by individuals who want to limit identification and access, as celebrities sometimes do. For example, famed reclusive celebrity Michael Jackson has been sighted entering and leaving hotels shielded by a cardboard box, at once gaining the effect of barring

sight while he also provides more of a spectacle for the general public and for those whose business it is to preserve such celebrities along with their tactics, paparazzi.

We have proposed to term this territorial preserve the shell, a more mobile and personal version of the stall (Goffman 1971:32–34) and used by the body in a manner meant to be as effective as a carapace in its ability to shield the frailties of the body in public places. The function of the shell is not simply to demarcate artefactually an individual's personal space. Rather, the shell is understood to have a necessarily protective function that both allows people with disabilities to achieve public interaction with others and allows others to have access, safe access, to people with disabilities. A shell such as the wheelchair, then, enables an individual to be both a participation and a vehicular unit. While the stall is typically a fixed space, the shell is not, especially since the shells we most commonly see in public in connection with people with MS are currently only of one sort, varieties of the wheelchair or the somewhat smaller scooter respectively).

4. *Possessional territory.* We modify this term of Goffman's to discuss how the existence of assistive devices (for example wheelchairs, wheelchair gear like special carryalls, canes, cane-chairs) forms both an extended bodily territory of articles felt to be more a part of the individual's body, and more valued at time for use as armour for the body more than a statement about the self. It is little wonder, given the uncertain severity and course of multiple sclerosis that an informant would sometimes choose a visible sign of general disability to take into public places when they did not, strictly speaking, know that they would need it. Assistive devices like crutches, "sticks," and canes could serve as indices of "trouble to come, preparing the unsuspecting public for anything that might happen." A young bank teller said: "They also are a way to get a wide berth so I don't get tipped over as easily." (Of course, the use of an assistive device might also advertise weakness in a way useful to human predators). Understandably, in addition to appearing in public with what were commonly known to be assistive devices, sometime an informant would do all that was possible to provide a functional equivalent masked in nondisabled trappings. One young college student carried a Native American staff rather than a cane, and wore specially made "normal-looking" boots to reinforce lower-leg stability and cover supporting hose.

5. *Body doubles*: Territories of the self involve much more than space to save, to denote use, to mark the intention of a body to return to claim space. The body itself exists in its present, physical integrity; and it also exists as an image or incarnation of itself, that is, as a body double. Here the double helps the self to adjust to or at least understand the body original. When the body in a public bathroom looks in the mirror, it uses this possibility as a convenience by which to check that all is well with the "real" body others will see and by which they may judge it. When a woman in a wheelchair on her way to give an address in a lecture hall sees her image, "airbrushed and hair just done and the wheelchair chrome shined," on posters plastered over a fence, her reaction is "one of alarm, then I was worried that the audience might be disappointed I didn't look as good as my picture." Here the image

is a distorted double, a body image that the self fears the body it now inhabits might not be able to achieve.

More than the threat to competence integrity, a threat to image integrity is involved. In a more basic sense, the body image has nothing at all to do with an individual's image well or badly produced or reproduced. It is also a way of simply fulfilling (or failing to fulfill) the basic criteria for bodies we consider, in whatever culture we live, to be "human." In this sense, the body image is also what allows us to pass by unnoticed in a large men's clothing store, unless we happen to be "apparently the only Little Person that these people ever saw." And it is what allows us to walk into a crowded conference hotel ballroom unremarked, unless we happen to "suddenly realize I was the only average-height man there, and just something peripheral, like I was a box or a car." This aspect of the image violates the basic expectations for form in a social gathering or among the unacquainted.

6. *Chaperones.* There is another way on which bodies can be doubled, and that is by their competence being overruled by the actions of an animate attendant or helper. Where the chaperones of, say, a royal court, were present in order to safeguard the always threatened virtue of their charges, the chaperones of the person with a disability are present to safeguard the always threatened public performances of their charge. Since the interactional climate in which a person with MS may find him or herself may change from mild to threatening in an instant, having a chaperone of the type we discuss available even when not immediately needed is often a wise course of action. An example of the sudden intrusion that can accompany MS would be the case, among our observations, of the well-spoken woman in the midst of a conference lecture about her very illness – who was surprised by a case of explosive diarrhoea that dribbled down her wheelchair, and legs – while answering an audience question about her day-to-day management of symptoms. Nor need chaperones always be human, nor their functions be less than precise. Both service and therapy animals can be surprisingly acute diagnosticians, in the process saving their principals from not only social improprieties but danger and death. (In Great Britain, dogs have been trained to anticipate epileptic fits, and to pin their owners to the ground so that owners come to no harm by falling.)

Depending on the situation's requirements and the person with MS's sense of her or his own health, she or he might choose to go out into the public realm accompanied by another person; the person could function not only as a companion but do for the body of the person with MS what the body was feared to be unable to do. The purest type of body double for the person with MS was a personal attendant, whose primary function was felt to be exactly this sort of fulfillment of competence claims – for another body. Family members and other loved ones were also reported to be dragooned or willingly to accompany informants. The enthusiasm of children could be particularly touching, as in the case of the child mentioned in the epigraph who wanted to serve as a "human crutch"; or the child could be quite willing to stand in for the parent's lapses but have his own agenda: "Our five-year-old always wants to help me by pushing the chair when we go shopping – but I know he does it because he likes to race down the hill to the Safeway." Whether judged pure of heart or owning the heart of a future thrillseeker, there are undoubtedly reciprocal exchanges possible, from doing a good deed to taking an illicit ride. We want to be individuals, as different and unique (within boundaries) as we can. In current society and in past centuries in Anglo-American cultures, women, the more tightly controlled in terms of appearance norms, have been counselled to make sure they do not end up wearing the same dress or suit to a formal function or business gathering, and even, according to some younger informants, to college class.

Precise imitation of the body-actions of another are done most often to ridicule, as illustrated in this story by a man who lives on disability who spoke of his high-school years:

> A teenage boy went to so much trouble, he was always after me, but he went and rented a wheelchair and he and his friends, they waited for me after school.... I never seen this guy so worked up, 'cause he did this imitation of me, he dressed a sort of like me [and] he started whooping and jumping around, walking like a cripple, then he get back in the chair and try to rush me. He even got this whippy dog – I got a service animal, Fargo. He is big and he is well trained.
>
> Kinda, I thought, [he was] creepy. It was, like it was unbelievable someone would go to so much trouble. [The other boy] dresses up like to try to kill me. It was like the Good and the Evil Twins.
>
> So my [service] dog bit his dog's leg half off. Fargo knew which one in which wheelchair was me.

Imitation is not always the sincerest (or safest) form of flattery: the very attempt at duplication, if recognized, implicitly marks the principal actor's actions as incompetent, poorly chosen, ridiculous, and laughable.

Conclusions

We have presented a series of troubles in public interaction that people with disabilities have encountered. We have presented them as if these are adjustments necessitated by "the infirmities of individual bodies." In fact, however, the various adjustments and armourings that we have discussed are in important ways necessitated by the character of the environments, physical and social, in which persons with disabilities must go about their business in the public realm. Were there shelters, such as bus shelters (for example), arrangements such as the huddle might be less necessary. Were there an etiquette promulgated that does not involve still allow patronizing verbal enmeshments (see the Post, Easter Seals, and Mitchell volumes, for example), the verbal parryings and swordplay that can tax the patience and the energy of people with disabilities might be eliminated. One goal is to disseminate knowledge of what many people do not suspect or what remains out of their awareness, that is, the everyday troubles and the micropolitics of these troubles of people with disabilities in public places. Partly we do so with good academic reason: there is a body of literature that substantiates events that constitute events that happen to people with disabilities that are much worse than many of the everyday occurrences we have mentioned here, and those events can now be considered, under today's social parlance of social problems, "hate crimes" against people with disabilities.

While we understand that Goffman correctly trained his observations in territorial metaphors on getting and keeping, getting away and keeping away, and verbal jousting, we think it worthwhile to "snipe at [this] target" from the point of view of vulnerable or vulnerable-seeming individuals in public. As Goffman often covertly indicates that the individual self must present a body that is all too likely to be seen as a target and guardian marker, and utilizer of possessions as well as of the body, we are also intrigued in the ways that at least some of potential targets manage, and often escape, even being defined as vulnerable. Where Goffman's interactants seem to be drawn from a nation of tradespeople, concerned most with possession and ownership, ours are drawn from a nation of soldiers, whose fight for beachheads such as a seat on a bus or a seat in a college class, is a fight which must be undertaken daily (see, on public-place hate crimes and abuse against people with disabilities Consortium for Citizens with Disabilities 1999; Sherry 2003, 2000; Sobsey 1994).

Acknowledgements

We are grateful to our informants for the opportunity to represent their experience. We are also grateful to Dennis Waskul and Phillip Vannini for their advice on earlier versions, which we have incorporated at several points without explicit credit and shamelessly verbatim.

References

Consortium for Citizens with Disabilities. 1999. "Disability-Based Bias Crimes." [Dated June 10, 1999; retrieved online November 15, 2005].

Easter Seals. "Resources. Disability Etiquette." http://www.easterseals.com. [Retrieved 2005].

Featherstone, Mike, Mike Hepworth and Bryan Turner, eds. 1991 *The Body, Social Process, and Cultural Theory*. London: Sage.

Frank, Arthur W. 1990. "Bringing Bodies Back In: A Decade Review." *Theory, Culture, and Society*, 7:131–162.

_____. 1991. "For a Sociology of the Body: An Analytical Review." in Mike Featherstone, Mike Hepworth and Bryan Turner, eds. 1991 *The Body, Social Process, and Cultural Theory*. London: Sage. pp. 36–102.

Gardner, Carol Brooks. 1992 "Kinship Claims: Affiliation and the Disclosure of Stigma in Public Places." *Research on Social Problems*, 4:203–228.

_____. 1995. *Passing By*. Berkeley: University of California Press.

Goffman, Erving. 1971. *Relations in Public*. New York: Basic Books.

_____. 1963. *Stigma*. Englewood Cliffs, NJ: Prentice-Hall.

Manning, Philip. 1992. *Erving Goffman and Modern Sociology*. Stanford, CA: Stanford University Press.

Mitchell, Mary. *The Complete Idiot's Guide to Etiquette.* New York: Alpha Books.

Sherry, Mark. 2003. 2000. "Hate Crimes Against People with Disabilities." *Social Alternatives*, 19, 4 9(October):23–30.

_____. "Don't Ask, Tell, or Respond: Silent Acceptance of Disability Hate Crimes." in Dawn Ontario: Disabled Women's Network of Ontario. http://dawn.thot.net/ disability_hate_crimes.html. [Posted January 8, 2003. Retrieved September 6, 2004.]

Sobsey, D. 1994. *Violence and Abuse in the Lives of People with Disabilities: The End of Silent Acceptance?* Baltimore: Paul H. Brookes Publishing Company.

Chapter 7

Opera and the Embodiment of Performance

Paul Atkinson

Paul Atkinson utilizes a dramaturgical framework to analyze the embodied craft of opera performance. Atkinson clearly illustrates a dramaturgical body which is fashioned of gesture. Based on his ethnographic work with the Welsh National Opera, Atkinson illustrates how, through tedious repetition, opera embodies gesture to stylistically convey meaning in a performance that is both a visual and musical: "Words, music, and bodies are brought into conjunction, and bodies are coached to move and interact in the physical space of the stage." Atkinson's analysis informs much more than opera, it is a lens into "the complex relations between embodied gesture, intentions and motives, emotions and reactions, characters and actions."

Symbolic interactionism lends itself well to the study of theatre and music-theatre. The interactionist tradition is in many ways perfectly congruent with the interests of singers, actors, producers, stage managers and others who are engaged in the practical work of theatre. There is a direct parallel between the task of the producer and the work of the interactionist ethnographer: both are preoccupied with the close observation and interpretation of action; both attempt to make sense of talk, gesture and conduct; both are thoroughly committed to taking the role of the other, and making sense of the social action they observe (Atkinson 2004a). The producer acts like a symbolic-interactionist interpreter – providing analyses of meaningful symbols and gestures. The performer's body is then socialized into the world constructed by the producer's interpretative frames of reference. The embodied work is crystallized and sedimented through the repetitious work of shaping and honing a performance. Memory is embodied through repeated gesture. The disciplined and rehearsed body of the performer is one of the most significant resources in the conduct of dramaturgy. In this chapter I explore some of these issues to make sense of the embodied work of operatic performance, drawing on my ethnography of the Welsh National Opera Company (Atkinson 2004a, 2004b, 2005).

This chapter brings together two themes in the interactionist tradition: dramaturgy and gesture. It may seem self-evident that music-theatre would invite and illuminate a dramaturgical perspective. Despite the centrality of dramaturgy to the broad interactionist tradition (Goffman 1959, 1974, Burns 1972, Lyman and Scott 1975) there have been few studies of theatrical work and performance and the sociology of the theatre itself has remained under-developed (Tota 1997). The dramaturgical metaphor, however, applies insights from an under-researched domain (the theatre) to make sense of everyday life. My ethnography of an opera company explores the everyday work of music-theatre itself. In the relative absence of studies of the theatre, one is forced to rely more on the reflective accounts of "insiders," such as Stanislavski (1967, Stanislavski and Rumyantsev 1998), or popular "backstage" accounts (e.g. Higgins 1978, Lenton 1998, Mosse 1995), than on the accounts of ethnographic observers. There have, of course, been studies of performance from within the interactionist tradition (see Denzin 2003), from other disciplinary origins (e.g. Bauman 1984, Hughes-Freeland 1998, Turner 1987), and the physicality of performance has been highlighted by ethnographic studies of dance (e.g. Wulff 1998, Buckland 1999). Indeed, performance and theatricality represents one of many fruitful areas of synthesis between the interactionist and other traditions in the social sciences.

The physical enactment of performance is dependent on the embodied *gesture* (Mead 1934, 1938, Strauss 1991). The semiosis of physical gestures, mutual orientation, and spoken interaction is central to the interactionist tradition (cf. Strauss 1993). In theatre, as in everyday life, the body is a vital resource in the creation of character, situation, emotion, and response (Shepherd 2005). When we are dealing with music-theatre, such as opera, the corporeal physicality of theatrical work is even more apparent: opera is intensely physical (Abel 1996). The gesture is of central significance in the embodiment of music-theatre. The bodily gesture is not a mere accompaniment to spoken discourse, and it is much more than a simple expressive repertoire. One cannot conceive of either people or symbolic interaction in the absence of embodied gestural action (Kendon 1997). Likewise, it is hard to envisage staged performance in which the gesture is not a fundamental aspect of the performer's craft: embodied craft knowledge makes possible the performance of actors, singers, dancers, musicians, and others.

Music is vividly gestural in quality. DeNora's (2000) account of music in everyday life shows how music entrains physical action and emotional response. Musical genres include their own musical gestures with conventional connotations of suspense, tension, or desire. The embodied work of the virtuoso is performative beyond the music itself. The orchestral or operatic conductor embodies music's performative quality and charismatic authority. The conductor provides a visual focus of shared attentiveness not only for the performers, but also for the audience. The collective attention of the string quartet depends on shared physical work, from the up-beat of the leader's violin bow, to members' shared breathing. Singers "sing" with the hands, arms and face, as well as the voice. The professional recital singer displays a characteristic gestural repertoire: the hand on the piano, the free hand that rises and falls, the arm that reaches out towards the audience and drops in resignation or resolution.

In opera the gestural quality of acting is often incompatible with the habitual gestures of singing. This contrast is immediately visible in the operatic rehearsal studio. It is common for the singers to "sing through" a scene before they work with the producer; they stand at the piano, often looking at the score, while the repetiteur plays, and the conductor directs them. As they do so, the principal singers act "like singers," using hands and arms to accompany their sung performance. Their hands are raised as the pitch of their voice rises. Gestures accompany musical climaxes. Points of musical energy and tension are reflected in bodily tension and effort. In contrast, when the singers come to "act" the operatic scene they often have to substitute these "singerly" gestures for "dramatic" ones. Producers want singers to do less rather than more by way of embodied, gestural work, and to eliminate anything that reflects the conventional gestures of singing – such as the dramatic sweep on the arm that so often accompanies a big operatic "moment." In practice, operatic performance is a compromise between the gestures of singing and acting.

Even when producers encourage a more graphically gestural style – or indeed when the operatic drama calls for more thoroughly physical action – they are at pains to ensure that singers do not rely merely on the habitual gestures of operatic singing. They often attempt to eliminate over-generalized gestural quality of much singing. The directorial style of many producers, therefore, consists of the attempt to engender specific actions that accurately, pointedly, and plausibly construct their characters, and render visible their emotional states and dramatic intentions. This physical work involves the coordination of singers with one another, and is keyed to the music, which in turn provides one of the basic resources for the temporal and interpersonal management of joint action. In the following section I draw on the details of ethnographic observation in the rehearsal studio to document and discuss in greater detail aspects of the work that goes into the creation of an embodied performance.

Keeping Together

> Producer to singer: "Do you want to do that again?"
> Singer to producer: "No. *You* want to do it again!"

The above exchange took place during a studio rehearsal for Monteverdi's *L'Incoronazione di Poppea*, produced by David Alden. It partly reflects the repetitious character of operatic rehearsal. As I have pointed out elsewhere (Atkinson 2004a), it is no accident that one of the key people in the opera studio, the pianist, is called the repetiteur. Rehearsals often consist of protracted patterns of repetition, in which producers and performers mimic one another, in a dialogue of talk and gesture.

As McNeill (1995) has observed, one of the primordial forms of social order resides in the act of keeping together in time. Military drill and dance are among the social activities that most clearly exhibit this imperative. Music itself is a means to keep people in time with one another; music requires participants to keep in time. While action is not performed "to" the music – as if it were dancing or ice-skating – its sequencing, pacing, and duration is framed by the unfolding music. The music compresses and stretches action. Thus, the temporal aspects of music-theatre are multiple, involving as they do the disciplines of musical and dramaturgical coordination. The disciplines of tempo and rhythm are conjoined with the dramaturgical requirements of coordinated action. Singers and producers have considerable license in interpreting the opera's plot and characters, and they can develop the action in accordance with their emergent interpretations. Nonetheless, whatever staged action they wish to portray, the performers can only do so within the constraints of the music. When an opera consists of "closed" numbers, such as arias and ensembles interspersed with spoken dialogue or recitative, the relationships between music, words, and action may be relatively clear – at least in terms of their general shape – but when the opera is more fluidly constructed, such as the through-composed work of Wagner or Richard Strauss and many other twentieth-century composers, then the relationships may be more open and indeterminate.

There is, nevertheless, the elementary requirement that physical action on-stage is in accordance with the temporal flow of the music. Time and space, voice and body; together they define disciplinary regime of music-theatre. The time of narrated action and the time of the singing may not be the same – as we have seen – and thus the singer's embodied work must encompass an acute sense of timing. The work of producing an opera often rests on the producer's capacity to direct – and the singers' competence to respond with – bodily movements in time and space. The management of entrances and exits is an obvious, but nonetheless case in point. Bodies have to be got on and off stage, and those actions have to be cued to the musical score. The music cannot wait for the performer to make her/his entrance, or to find her/his spot on the stage.

Much of the work of opera production therefore lies in the physical coordination and temporal alignment of performers' bodies. This is especially apparent considering the work of the chorus. While by no means unique to opera, the presence of the chorus is an especially characteristic feature of this performing art. The work of the chorus presents the producer with particular demands. A body of bodies has to be arranged and distributed within the physical and symbolic space of the stage set. Managing the chorus is a skill of the experienced opera producer. Producers are often deemed less successful if they are judged inept in handling the chorus. A chorus of up to forty or more singers requires a good deal of physical management.

The physical work of rehearsal and performance is hedged by material and symbolic boundaries. Each production must take place within the physical spaces prescribed by the set design. The realization of that design in concrete and material reality creates simultaneous opportunities and constraints for the physical action of the opera, as well as expressive possibilities. Equally significant, opera also inhabits a symbolic space that is constituted by light and lines of perspective.

The rehearsal of the opera – like many similar activities including sports training and varieties of learning – depends upon the repeated, embodied enactment of desired outcomes. Rehearsal is thoroughly dependent on repetitious patterns of activity. There is, therefore, a repetitious dialogue between a world of embodied gestures and physical movements, and the commentary of performers and producers in the shared search for plausible and satisfactory representations of opera's narratives and characters.

Embodiment, Mimesis, and Expression

The creation of a role and drama is an emergent process in the theatre, as in everyday life. The process is also thoroughly embodied, as producers and performers attempt to perform physically and make visible the motives and intentions of the opera's characters. Plausible drama depends on the legibility of performers and their embodied presence on-stage.

The following example is derived from a studio rehearsal of Verdi's opera *Simon Boccanegra*. The rehearsal is of the Council Chamber Scene, a remarkable large-scale "set piece" that Verdi and Boito added to the opera when they revised and extended it in 1881. The action of the opera takes place in mediaeval Genoa. Like Venice, Genoa had an elected Doge and the Prologue shows the corsair (pirate) Simon Boccanegra being elected. The Council Chamber Scene is highly dramatic. The Senators assemble and the Doge hastens into the Chamber, clutching his business papers. Boccanegra proposes a peace settlement with Venice, Genoa's enemy and rival Italian maritime republic. His proposal is supported by a letter from the great Italian poet Petrarch, which Boccanegra reads, celebrating a vision of one united country (one of Verdi's allusions to the contemporary Italian political context and nationalist risorgimento aspirations). The Doge reads aloud the letter from the poet Petrarch urging peace between Genoa and Venice, but the Senators shout him down, reaffirming war.

After the principals have run through the scene once, David Pountney – the producer – gives a series of notes (producers "give notes" at the end of a rehearsal in order to correct things they do not like, suggest changes, and propose ways of improving the acting). His remarks are mostly addressed to Philip Joll, the baritone singing the part of the central character Simon Boccanegra, the Doge, himself. To Philip, David Pountney says, "It's not how we did it before. You should be coming on quickly – as if you're coming in from another meeting. Simon almost starts to speak before he gets on, looking at his papers." Then Pountney goes on to suggest that Joll should "look up, in a more reflexive way," when he says he has a more "generous" request to make of the Council. The conductor, Carlo Rizzi, makes a musical point about Joll's phrasing when he actually sings the word generoso, while Pountney suggests that at this point it is "too grand, not what you would get from a soldier." Rizzi adds again that the singing should be "subdued but intense." Pountney goes on giving further notes to Philip Joll:

> When you lose your temper, I want to see you doing it. He has a vision that no-one else has, for one country. He's in tune with this visionary man Petrarch. So when somebody knocks their idea down with silly remarks, you're very angry. I want to see that. You're a pirate.

Pountney is reminding Joll that Simon Boccanegra is a pirate when he becomes Doge. He continues, "Have your vision first. It's like 'I have a dream,' like Martin Luther King."

They start to run the scene again, Philip Joll starts singing. As he does so, David Pountney starts to put his hands together in front of him. He stops Philip. "Why don't you use your hands?" he says, and clenches his own fists by way of demonstration. "It's getting better," he adds. Pountney also suggests to Joll that he could use the papers before him more: looking at them, but not paying attention, and he suggests it could be like "the first item on the agenda is...," as if he is chairing a routine business meeting. They continue, to the point where there is an off-stage commotion from the populace of Genoa. David Pountney again stops Philip. "OK, so when this breaks out, Phil, I must see you hear it, I must see you hear it. You go on with your paperwork, but I must see you hear it. You are being very alert to what's going on around you."

They take a short break and then rehearse the scene again. David Pountney gives notes again. "Very good. Very good. When you lose it – when you lose your temper – look straight ahead. When you use your hands you must watch it. Don't make it too much. And if you look over here, it doesn't have any value.... *E la Venezia*: The point about this, Phil, is – if it were anywhere else it would be different, but it's the old enemy. You need to be aware of that when you say *Venezia*. It's like making peace with Germany."

Here we glimpse some of embodied dramaturgical work that goes into the conduct of rehearsals, and so into the creation of the opera production. In many ways the most illuminating comment from the producer is when he insists to his singer that he has to see the emotion his character is feeling. This is, of course, at the heart of all acting, and is by no means restricted to the work of opera; the physical expression of emotion is a key feature of the work of operatic singing as well as of acting more generally – although in operatic performance there are particular demands and constraints on embodiment. We also see how the producer models the physical gestures and actions that he envisages and wants the singer to emulate. From this extract, we also learn of the potential significance of the gaze. The producer draws the singer's attention to the direction of his gaze – suggesting that if he looks "straight ahead," it will be more effective than if he directs his gaze elsewhere. The gaze and the line of sight are of fundamental importance in realizing an opera. The performing space – in the rehearsal studio or in the theatre – is defined, metaphorically, by invisible frames of mutual orientation.

The following extract from the rehearsal of a different scene from *Simon Boccanegra* illustrates similar features. It is from the very beginning of the opera's Prologue, and takes place in a square in Genoa, in front of the church of San Lorenzo. Paolo – a leader of the plebeian faction – is in conversation with Pietro, another leading plebeian. They talk about the coming election of a Doge, and their desire to overturn the patricians by nominating their own candidate. Paolo proposes "the courageous man who freed our seas of African pirates and restored the flag of Liguria to its ancient glory" (the corsair Simon Boccanegra). Pietro agrees, in return for gold, position and power. Boccanegra himself enters, greets Paolo with an embrace and asks why they have asked him to come. Paolo outlines his proposal, but Boccanegra rejects it as madness. Paolo then points out that if he is Doge nobody will be able to refuse him anything, and he can marry Maria, the daughter of the patrician Fiesco, with whom Simon has had a love affair. Maria has given birth to his illegitimate daughter, and is now a prisoner in her family home. Boccanegra finally agrees to the proposal. The Prologue continues with Paolo and Pietro persuading the Genoese people to vote for Boccanegra, and a confrontation between Simon and Fiesco. Simon enters the Fiesco palace, which appears to be deserted, and the Prologue ends with his discovery that Maria is dead, while the square fills with a crowd hailing Simon Boccanegra as their new Doge: he has gained a throne and a tomb.

After the three male singers have run through the scene, Pountney gives them a number of directorial notes. He says to Paolo, "I haven't found the right way for you to appear.... I'd like it to be more enigmatic. Ooze out and just flow off." And to Pietro he adds, "When you make that move, just follow him off." He emphasizes that the moves between Paolo and Pietro need to reflect the music: to Paolo he suggests that he is making one of the moves too soon. He needs to make it look as if his suggestion to elect Boccanegra is "almost as if you have an afterthought." Between them they need to establish precisely when Paolo turns his body as Pietro exits. Pietro himself inquires, "Do you want me to leave earlier?" Pountney himself acts out how he wants the two singers to enact their movements, showing how he wants Paolo to insinuate himself into the set for his entrance. He displays a more sinuous movement. Paolo has been bustling onto the set in a rather more abrupt fashion. Pountney is trying to convey to him a more insidious entrance. David Pountney gives a note to Simon Boccanegra, sung by Philip Joll, saying that when he comes on, saying "*Un amplesso*" ("an embrace"), and holding Paolo: "This embrace has got to be very strong. Don't compromise. Don't hold back.... I don't get enough *bite* from it." The two singers go through the action again. Still Pountney wants the gesture to be stronger: "Philip, as soon as he's close, grab him."

Here the producer directs the physical embodiment of action and character. Throughout the rehearsal period, the producer kept trying to get Paolo to "act" differently. Indeed, the singer himself became frustrated and upset by his apparent inability to please David Pountney, who in turn seemed to get rather irritated with the singer. In this and similar rehearsal sequences, Pountney wanted the singer to express his conspiratorial, sinister character through his singing and physical presence. Although the singer tried repeatedly to follow the instructions and demonstrations he was given, he was not apparently able to do exactly what his producer had in mind. He seemed always too matter-of-fact in his demeanour, too "perky," rather than darkly insinuating or menacing. The problem was partly a reflection of the singer's fairly slight stature, which gave him a rather jaunty air. Likewise, Pountney repeatedly directed Philip Joll as Boccanegra to convey his personal authority through his physical acting. Joll is physically big, but did not always appear to be making the best possible use of his physical presence. In the example I have just summarized, Joll's "embrace" of his friend Paolo seemed too perfunctory, not sufficiently wholehearted. Pountney was obviously looking for a larger physical gesture.

This example illustrates a series of simultaneous interpretative processes. The intentions of the producer are themselves realizations of the implied intentions of the character(s) in question. These are translated into physical actions, which may be acted out by producers to demonstrate what they want. What is in the mind of the producer is projected to the actor, which must then be translated into embodied action that mirrors the producer's visions, actions, and/or verbal descriptions. This action in turn relates to the search for the character's intentions once more, in a joint attempt to locate these activities within a shared frame of dramaturgy, narrative, and character. There is, therefore, a repeated series of dialogues, expressed verbally and physically, exploring possible relationships between intentions, gestures, and other physical performances.

These embodied actions and processes are further illustrated in the following extracts from the studio rehearsals for *Tristan und Isolde* (Wagner), a revival being directed by Peter Watson who had worked on the original production. They are rehearsing part of Act III. Tristan is lying mortally wounded, attended by Kurwenal, awaiting Isolde's arrival. The set is very simple, defined primarily by a steep, curved rake. Much of the visual effect of the staging is generated by the lighting that defines the space behind and around this simple set – and the equally simple sets for the other Acts. Kurwenal says to Peter Watson that he is unhappy with his movements. He is towards the top of the raked curve; he says it is such a small space and feels very uncomfortable. It is clear from watching that he is tentative in his movements. Peter Watson replies, "I can assure you that it doesn't look a small space, with what's behind it. It is a complete optical illusion." Later in the scene, Kurwenal comes down-stage, down the slope, to be with Tristan. As the singers and the production staff discuss the scene, Kurwenal suggests that at a particular point, Kurwenal is "shut out" – it is really Tristan's emotion alone. He adds somewhat diffidently, "I don't want to interfere in the production." Tristan meanwhile is lying, propped up, on the raked set, where he has been lying and singing throughout the scene. He replies to Kurwenal's suggestion saying, "I can work with that." Watson suggests to Tristan that perhaps his gesture when he sings the name "Isolde" is "a bit too strong." Lawton (Tristan) says that perhaps he can pull himself into a more upright posture with one hand. Watson replies, "OK, we'll try that next time we do it." Watson and Kurwenal talk about the scene quietly while Anthony Negus, who is conducting the rehearsal, goes over to talk to Tristan (who is still recumbent on the set). They go over some details of musical phrasing. Negus suggests a different phrasing, but Lawton explains that he is phrasing it the way he is "because of the breath there." They discuss between them precisely where he should breathe, and Lawton sings the phrases to himself *sotto voce*.

Tristan, Kurwenal, and the producer then go on to discuss the next part of the scene. Tristan can recall how the scene was originally played. He says that when he sings "*Isolde kommt*" ("Isolde is coming") he falls back against Kurwenal. A little later Peter Watson says, "I know Tristan does something here, but I can't remember what." Jeffrey shows him what he does. He throws off the blanket that he has been wrapped in, staggers across the set and throws himself down. "At this point," he says, "the orchestra wonders where the hell I'm going. They brace themselves," adds one of the others. They continue to rehearse. As they do so, Jeffrey again draws on his previous work in the role. He shows Kurwenal "How I do it," and how he starts to fall forward, so that Kurwenal needs to grip his shoulders, to hold him up. Jeffrey then sings through from "*Isolde kommt...*" to "*Kurwenal, siehst du es nicht?*" Kurwenal bends over Tristan as he raves in despair. Finally Tristan throws himself down. "Don't ask me to do that again!" he says. To Kurwenal, Lawton says that everything was fine as he was crouching over him, except that at one point he needed to take a deep breath and did not have enough room to do so.

These fragments from Tristan und Isolde help us to understand some of the physical work of operatic performance. We see examples of singers who grapple with the physical constraints of staging and acting. Tristan has to spend a great deal of the scene lying on the stage or huddled at the foot of the raked slope. Indeed, he only gets up once in order to slump down in a different spot. He therefore has to sing from this more-or-less horizontal posture. Moreover, he had the physically demanding task of managing a small foot-hold screwed to the sloped part of the set, to prevent him sliding down-stage – itself physically demanding. The singer's final exclamation of "don't ask me to do that again!" was heartfelt. The demands on singers include the physical requirement to sing *and* breathe. Postures and positions must sometimes be adapted in order to accommodate the basic bodily exigencies of operatic singing, which is in itself a physically demanding activity. In doing all this, the performers are, of course, performing within the physical constraints of the stage set; the set defines the space in which they can move and act. They must adapt and fit their physical movements to the space. In the case of Tristan and Isolde, the steeply sloped feature meant that keeping one's balance needed considerable physical effort. While Tristan has little or no "action" to perform in this section, there are several key moves to be accomplished accurately. Gestures have to be "right:" enough to convey the character's emotional response, not so much as to appear exaggerated. Moreover, they have to be cued to the words-and-music simultaneously.

This process is not merely a gestural dialogue of bodies in interaction, or physical mimicry. There is also a dialectical relationship between words and actions. Rehearsals are characterized by the search for interpretative frames of reference through which producers and performers can make sense of the words they find in the libretto, the action of the opera, the music that pervades the work, and their understanding of how to put these things together. Bodies and intentions, words and actions are brought into a dialogic relationship in rehearsal.

The creation of action is an intensely physical, embodied activity. The world of stage action is not just one of words and music. It is thoroughly encoded in a repertoire of gestures. Protracted participation and observation of a series of operas suggests a number of things about the gestural quality of operatic production and dramaturgy. It is clear that each producer has a characteristic embodied presence, and that to some clearly perceptible degree, each staging is a projection, through the performers, of his of her own physical presence. I have described this process more fully elsewhere (Atkinson 2005). Each producer has a distinctive way of being-in-the-world, and of-being-on-stage. Each has a characteristic way of standing, gesturing, and moving. The tilt of the head, the posture of the back and shoulders, the expressive use of gesture – these are all constitutive of how the director embodies not just himself, but also his/her display of how performers should approach a scene. When the producer envisages a scene and blocks the action within it, she or he is projecting into it her or his own embodiment as well as engaging with the physical presence of the performers. Throughout a rehearsal period producers repeatedly demonstrate their own physical interpretations of what they desire and think possible.

Each singer is not a physical *tabula rasa*. Just like each producer, each singer has her or his own idiolect of gesture. Each body provides a unique repertoire of physical competences and possibilities. Just as each singer brings a unique voice to the part, so she or he brings a unique body too. The body is simultaneously a set of resources and a set of constraints over what expressive gestures and practical actions can be accomplished. Each individual singer thus brings to the part a unique gestural style that reflects her or his own embodied identity. If one observes the same singers in different roles – especially if one has the ethnographic privilege of seeing the same singers create different roles through the rehearsal process, one can readily see how each "new" role reflects "the same" resources of the body and its performative possibilities. Each singer, however much he or she may attempt to act out the producer's directorial wishes, does so in accordance with a repertoire of gestural resources. The same characteristic turn of the head that signifies the receipt of an insult or rebuff; the same step backwards that indicates surprise, shock, or revelation; the same little gesture of hands clasped at the waist to accomplish nervous innocence and anxious anticipation; the same clenched fist that enacts resolve, anger, and vengeance; the repeated hunched shoulders of existential despair and crushing responsibility. This is not a reflection of dramaturgical incompetence or limitation. On the contrary, the most accomplished of actors – whether in opera, film, television or the stage – manifestly have a split performance. Each plays the role. Each also enacts her or his presence and skill as a performer. Audience members always know that they are not simply watching a character act out the drama; they also know they are watching a particular performer's version of that role. In the opera house, one is never oblivious of the fact that one is witnessing Bryn Terfel's Wotan, or Renée Fleming's Thaïs. This applies especially to "stars," but is true of all performance artists (Barba 1995). Of course, this brief summary hardly does justice to the nuances and complexity of role-playing and performance. It is not necessary to be involved in theatrical work to be engaged in the construction of a "persona" (Fine 1983, Waskul and Lust 2004). The degrees of engagement, distance, playfulness and so on are multiple, as are the frames of rehearsal and performance.

Conclusions

As I have emphasized throughout this chapter, the accomplishment of opera is profoundly physical work. Operatic singing, which demands a highly developed, physically supported voice, is more taxing than most forms of singing. Singers themselves compare their vocal work with that of athletes. The production of the voice depends upon the management of the body and control of the breath that is very different from the everyday production of singing. The amplitude of sound produced by a solo singer – to say nothing of the sound produced by an operatic chorus – is testimony to the energy expended. The physicality of operatic singing by no means exhausts the embodied work that performers must undertake.

Operatic performers need to engage in a regime of embodied physical gesture. Words, music, and bodies are brought into conjunction, and bodies are coached to move and interact in the physical space of the stage. Music facilitates physical movement. It also provides inexorable temporal frames and limits to what movement is possible. The opera singer is faced with the same sort of physical, gestural demands as is the 'straight' actor. They must both find and negotiate ways of being-on-the-stage that make visibly meaningful the actions of their character, respond to the actions of others, and create dramatic narrative. It is not necessary in either genre that these actions should be naturalistic. Indeed, opera may be performed in a variety of dramatic genres, some naturalistic, others highly stylized. Producers – especially in opera – construct their own visual and dramatic idioms that simultaneously constrain and generate the actions of their performers. There is, therefore, a mimetic aspect to the embodied work of the singing-actor. This depends not merely on the mimesis of everyday codes of action and gesture. It is refracted through a mimetic relationship with the producer's embodied work.

We have reversed Goffman's analytic spyglass. To return to the beginning of this chapter, we have examined the everyday life of dramaturgy, in contrast to Goffman who documented the dramaturgy of everyday life. Between them sociological commentators like Goffman and theatrical innovators like Stanislavski provide complementary, mutually illuminating accounts of the complex relations between embodied gesture, intentions and motives, emotions and reactions, characters and actions. We need therefore to pay close attention to the work of professional performance as well as to the performative aspects of everyday life.

References

Abel, Sam. 1996. *Opera in the Flesh: Sexuality in Operatic Performance*. Boulder CO: Westview Press.

Atkinson, Paul. 2004a. "Performance and Rehearsal: The Ethnographer at the Opera," in C. Seale, G. Gobo, J.F. Gubrium and D. Silverman (eds) *Qualitative Research Practice*. London: Sage, pp. 94–106.

_____. 2004b. "Performance, Culture and the Sociology of Education," *International Studies in Sociology of Education*, 14, 2:149–167.

_____. 2005. *Everyday Arias: Making Opera Work*. Walnut Creek CA: AltaMira.

Barba, Eugenio. 1995. *The Paper Canoe: A Guide to Theatre Anthropology*, trans. Richard Fowler. London: Routledge.

Bauman, Richard. 1984. *Verbal Art as Performance*. Prospect Heights IL: Waveland Press.

Buckland, Theresa (ed.). 1999. *Dance in the Field: Theory, Methods and Issues in Dance Ethnography*. London: Macmillan.

Burns, Elizabeth. 1972. *Theatricality: A Study of Convention in the Theatre and in Social Life*. New York: Harper and Row.

DeNora, Tia. 2000. *Music in Everyday Life*. Cambridge: Cambridge University Press.

_____. 2003. *After Adorno: Rethinking Music Sociology*. Cambridge: Cambridge University Press.

Denzin, Norman. 1992. *Symbolic Interactionism and Cultural Studies: The Politics of Representation*. Oxford: Blackwell.

_____. 2003. *Performance Ethnography: Critical Pedagogy and the Politics of Culture*. Thousand Oaks CA: Sage.

Edmondson, Ricca. 1984. *Rhetoric in Sociology*. London: Macmillan.

Fine, Gary Alan. 1983. *Shared Fantasies: Role-Playing Games as Social Worlds*. Chicago: University of Chicago Press.

Foster, Gwendolyn A. 2000. *Troping the Body: Gender, Etiquette, and Performance*. Carbondale: Southern Illinois University Press.

Goffman, Erving. 1959. *The Presentation of Self in Everyday Life*. Garden City NY: Doubleday.

_____. 1974. *Frame Analysis: An Essay on the Organization of Experience*. Boston MA: Northeastern University Press.

Higgins, John. 1978. *The Making of an Opera: Don Giovanni at Glyndebourne*. New York: Atheneum.

Hughes-Freeland, Felicia (ed.). 1998. *Ritual, Performance, Media*. London: Routledge.

Kendon, Adam. 1997. "Gesture," *Annual Review of Anthropology*, 26:109–128.

Lenton, Sarah. 1998. *Backstage at the Opera*. London: Robson Books.

Lyman, Stanford M. and Scott, Marvin B. 1975. *The Drama of Social Reality*. New York: Oxford University Press.

McNeill, William H. 1995. *Keeping Together in Time: Dance and Drill in Human History*. Cambridge MA: Harvard University Press.

Mead, George Herbert. 1934. *Mind, Self and Society*. Chicago: University of Chicago Press.

_____. 1938. *Philosophy of the Act*. Chicago: University of Chicago Press.

Mosse, Kate. 1995. *The House: Inside the Royal Opera House, Covent Garden*. London: BBC.

Napier, A. David. 1992. *Foreign Bodies: Performance, Art, and Symbolic Anthropology*. Berkeley CA: University of California Press.

Shepherd, Simon. 2005. *Theatre, Body, Pleasure*. London: Routledge.

Stanislavski, Constantin. 1967. *On the Art of the Stage*. London: Faber and Faber.

Stanislavski, Constantin and Rumyantsev, Pavel. 1998. *Stanislavski on Opera*. London: Routledge.

Strauss, Anselm. 1991. "Body, Action-Performance, and Everyday life," in Anselm Strauss, *Creating Sociological Awareness*. New Brunswick NJ: Transaction, pp. 385–95.

_____. 1993. *Continual Permutations of Action*. New York: Aldine de Gruyter.

Tota, Anna Lisa. 1997. *Etnogrtafia dell'Arte*. Rome: Logica University Press.

Tulloch, John. 1999. *Performing Culture: Stories of Expertise and the Everyday*. London: Sage.

Turner, Victor. 1987. *The Anthropology of Performance*. New York: PAJ Publications.

Waskul, Dennis and Lust, Matt. 2004. "Role-Playing and Playing Roles: The Person, Player, and Persona in Fantasy Role-Playing," *Symbolic Interaction*, 27 (3):333–56.

Wulff, Helena. 1998. "Perspectives Towards Ballet Performance: Exploring, Repairing and Maintaining Frames," in Hughes-Freeland, Felicia (ed.) *Ritual, Performance, Media*. London: Routledge, pp. 104–20.

Chapter 8

Samba no Mar: Bodies, Movement and Idiom in *Capoeira*

Neil Stephens and Sara Delamont

In this chapter Neil Stephens and Sara Delamont examine bodies in capoeira, *a Brazilian dance and martial art. Drawing from Arthur Frank's typology, Stephens and Delamont magnify how, in* capoeira, *bodies are fashioned of discipline and control. Yet this discipline and control is a dramaturgical effect of a scene that comes off; teachers and students necessarily express and impress themselves upon others by means of sign vehicles, some of which are specific to* capoeira *but most are broadly conventionalized and reflective of the ways in which we all dance and kick our way through everyday life.*

"Samba no mar – dance in the sea," is sung to accompany *capoeira*: a dance and martial art practiced and performed to music. Owing to widespread popularity of martial arts in Europe and America, many men and women acquire various degrees of skill in disciplines such as *aikido, karate, tae kwan doh*, or *capoeira* derived from a very different cultural origin. Brazilian *capoeira* is the empirical focus of this chapter, and our analysis primarily contrasts the bodies of experts and novices, drawing on fieldwork in three British cities. In classes, at public performances, and when experts demonstrate advanced skills, disciplined bodies are displayed for emulation, admiration, and education. We illustrate how bodies in *capoeira* are sign vehicles (Goffman 1959) by which masters and student express and impress; control, discipline, emulation, admiration, and desire are embodied in ritualized play and performance.

We start with an extract from our fieldnotes. In the traditions of *capoeira* teachers give their students a nickname, often in Portuguese. For the purposes of this chapter, Delamont is *Bruxa* (witch), Stephens is *Trovao* (thunder).[1]

1　As practitioners of *capoeira* we have real nicknames, but publish with pseudonyms. We select *Bruxa* and *Trovao* for various reasons. In European folklore witches are often jealous old women, so *Bruxa* seems appropriate. *Trovao* invokes *Xango*, the Yoruba God of Thunder, an important figure in *Candomble*, the African-Brazilian religion. We also use pseudonyms for teachers and students. Achilles teaches in two British cities with universities, called here Tolnbridge and Cloisterham. Male students' nicknames such as Hathi and Darzee come from Kipling's *The Jungle Book*.

It is a Sunday morning in late November in Cloisterham, a British university city. Chilly and overcast, though not actually raining or snowing, it is not really cold, but not good weather either. The streets are largely empty. In a redundant church, converted to a dance studio, about a hundred and twenty people are, for all practical purposes, not in Cloisterham at all, but in Brazil. Most of them are singing "Samba no mar, marinheiro" (Dance in the sea, sailor), the chorus of the song being sung by Orestes, a tall African-Brazilian man. He, dressed all in white, with his skin gleaming and his hair in dreadlocks, plays an African-Brazilian instrument, a *berimbau*, at the far end of the hall. Around him are six other Brazilian men and one woman, also in white, playing other *berimbaus*, drums, agogos or *pandeiros* (tambourines). At the far end of the hall from the Brazilian *bateria* (group of musicians) is a raised seating area. Spread around among the seats are about fifteen spectators, one or two resting, a few nursing injuries or hangovers, a few the friends and relations of the students practising. In the body of the hall are about a hundred young people, mostly white, mostly in white t-shirts and trousers, like the Brazilians, including *Trovao*, practising attacks, defences and escapes under the instruction of Xenokrates, a tanned Brazilian, also with dreadlocks. The class is due to end in about thirty minutes time, and the man in overall charge, a tanned Brazilian called Achilles, tips used paper plates and cups into a black plastic rubbish sack held by a much older white woman. Achilles seizes half a mango, waves it at the woman and says "Hey *Bruxa* eat this mango!" Around them, the chorus rises "Samba no mar, marinheiro, Samba no mar" and a hundred people cartwheel, launch kicks at each other, and sway in time to the music. The woman obediently puts down the rubbish sack, and starts to eat the mango, offering some of it to a passing child and some to *Luckannon* and *Lunghri*, two British men she knows. "Samba no mar, marinheiro," the class sing, "Samba no mar."

Here Delamont (*Bruxa*) has abandoned writing observational fieldnotes to help the organizer Achilles clear up the breakfast buffet provided for the teachers. Stephens (*Trovao*) is a *capoeira* student and *Bruxa*'s co-author (Stephens and Delamont 2006; Rosario, Stephens and Delamont 2006). *Trovao*'s teacher, who appears in our publications as Achilles, chooses to be named as Claudo Campos Rosario who is an instructor in the Beribazu group. He has been in *capoeira* since 1991.

This master class in Cloisterham was the penultimate event in a festival. Achilles, the Brazilian *capoeira* teacher in Cloisterham and Tolnbridge, had organized the festival for both cities. Training on Sunday morning included about three fifths of all the students involved. Normally they learn only from Achilles, but during festivals, other teachers from all over the UK, Europe, and from Brazil are invited. Twenty-seven teachers were at this festival. It was the third festival *Bruxa* had attended, and *Trovao*'s fourth, where he was awarded his second belt – the *azul-marron* (blue-brown). Festivals include master classes, parties, demonstrations, lectures, dance classes, music lessons, and folk-cultural forms such as *maculele*,[2] the baptism[3]

---

2   A dance done in grass skirts, with wooden sticks that are clashed noisily together.

3   The symbolism of the term baptism is explicit in *capoeira*: the novice is welcomed into a *capoeira* "family" with a new *capoeira* name. A student, who has trained conscientiously for a few months, is put forward to a baptism (*batizado*), where they play with a master, are ceremonially knocked to the ground, and given their first belt (*corda*). Brazil is a Roman

of novices into *capoeira* (when their nickname is given), and the testing of more experienced players who graduate to the next, higher, belt.

"Samba no mar" takes us to the heart of *capoeira* bodies. In contrast to most martial arts, where the body is disciplined to be rigid and hard (Ashkenazi 2002; Donohue 2002; Holcome 2002; Twigger 1999), in *capoeira* the body is sinuous and rhythmic. Images of the sea, of sailing, of marine creatures, and of the sea goddess *Iemanja*, are part of symbolism and culture of *capoeira*: students are also taught a stylized fisherman's dance. Images of the archetypal Brazilian dance, the samba, are even more prevalent: students are encouraged to take samba classes to improve their *capoeira* agility and beauty. The exotic, the dance, the marine imagery – all convey important aspects of our symbolic interactionist analysis of bodies in British *capoeira*, which are central to the dramatic and artful fashioning of *capoeira* embodiment. Indeed, *capoeira* is played, danced, fought to the music of the *berimbau*. Browning (1995:87) writes of its "elegance" as "excruciating," Schreiner (1993:43) enthuses that "the *capoeira* dancer is, at one and the same time, artist and athlete, performer and poet." *Capoeiristas* have disciplined bodies, capable of twisting, leaping, kicking, and folding themselves into small spaces with great flexibility.

In *capoeira*, bodies are symbols of Brazil, of sensuality, of fitness, of beauty, and of aggression. The *capoeira* expert's body is a sign-vehicle, Goffman (1959): presented to others as a sign of expertise and authority in the art. The expert's body is the means by which he earns his living and its presentation is carefully planned. For *capoeira* learners, the disciplined body (Frank 1990, 1991) of the teacher is a sign and object of emulation and admiration. The expressive and impressive drama of the teacher's body is an engrossing performance for learners who train to transform their bodies to their individual version of the teacher's body. By these disciplined and dramaturgical rituals and performances, *capoeira* students perform action on their bodies (Strauss 1993).

Bodies in *Capoeira*

The study of *capoeira* is, inevitably, the study of bodies. Two types of body are central to analysis: those of instructors and students. Instructors have bodies which are highly disciplined objects of emulation and admiration. *Discipulos* (students) have a wide range of bodies, but if they are in serious training, they desire to emulate their master's body. They observe teachers closely to see which moves they can adapt to their own game, and practice to change their bodies so they can also perform those moves. In the following reflection on expert bodies and skills, *Trovao* who had been to a festival with visiting teachers, told *Bruxa* what she had missed:

> They were all good, but some of them were OUTSTANDING! I mean – Achilles, was way up within the top, maybe the best three, because there were a lot of people that were

---

Catholic country, and the concept of baptism is treated in *capoeira* as a parallel to a Catholic baptism.

high graded, but, they were older so, a bit less sort of flexible. Probably the best one was a
fella, Ajax, that's what he was called. When he wanted to show off, he would start off by
… by just jumping on his head and then he'd slide the length of the *roda* on his head. He
had a shaved head. Then he would just stop – and just not move, still upside down, when
the other person's thinking "What on earth do I do?" Then he'd kind of go up on one arm
and he'd – aahh – he was, he was insane. And it was just a normal game.

Here *Trovao* reports pride in the body of his teacher, Achilles, and his enthusiasm
for the bodily skills of Ajax *in a normal game*. Clearly, *Trovao* is impressed by the
performance of Achilles and Ajax. Moreover, for a novice, Ajax's abilities – not in
a special display, but in an ordinary game – are displayed for emulation. *Trovao* and
his fellow students, who had not seen many experts before this festival, subsequently
set out to emulate the performance of the masters they saw: "You go there to watch
them, to do what they do."

A superficial exposure to *capoeira* can be misleading. The music, mixed classes,
and gaiety, can appear spontaneous and even undisciplined. A casual observer could
think that *capoeira* bodies are not disciplined compared, for example, to those of
karate (Ashkenazi 2002) or other Eastern martial arts (Donohue 2002; Holcombe
2002). A closer study, or participation, reveals that behind the fluent performance
are hours of drill and practice; skilled *capoeiristas* present highly disciplined bodies.
Precisely because the bodies of experienced *capoeira* players display discipline, and
because much of the teaching consists of drill, albeit drill to enjoyable music, classic
symbolic interactionist analysis of the disciplined body can be applied.

The disciplined body is an ideal type, which Frank illustrated with examples from
military drill, medieval holy anorexia, and professional dance (Frank 1990, 1991).
The disciplined body is fashioned in the performance of *dramatic ritual*. As Frank
details, the disciplined body is located on four dimensions: other-relatedness, self-
relatedness, desire, and control. The disciplined body is regimented, and displays
predictable skills; there is a high degree of control. On the desire dimension, the
disciplined body either lacks desire, or produces it. As far as other-relatedness is
concerned, the disciplined body can be constituted through its relations with others
(dyadic) or focused inwards upon itself (monadic). If the disciplined body dissociates
itself from its own corporeality it will be low in self-relatedness, if focused upon it,
high.

We hinge our examination of the dramaturgical body using Frank's seminal
analysis, focusing squarely on two distinct bodies in *capoeira*: the disciplined and the
becoming disciplined. Using Frank's four dimensions, we contrast the dramaturgical
performances of the expert disciplined body of the *mestre*, or near master, and the
many undisciplined, or partially disciplined bodies of the students in the classes.

Self-Relatedness: Masters' Bodies

Frank argues that the self-relatedness of the disciplined body is either comfortable
with its own corporeality or dissociated from it. For the purposes of our analysis we

draw from Goffman (1959) to suggest that comfort or disassociation with the corporeal body is a dramatic effect of a scene that comes off, not the cause of it. *Capoeira mestres display* public comfort with their disciplined, corporeality. Instructors have bodies of very different sizes and shapes, races, and ages but all display themselves as "at home" in their bodies; all convey easy grace when resting, sensuality when dancing, amazing agility, and considerable strength when teaching and performing for the public. Instructors display satisfaction with their own corporeality when they play or perform, when they teach moves and when their bodies are at rest, though their mastery of rhythm; their hair, skin, tattoos, clothing; and their balance, pace, energy and exuberance are all brought together into one disciplined and embodied performance. When teaching they display satisfaction by the ease with which they demonstrate the movements the students must practice, mimic, and learn. At rest they display satisfaction through their muscles, skin, tattoos, and clothing.

Play and Performance

Capoeira is performed to music. While music may be employed to accomplish numerous dramaturgical intents, in the case of *capoeira* music is literally instrumental to performance. The music provides rhythm, which is all about time and "keeping time." Music, in this disciplined sense, is a mode of order that people play at and play with. Manifestations of rhythm include singing, playing instruments, and samba. Masters display satisfaction with multiple aspects of their corporeality as singers, because they lead the singing in the *roda*. They sing the verses solo and may extemporize about the events of the *roda*. Then they play the instruments, especially the *berimbau*, for *capoeira* sessions, both during practices and lessons, and always for *rodas*. The *berimbau* is played with the gourd pressed to the player's stomach, or lifted off it, so the body of the musician is a vital part of the production of the sound. Their mastery of different styles and rhythms sets the pace of the *capoeira*, and therefore they display musical competence on a bodily-based instrument. When samba is included, masters do the drumming and determine the way the dancing is to be done. Their bodies encapsulate the rhythm and the "Brazil-ness" of samba: they display an apparently unselfconscious sensuality.

Leading the Class

Perhaps most important, however, is the master's performance of self confidence and energy in leading the class: he can do all the moves at high speed and land smiling (Delamont 2006). He demonstrates how the kicks, throws, and takedowns are accomplished; either by attacking the students, or, much more usually, by stopping short of landing a kick, throwing the opponent, or taking down the fall guy. The latter is a much admired skill because it demands bodily control. All students understand, however, that their *mestre* could throw them at any moment – without any difficulty and laugh while doing so. In Britain *capoeira* is normally a non-contact activity; students do not routinely knock each other down, but the teacher has both the skills and the authority to take down any students he chooses. At the *batizado*, as *Trovao* explains to *Bruxa*, "The *mestre* is meant to trip you to the floor, and then you've been put in your place but you've also come into the world." In routine demonstrations at classes, Achilles is "the only one who can do takedowns." When students join *capoeira* they become the disciples of a master, and cede him the right to throw them. As the master plays the lead *berimbau*, and the rhythm of the lead *berimbau* determines the speed and style of the play, the teacher's control is expressed through the authority of the *berimbau*.

Adornment

In addition to these embodied disciplinary skills, as previously mentioned, the master's body is directly implicated in his presentation of self; his hair, skin, tattoos, clothing, his balance, and exuberance are not only part of his self presentation but also create and sustain the success of the classes. Masters frequently either wear dreadlocks, or have shaved heads. The former is symbolic of an "African" self-presentation, echoing the history of *capoeira* in the era of slavery. Their skin is glossy: if they are not African or African-Brazilian, then they aim to be tanned. For Brazilians, life in northern Europe has the disadvantage of long winters and wet summers that make it hard to keep tanned. Visits to Brazil, or to sunnier holiday areas such as the Canary Islands, are made. Achilles spent a six week period in Brazil one winter and came back to Tolnbridge very brown: after about twelve weeks in the UK he announced one evening, "I came back here strong and brown: now I am weak and pale." A British student put his pale arm next to Achilles's, to show that Achilles's was still, by UK standards, tanned and everyone laughed. However it was true that Achilles was no longer the deep brown he had been, and that *he* felt himself less *well* for it. Similarly Perseus, a light-skinned African-Brazilian, said to *Bruxa* before going to a festival in Southern Italy, "I'll get some sun on my pale skin: I need to stop looking so pale." This was only partial jest: Perseus wanted to expose his body to a strong sun. Tattoos (Fisher 2002) are commonly seen in *capoeira* classes, on pale skinned masters' bodies. Masters display their status with their clothing: if they wear the white uniform their *cordas* are the highest in the room. Their t-shirts are advertisements for themselves, for their revered teachers, or for festivals at which they have been the stars. Achilles might wear a t-shirt that said "Bellagio Festival 2004: 3rd *Batizado*" and a list of the masters who had arranged that *Batizado*. Alternatively he might wear a t-shirt that said "*Capoeira* Club of Cloisterham" and the name of his lineage across the top, and "Instructor Achilles" across the bottom, with a picture of flying players between the two lines of writing. In either case, his prowess is worn on his body. Week to week students can see events where *their* teacher has been an honoured guest, and the history of their lineage and their teacher's prowess, displayed on his body.

Self-Relatedness: Students' Bodies

Students vary in their expressions and impressions of comfort or dissociation with their corporeality – both in general and in relation to the ideal, disciplined body of the *capoeirista*. Students vary across the three analytic domains of music, of bodily self-presentation, and self-confidence. However they are always inferior to instructors. Musically, even the best students are less skilled on the instruments, know the choruses of only a few songs, are more likely to lose control of the rhythm, and might even stop singing and clapping when concentrating on their training and *capoeira* play. Unless Portuguese speaking, students are generally insecure about singing. Non-Brazilian disciples frequently display self-consciousness when dancing. Downey (2005:125–129) discusses the Brazilian stereotype that Europeans have a *cintura dura*, a "hard waist" and therefore find traditional Brazilian dance and *capoeira* challenging.

Students vary in their adherence to the official clothing rules. Novices are visibly distinct because they dress in "ordinary" clothes. More experienced students may wear *capoeira* kit that is crumpled, grubby, ill-fitting, and unflattering (except on special occasions), or immaculate in a freshly laundered "correct" kit. Students wear many hair styles in *capoeira* classes, from dreadlocks to short back and sides among men; among women, hair is usually tied up or back for class for functional rather than aesthetic purposes. Few students have the tans or glossy oiled skin common among instructors except when they have groomed themselves for public performances.

Students display a wide range of capabilities and a correspondingly wide range of satisfaction or dissatisfaction with their abilities and fitness levels. Students never present themselves with the air of effortless self confidence, energy, and smiling competence of instructors. Most look as if they are enjoying themselves, but also give-off signs of exhaustion, incompetence, and even incomprehension. When instructions include difficult moves (bridges, back flips, hand stands, head stands, and the *queda de rins* for example) they are often greeted with rueful glances as students try to comply. Even advanced disciples enact dissatisfaction with their inability to master specific moves, such as the back flip, or to feel and see improvement in their game. Regular students are self-critical and will discriminate between *capoeira* skills they have some grip on, and those they have yet to master.

Other-Relatedness: Masters and their Students' Bodies

Frank (1990, 1991) differentiated the disciplined body focused upon itself (monadic) from that constituted around relationships with others (dyadic). In *capoeira* classes masters stress regularly that the body *cannot* be monadic: the player should always be focused upon an actual or potential opponent. Like a classic Meadian (1934) conversation of gestures, the player must always be ready to answer the question posed by their opponent: to defend against attacks, and attack in their turn. Instructors work hard to teach learners to recognize that the point of *capoeira* is to play an opponent in the *roda*, and practice is a rehearsal for such play. The commonest exhortation in class is that students should always look at their opponent, or when practising a move, look in front where an opponent would be. This constant gaze on the other is achieved when not facing him or her by looking over the shoulder, between one's legs, or up from a handstand. In *capoeira* you do *not* look at your hands or the floor when doing handstands or cartwheels – you look at the opponent if playing a game and during paired practice, and you focus on the place where he would be when practicing alone. The *capoeirista* acts reflexively on himself, in addition to the dialogue between players in the Meadian sense. Cooley's (1902) notion of the "looking glass self" is, both metaphorically and literally, present in *capoeira* play.

Akin to Mead's conversation of gestures, Achilles uses the interesting metaphor of "question and answer" while, akin to Cooley, other instructors talk of "mirroring" the opponent. Cadmus's classes contain the recurrent instruction, "Don't look at the floor." Achilles regularly yells out exhortations such as "Look to the front," "Look for the guy" (the person you are fighting) and "You need to *look*." One kick starts with the player bending over and putting his hands on the floor, and when this is practised, Achilles routinely yells "Look between your legs." While preparing to deliver this kick, the player is vulnerable, and must watch his opponent. Perseus asks periodically during paired practice: "How many of you can see your opponent all the time?…either centrally or peripherally." In this way *capoeira* is the antithesis of body-building (Monaghan 1999). *Capoeira* bodies are prepared to play, dance, and fight with other people who have *capoeira* bodies. They may provide private satisfaction to their owners, but the work that goes into their production is dyadic and transactive.

Some students strive to perform a monadic disciplined body. Such *capoeiristas* appear more concerned with what *their* body can do than responding to "questions" posed by their opponents. Such people may be technically good at isolated moves but are not regarded as good *capoeiristas* by teachers or students, because *capoeira* play is essentially a dyadic activity in the *roda*. Shere Khan described a poor player who just displayed moves rather than interacting with his opponent: "You're not playing with him, you're just playing alongside him;" all the listeners agreed that this is inadequate *capoeira*.

Lunghri, one of Achilles's most enthusiastic students, reports his best quality as follows:

> I'm not technically good, I'm not good at doing the movements individually but I find that my strength is that I do think about what I'm doing and where I put myself in the game. The majority are not really thinking about what they're doing. But Achilles is now – he's trying to teach us ways of thinking along the lines of controlling the game, when you're playing *capoeira*, you're not just reacting, you're actually starting to control the other person.

Instructors draw distinctions between different aspects of other-relatedness in *capoeira*. These are made explicit in class, especially when students are preparing to play in contexts other than regular lessons. There are two different "others" for whom students perform: the lay public, and *aficionados* such as visiting *mestres*. The distinctions drawn between *capoeira* inside "the academy" (in private) and that done at performances or in the street (in public) is marked by clothing and playing style. White clothing is worn in lessons; coloured street trousers are worn outdoors when *capoeira* is done for personal pleasure. Demonstrations are often done in the white kit, but men sometimes strip to the waist.

More important than the choice of clothing, however, is the differentiation marked by the style of the play. In demonstrations students are asked to do "flashy" kicks and leaps, and the *mestre* himself does gymnastic feats. In class the teacher is more likely to stress skilful moves that may not be "showy" or impressive to the uninitiated, and he may not perform anything complex or elaborate at all. However, during a public performance the skills of the teacher and best students are showcased. For the more advanced students, being chosen by the teacher to perform at displays is a privilege and an affirmation of their relative skill. When Perseus chose Mowgli and Andromeda to carry real machetes in a *maculele* display, while everyone else danced with wooden sticks, it was a public sign that they were the best students.

Turning from dyadic relations between students and lay audiences to the dyadic relations between students and their most informed audience, visiting *mestres*, there are conventions about clothing, who plays, and playing style. Dress at *batizados* is carefully planned. White trousers are required, and t-shirts designed specifically for the event are worn. The cost of the event includes a t-shirt, which the *discipulos* being baptized or moved up a *corda* are required to wear, as are other club members who are more peripherally involved. *Trovao* explained to *Bruxa* how he learnt this rule at his *batizado*:

> Achilles had been going on for weeks in advance that we all had to have the *abadas* [trousers]. So everyone had to have *abadas*. And then the t-shirts Achilles gave out in the morning. I already had a white t-shirt on, I didn't realise you had to wear that specific one, not for the training session, and I carried on just wearing my white one. And then Achilles came up to me "*Trovao* what are you doing? Where's your t-shirt?" and so obviously you had to wear this particular one to celebrate our *batizado* – I thought we were just having it, I didn't think we had to wear it specifically then.

At a subsequent *batizado*, *Trovao* and *Bruxa* saw a student, Baloo, in an ordinary, grubby t-shirt who was prevented from entering a *roda* by Achilles. Another student pulled him off the stage and took him to get the special, commemorative t-shirts produced for that *batizado*; only then could he join his club mates on stage and play. Baloo was not due to get a new higher *corda* and had not realized that he was forbidden to do any *capoeira* unless he was properly dressed. The t-shirts are a significant aspect of students' other-relatedness. The teacher's t-shirts are part of his performed dyadic relatedness. At festivals, the local organisers often produce special t-shirts for the visiting teachers to wear during the event, so they stand out from the crowd. At Perseus's 2004 *batizado* the students had white t-shirts, while the visiting teachers had turquoise ones: at one of Achilles's events the students got emerald green t-shirts, the masters yellow ones. Even ignorant spectators could therefore see the status of the players.

Players who have the kit, and earned a *corda*, walk into class, train, and play in the *roda* display more confidence than those in ordinary clothes, or as yet without a belt. Students with the higher *cordas* may be taught separately. Guest teachers who wish to divide the students into subsections will use the presence of a belt to make that division:

> When Meneloas visited Perseus's group for a master class, he divided it into two halves saying "Beginners over there, intermediates here." He then scanned the "intermediate" group, all but one of whom had blue, or blue and brown belts on. Meneloas looked at Perseus, querying with his eyes if the unbelted student, Ferao, had chosen the wrong sub-group. Perseus signalled that Ferao *was* an intermediate student, and Meneloas went into teaching a complex sequence of moves.

Inside the private sphere of the regular practice session everyone, however bad a player, is given time and space to try their *capoeira* moves; better students are required to help and encourage less experienced ones (Reis 2005). During a *roda* in ordinary classes students are routinely ordered to adjust their play to the skill level of their opponents, that is, to be genuinely dyadic in the *roda*. Orders are issued such as: "Play gently with the beginners," "make no kick really strong," "use the *ginga*, not just kicks," or "practice the moves we have trained today," and "relax and enjoy the game in the *roda*." In other words, in the *roda* that ends the training classes, enjoyment and practice are to govern the play, but in a dyadic way. Advanced players must play in ways that will help beginners to learn, not be selfish or expose them to danger.

Control: Masters' and Students' Bodies

Control is the most obvious dimension where the *mestres* and instructors are differentiated from the students. Experts have highly controlled bodies: they know exactly where their cartwheel (*au*) will take them, and where they will land after it. On the control dimension, the disciplined body is regimented and predictable. *Capoeira* appears spontaneous and free-flowing to a casual observer. In fact, that impression is achieved by master players who have trained for many hours and are able to perform their gymnastic feats with a precision that is predictable (although dyadic).

Students are learning to control their bodies whenever they perform *capoeira* moves, and have an agenda of moves they cannot perform at all. Many of them also lack enough understanding of *capoeira* to appreciate the value of moves they are taught.

It is in the sphere of the teacher's authority over the body of the student that the regimentation becomes most apparent. The *mestre* has social control over the bodies of the students. In the following extract, *Trovao* reflects on how, at *batizados*, the masters demonstrate their own bodily superiority and their physical, social, and moral control over the bodies of the *discipulos*. He explains how the masters tricked the beginners:

> You and the *mestre* cartwheel in, and you start playing. This is the first time we beginners just saw a lot of the kind of the humour element of it all, through the weekend as a whole: and sometimes they'd do tricks, play jokes, like they'd touch the *Berimbau*, then they'd get us beginners to cartwheel and then the masters would just sort of stand up and touch their chin as the person flies into the roda looks round and....Like, – "what are you *doing*?" (laughing) You know, "Come on, we haven't started", and, and they'd do tricks like that.

Here *Trovao* is explaining how, when a beginner is tested, the master would deliberately tease the novice, by only pretending to start the contest. The apprehensive beginner would cartwheel into the centre of the *roda* expecting to embark on a paired routine, only to find that the master was standing watching his or her fumbling movements, not playing at all.

In the next comment *Trovao* is explaining that the *mestre* who plays with a beginner at his *batizado* determines how long the game will last and when the belt will be given (if the beginner has not been thrown or taken down in the ring, how they will be tricked into taking a fall at the end):

> The *mestres* play and then I don't know how they decide to stop but they just decide to shake your hand and take you over to the foot of the *berimbau*. And they actually tie the *corda* around you. And if the *Mestre* hadn't managed to trip you up, they put the *corda* over your head, as if they're gonna put it round your neck, and then they drop the *corda* to below your knees and pull your legs away from underneath. So they get you in the end.

Desire

The *capoeira mestre* has a body which is an object of desire in two ways. First, the serious students desire the body of the *mestre* in the sense of emulation: they want a body that performs like that of the *mestre*. Students try to emulate the *mestre* who can walk on his hands the length of the gym, can spin on his head, and can perform a sequence of complex moves without apparent hesitation or even conscious planning. This is the official desire of the *capoeira* organizations: that people should train to achieve a body that can perform these fantastic feats. Students also desire the experts' singing voice, percussion skills, dance rhythms and instinctive instantaneous responses to the game. Male students want the upper body strength, tough feet, agility, and balance of their male teachers. Female students, who are regularly told that women are equal in *capoeira*, that women are better at playing beautifully, and that they can proceed up the grades, want the skills, but do not lift weights or desire the muscle mass. For both sexes the desired body is less like a body builder and more like a ballet dancer, breakdancer, gymnast, or circus performer. Where *capoeira* is taught in the same gyms used by body builders, the *capoeira* men show no visible interest in the equipment or the nutritional supplements that are prominently displayed. Indeed, in one fitness centre, Perseus teaches *capoeira* in the "ladies" gym, while the male body builders are on another floor. Two of his elite students, Raksha and Mowgli, exercised to develop upper body strength for the one-handed handstand that figures in *capoeira*, but both stated that they did not want 'deformed' bodies like those of the body builders who used the same gym.

There is also another dimension to desire: the *mestre*'s body may also be an object of sexual desire. Good *capoeira* is sensual. Players move their bodies beautifully, in time to the music, in partnership with their opponent. Any skilled player can arouse a sexual desire in the audience by the beauty of their play. Lewis (2000:546-7) writing of Brazil comments:

> *Capoeira* is still primarily a man's game, and *capoeira* players are macho men.... Singing, drumming and dancing skills are said to make a man a good lover as well, and tales of virility and sexual conquest are endemic in the *capoeira* world.

Nestor Capoeira (2002:51–56) argues that the modern *capoeira* teachers in Europe can live a contemporary version of the *malandro* tradition. The *malandro* is a Brazilian man who dresses sharply, lives by his wits in a twilight between the legal and the illegal, between the respectable world and the violent criminal world, can use, but not be a victim of, alcohol, drugs, violence, and sexual energies. It can be used admiringly or disparagingly (Da Matta 1995). The very skills that make great players in the *roda* are, Capoeira (2002) argues, magnetic for European women.

In Britain *capoeira* classes often include samba, and at special events Brazilian dancing is also taught and enjoyed. As the students learn *capoeira* and get fitter, they are also developing their abilities to move fluently to music and, indeed, to dance. In our fieldwork we saw students becoming more comfortable with the sensual aspects of their bodies and their movements as their *capoeira* skills grew. The culture of the classes also includes very "un-British" hugging and kissing as part of the "Brazilian" ambience. There is a developmental process whereby the embodied self presentations of the more advanced students are moving closer to that of the teachers, in *capoeira* skills, and in relaxed use of their bodies in heterosexual peer interaction and dance.

Conclusions

Our analysis has explicitly employed Frank's ideal type, the disciplined body, in specific reference to *capoeira* teachers and students. The *capoeira* teacher's disciplined body has high physical capital which is reflected out onto the bodies of the students, who attempt to emulate them. The *capoeira* students are taking action *on* their own bodies, in a social structure built around embodied performance. However, more than a simple application of Frank's conceptualization, we have also detailed how discipline is embedded within ritualized dramaturgical performance. As Waskul and Vannini suggest in the introduction to this volume, the dramaturgical body is embedded in social practices: "people do not merely 'have' a body – people actively *do* a body. The body is fashioned, crafted, negotiated, manipulated and largely in ritualized social and cultural conventions." Both dimensions of the dramaturgical body are illustrated in our analysis of *capoeira*. On one hand, both teachers and students necessarily express and impress themselves on each other, as well as various audiences that witness their performances. On the other hand, it is also in these dramatic body-rituals that *capoeira* students and teachers reveal themselves as constituents of a moral order: the bodies of teachers and students are coproduced and bound by encultured rituals that are simultaneously personal and communal.

Acknowledgements

We are grateful to Rosemary Bartle Jones for word-processing the chapter. Our ideas have been clarified by Gary Alan Fine, Ben Fincham, Jonathan Skinner, John Evans, and Susie Scott. Rodrigo Ribeiro, in true academic comradeship, has cartwheeled into *rodas* in Tolnbridge to share his Brazilian insights into a British phenomenon, as well as his social science observations, which we appreciate.

References

Almeida, Bira. 1986. *Capoeira: A Brazilian Art Form*. Berkeley: North Atlantic Books.

Ashkenazi, Michael. 2002. "Ritual and the Ideal of Society in Karate." In D. E. Jones (ed.) *Combat, Ritual, and Performance*. Westport, Conn.: Praeger.

Assuncao, Matthias R. 2005. *Capoeira: The History of an Afro-Brazilian Martial Art*. London: Routledge

Browning, Barbara. 1995. *Samba: Resistance in Motion*. Bloomington, IN: Indiana University Press.

Capoeira, Nestor. 1995. *The Little Book of Capoeira*. Berkeley: North Atlantic Books.

_____. 2002. *Capoeira: Roots of the Dance – Fight – Game*. Berkeley: North Atlantic Books.

Cooley, Charles H. 1902. *Human Nature and the Social Order*. New York: Scribners.

Crossley, Nick. 2004. "The Circuit Trainer's *Habitus*." *Body and Society*, 10:37–70.

Da Matta, Roberto. 1995. *Carnivals, Rogues and Heroes*. Notre Dame: University of Notre Dame Press.

Delamont, Sara. 2005a. "No Place for Women Among Them? Reflexions on the *Axe* of Fieldwork." *Sport, Education and Society*, 10, 3:305–320.

_____. 2005b. "Where the Boys Are." *Waikato Journal of Education*, 11, 1:7–26.

_____. 2006. "The Smell of Sweat and Rum: Authority and Authenticity in *Capoeira* Classes." *Ethnography and Education*, 1, 2:161–175.

Donohue, John J. 2002. "Wave People: The Martial Arts and the American Imagination." In D. E. Jones (ed.) *Combat, Ritual and Performance*. Westport, Conn.: Praeger.

Downey, Greg. 2005. *Learning Capoeira*. New York: Oxford University Press.

Fisher, J. A. 2002. "Tattooing the Body, Marking Culture." *Body and Society*, 8:91–107.

Frank, Arthur W. 1990. "Bringing Bodies Back In." *Theory, Culture and Society*, 7:131–162.

_____. 1991. "For a Sociology of the Body." In Michael Featherstone, Michael Hepworth and Bryan S. Turner (eds) *The Body*. London: Sage.

Goffman, Erving. 1959. *The Presentation of Self in Everyday Life*. Garden City, NY: Anchor.

Holcombe, Charles. 2002. "Theater of Combat: A Critical Look at the Chinese Martial Arts." In D. E. Jones (ed.) *Combat, Ritual and Performance*. Westport, Conn.: Praeger.

Lewis, J. Lowell. 1992. *Ring of Liberation*. Chicago: The University of Chicago Press.

_____. 2000. "Sex and Violence in Brazil." *American Ethnologist*, 26:539–557.

Mead, George Herbert. 1932. *The Philosophy of the Present*. Chicago: The University of Chicago Press.

Monaghan, Lee. 1999. "Creating 'The Perfect Body'". *Body and Society*, 5:267–290.

Reis, Andre L.T. 2005. *Capoeira: Health and Social Well-Being*. Brasilia: Thesaurus Editor de Brasilia Ltd.

Rosario, Claudio Campos, Stephens, Neil and Delamont, Sara. 2006b. "I'm Your Teacher, I'm Brazilian!" Paper in progress.

Sassatelli, Roberta. 1999. "Interaction Order and Beyond: A Field Analysis of Body Culture Within a Fitness Gym." *Body and Society*, 5:227–248.

Schreiner, Claus. 1993. *Musica Brasileira*. London: Marian Boyers.

Stephens, Neil and Delamont, Sara. 2006. "Balancing the *Berimbau*." Forthcoming in *Qualitative Inquiry*.

Strauss, Anselm. 1993. *Continual Permutations of Action*. New York: Aldine.

Twigger, Robert. 1999. *Angry White Pyjamas*. London: Phoenix.

PART 3
The Phenomenological Body: Body as Province of Meaning

Chapter 9

Corporeal Indeterminacy: The Value of Embodied, Interpretive Sociology

Lee F. Monaghan

Interactionist and phenomenological approaches to embodiment posit corporeality as a symbolic universe within which active subjects constitute shared meanings of bodies through their bodies. The constitution of self, body, meaning, and society is an embodied affair primarily because such processes depend on intentionality and therefore, as Lee Monaghan suggests in this chapter, on "particular ways of experiencing bodies, specific cognitive styles, and forms of sociality that jar with other 'taken-for-granted' modalities of embodiment." For Monaghan this process is therefore quintessentially "mortal" in that it is open to befuddlement and reconfigurations, inevitably limited in its potential for shared understanding, and ultimately "open" in its indeterminate predisposition. Mortal embodiments, both as objects of analysis and as interpretive subjects, cannot but engage in a type of analytical inspection that is therefore finite; circumscribed by an "unavoidably ambiguous, messy..., and complex" process of embodiment. Such is the nature of interpretive sociology for Monaghan: its embeddedness within embodiment, and the uniqueness of its value as a mortal undertaking.

From Perfect to Imperfect Bodies and Back Again

Outlining the sociological implications of the thought of G. H. Mead, Blumer (1966:539) states that any object in the social world is not a self-existing entity with an intrinsic nature. Rather, its nature is dependent upon the action and orientation of social actors towards it: a star would have different meanings for a sheepherder of antiquity and a modern astronomer, a tree would mean something different to a botanist and a lumberjack. This pragmatic symbolic interactionist argument, which is compatible with social phenomenology (Schutz 1962), may be extended to human corporeality. Ideals of physical perfection, for instance, are inextricably tied to people's shifting actions and orientations within different interpretive communities: a case of beauty being a contingent social judgment that is inter-subjectively constructed and perceived through the eyes of beholders rather than a solipsistic beholder. In contemporary Western culture, Ruben's voluptuously beautiful woman, or the powerful Japanese Sumo wrestler, are negatively labelled "obese" or even "morbidly obese" using calculations of weight-for-height, or Body Mass Index (BMI, Kg/m^2). Yet, in particular times and places such bodies epitomize physical perfection; they are or have been credited and valued rather than "discredited" and stigmatized (Goffman 1968).

However, comparing socially contingent perceptions of stars, trees, and human bodies only goes so far. Important differences exist between objects of the "natural" world and human bodies (which, even in death, ambiguously straddle the nature-culture divide). Lived bodies are also embodied subjects (Williams and Bendelow 1998); we have bodies but we are also bodies (Turner 1996). This picture of the embodied social agent fits well with Mead's picture of the human being. For Mead, we are organisms with a self, meaning we are objects to ourselves and objects of our own actions (Blumer 1966:535). Through symbolic interaction, we are capable of reflexively (re-)forming definitions or "typifications" (Schutz 1962) of our own and other people's corporeality. Such processes include working upon and actively reforming the very corporeal matter of "unfinished" bodies (Shilling 2003), as well as supposedly innate drives such as sexual interest. Blumer (1966) was writing before the "somatic turn" in the social sciences, but his Median argument extends to human bodies and embodied selves.

Embodied sociology, which productively engages classic social thought (Shilling 2003), may therefore be used to re-read interactionist and other "meaning and action" approaches. To slightly modify Blumer (1966), human bodies are not simply objects in the social world with an intrinsic nature; rather, their meanings are dependent upon the actions and orientations of people towards them/selves. In short, people, as body-subjects, co-constitute shared yet fragile symbolic universes that reflect, and are a product of, embodied definitional practices and interactions. Some of these meanings are welcomed. They constitute a velvet glove for massaging bodies and egos, but an iron hand also often exists within. Depending upon people's shifting locations, interpretations and definitions of the situation, social divisions such as class, gender, ethnicity, age, ability, and other axes of power are inscribed upon, and worked through, relational bodies with inflationary and deflationary effects.

The central argument in this chapter is that human bodies are essentially indeterminable. This does not mean bodies escape inter-subjective meanings, or they cannot be clearly measured and counted. What is being stated here is that social agents meaningfully engage in processes of re-interpreting and re-signifying the brute materiality of fleshy bodies. Correspondingly, there are particular ways of experiencing bodies, specific cognitive styles, and forms of sociality that jar with other "taken-for-granted" modalities of embodiment. Mortal human bodies co-constitute (even if only in imagination or fantasy) and embody "finite provinces of meaning" (Schutz 1962), rendering biological bodies social bodies through and through. During these embodied processes, people may befuddle and reconfigure supposedly clear corporeal descriptions, typifications, "natural" drives, and experiences. As noted, dominant definitions of bodily perfection, goodness, and virtuousness may be challenged and inverted: "fatness" may be eroticized and enjoyed while the extreme muscularity and vascularity (prominence of veins) displayed by elite competition bodybuilders may be rewarded (Monaghan 2001a). Alternatively, people endowed with ample economic, social, and cultural capital may partially or totally eclipse the "imperfect" physicality of the self while remaining corporeally grounded. Embodied, interpretive sociology plays an important role in understanding these social processes. Among other things, this type of sociology provides a humanistic perspective to debates that seek to pathologize differentially endowed bodies, stripping people of dignity and respect all in their supposed best interests.

Embodiment is unavoidably ambiguous, messy (sometimes literally), and complex. Lived bodies are ongoing practical accomplishments that are irreducible to any single discourse or practice (Williams and Bendelow 1998). We are embedded within, embody, reproduce, and modify multiple fields of interaction and interpretation. Even within a given historical period, taken-for-granted meanings of human corporeality and embodied actions are never immutable, fixed, or determinate. Undoubtedly, hierarchies of knowledge and credibility disparagingly mark, as well as favourably remark upon, individual and collective bodies. Some bodies are rendered more "acceptable," "appropriate," or "correct" than others. However, even hegemonic definitions – expressed through organizational bodies, their representatives, and others – are never immutable, unshakeable, and incontestable. Diverse groups, subcultures, and dissenting voices may and often do resist and re-frame the meanings of bodies and embodied actions (e.g. eating, sex, drug-taking, and violence). In this chapter, I maintain that embodied, interpretive sociology makes sense of these processes. Such an approach treats lived bodies as the source, location, and medium of society (Shilling 2003), and is fully compatible with interactionist and other "meaning and action" perspectives.

This chapter draws from three of my own studies in embodied sociology. These ethnographies explore social meanings and practices in relation to bodybuilding, nightclub security work and bodyweight (the obesity debate). Theoretically, I often use social theorists such as Schutz and Goffman when making sense of worlds and situations that may appear anthropologically strange from without. Though similar to other British sociologists indebted to interactionism, my approach is eclectic (Atkinson and Housley 2003). Indeed, interpretivism may be usefully complemented with a critical realist understanding of macro-social structures that extend beyond specific individual or group definitions of the situation (Williams 2003). However, given the primary focus in this section of the book on the body as a "province of meaning," in this chapter I underscore the value of Schutzian phenomenology.

Similar to symbolic interactionism and pragmatism, phenomenology is "good to think with" when contributing to social studies of the body. Yet, while classic social theory, ranging from Durkheim to Goffman, has been re-read in corporeal terms (Shilling 2003, Williams and Bendelow 1998), Schutz has largely been marginalized or ignored. This is unfortunate. Schutz's writings on, for example, systems of typification and relevance, and the social distribution of knowledge, make sense when researching the body in everyday life (Nettleton and Watson 1998) *and* the embodiment of everyday or night life. This argument is empirically grounded with reference to: (1) bodybuilding ethnophysiology and ethnopharmacology; (2) heterosexual risk in Britain's nighttime leisure economy; and, (3) a critical, gendered take on the obesity debate.

Studies in Embodied Sociology: Phenomenological Insights from Three Ethnographies

Bodybuilding, Drugs, and Risk

In the early 1990s the British and US media contributed to a moral panic about bodybuilding, steroids, and violence (Dobash *et al.* 1999). Male bodybuilders putatively risked themselves and, more worryingly, female partners and the public, through steroid-induced psychosis or 'Roid-Rage. In such a context, bodybuilders risked social censure for alleged drug abuse, uncontrollable aggressive violence, and transgressing everyday conceptions of the body acceptable (the bourgeois civilized body). Bodybuilding and its practitioners, long viewed with suspicion anyhow, were presented in a highly disparaging light. However, such representations were the product of cultural stereotyping rather than systematic social science.

Ethnography conducted among bodybuilders in South Wales in the 1990s provided an empirical basis for exploring such issues and the *meaningfulness* of "risky" bodies and embodied practices (Monaghan 2001b). That is, a social world comprising shared meanings and actions pertaining to bodies which were irreducible to illicit drugs or individual personality traits. This life-world may have been the focus of sensationalized, moralized, and "masculinity in crisis" readings that largely discredited muscle-building. Yet, bodybuilders, and other group members with whom I talked, inter-subjectively constructed "finite provinces of meaning" upon and through which they "bestow[ed] the accent of reality" (Schutz 1962:341). Interestingly, these bodybuilding life-worlds comprised sophisticated ethnophysiological and ethnopharmacological stocks-of-knowledge, i.e. subcultural relevances pertaining to types of "perfect" muscular body and normalized drug *use*. Non-participants may have trivialized these relevances but they were defined as real by bodybuilders and they were real in their consequences.

The preceding point is important. Finely spun subcultural norms inform drug usage, and mediate drug-related experiences, with the goal of minimizing harm while maximizing benefits. This relates to the physicality or physiology of the material body but also, given putative steroid effects on mood and behaviour, the body as a mindful/emotional/relational entity. Here, a parallel may be drawn with Becker's (1967) interactionist research on various drug subcultures. In that work, so-called "drug psychoses" are attributed to the fears and anxieties of the novice. Participation in drug subcultures minimizes such occurrences because others provide alternative definitions. Similarly, for steroid-using bodybuilders, in-group definitions were instrumental in mediating drug-related experiences. They were also instrumental in constructing a sense of responsibility to self and others, thus helping to sustain an activity that was labelled as "risky" from without.

This relates to the argument that bodies are finite provinces of meaning, as well as body-subjects who co-constitute and express such meanings. The first proposition concerns the social and organic grounding, durability, changeability, and ultimate mortality of lived bodies. We are born into an ongoing social world and, through the lifecourse, grow, mature, decay, and die (though bodybuilding often has a postmodern appeal by allowing aged and ageing bodies to embody an image of youthfulness) (Monaghan 2001c). Until science fiction becomes fact, we remain finite as lived, corporeally grounded subjects. Our awareness of our mortality, according to Schutz (1962), constitutes the fundamental anxiety. We live knowing we will die. We also know our lives may change radically due to disease, illness, and injury. Volitional risk-taking, such as illicit drug-taking, therefore occurs within the context of *possible* danger to life, limb, and other aspects of finite bodies. Viewed from without, taking illicit steroids and other muscle-building drugs is foolhardy. It is assumed to be the product of an inadequate personality (Klein 1993) and the principle etiology for negative mood changes and uncontrollable violence (Pope and Katz 1990). However, phenomenology offers a more appreciative understanding and overcomes some of the blind spots associated with correctional research. For example, it is possible to identify socially distributed ethnopharmacological knowledge, comprising a taxonomy of anabolic and androgenic steroids, different administration routes, effects, strength, and toxicity (Monaghan 2001b:98). Of course, here we are moving from the brute materiality of physical and socially censured bodies to body-subjects who practically accomplish symbolically meaningful universes.

It is more appropriate, therefore, to focus upon body-subjects as finite provinces of meaning. People embody and reproduce the shared presuppositions of a field or habitus through social learning processes comprising habit and exercise. Bourdieu *et al.* (1991) discuss this in relation to the love of art, and this may be extended to (drug-using) bodybuilders who acquire an ethnophysiological appreciation of "extreme" muscularity and other prized aspects of pharmaceutically enhanced, competition standard physiques. These meanings, reflecting and informing socially cultivated taste and distinction, are not widely shared outside their subculture. The meanings of "the muscular body" (which are pluralized by participants and considered highly heterogeneous), alongside the techniques required to build and sculpt and appreciate such living art, are finite and indeterminable to others who struggle to make sense of these "pathological" forms and actions. These subcultural relevances are, by definition, not part of the non-affiliates' mental and corporeal schema through which they interpret the world and endow it with sense and meaning. Bodybuilding "systems of relevance" (Schutz 1970) are alien to "outsiders" just as championship standard physiques are themselves considered alien-like by those who are close to, but not within, the cult of muscularity (Monaghan 2001a).

I will briefly elaborate upon this formal sociological statement, making reference to my own bodily participation in the fieldwork process. As stated by Coffey (1999), within ethnographic literature relatively little is made of the embodied nature of the fieldwork task. In offering reflexive methodological commentary, I am aware from my own shifting perceptions of and with the body that what I once considered "muscular" as a non-participant radically changed after I became practically immersed in gym culture over several years. This was a slow process and one that I only fully realized when I saw a film, for a second time, starring Jean-Claude Van Damme. Before learning to see bodies as bodybuilders see them, I considered Van Damme, popularly dubbed "the muscles from Brussels," heavily muscular. However, after spending a few years in bodybuilding gyms, I realized that while Van Damme was lean and athletically muscular he was not muscular *relative* to those who develop competition standard bodybuilding physiques. (These include types of muscular body that are displayed at local level, amateur competitions.) Similar to Becker's (1963) neophyte to marijuana, I learnt in a very corporeal sense that becoming a bodybuilder is dependent upon processes of symbolic interaction, redefinition, and the emergence of motives and dispositions. It is an aesthetic education. It also became clear to me that the psychiatrist's concept of "muscle dysmorphia" or "reverse anorexia" (Pope *et al.* 2000) is ethnocentric when applied to bodybuilding. If a bodybuilder claims he is not that muscular then he is probably offering a realistic appraisal of his physique relative to others he routinely sees at the gym, at competitions or in bodybuilding magazines. He inhabits a different symbolic universe comprising learnt ways of looking at and appreciating extremely muscular bodies. To claim he has a body image disorder involves negatively judging one culture from the standards of another, similar to nineteenth century colonialists who misperceived native life. Types of pathologizing "excuse-account" (Scott and Lyman 1968), like muscle dysmorphia or gender inadequacy, may have situational efficacy for some gym members in some circumstances. However, they are neither necessary nor sufficient conditions for bodybuilding. Also, bodybuilders I talked with overwhelmingly justified rather than excused their putatively "deviant" muscle-building activities (Monaghan 2002a).

To slightly modify Goffman's (1989) arguments, any group of people, whether prisoners, primitives, bodybuilders, or ballerinas, have their own ways of perceiving, experiencing, and living with and through their own and others' bodies. These ways are normal and reasonable once you get close to them. Clearly, this is not necessarily reflected upon and deliberated in everyday life. Embodied worlds are "permeated by appresentational references which are simply taken for granted" (Schutz 1962:328) by social agents when undertaking routine practical activities with, among, and through bodies. Whether aspects of the body (e.g. a weak muscle group), or actions pertaining to the body (e.g. selecting and administering types of drug), are the foci of polythetic (extended) attention depends upon members' systems of relevances, such as level of interest, and socially distributed stocks-of-knowledge (viz. ethnophysiological and ethnopharmacological knowledge). In short, recipes of action, ways of doing things, are the product of embodied life-worlds, comprising presuppositions that are constructed, expressed, shared, learnt and modified by relational bodies. Of course, stocks-of-knowledge and recipes for action may be shared with others differentially located in space and time. Modes of communication include written media, which have different directions of travel and influence depending upon the structures of the life-world and the status of social actors as predecessors, contemporaries or successors (Schutz 1962).

This theorizing, pertaining to lived bodies, embodied perceptions, and corporeally grounded actions, is empirically informed. Regardless of the reader's particular substantive interests, ethnography on bodybuilding, drugs, and risk provides meat to the conceptual bones of more abstract theory. Such theorizing includes writings on modernity, the body, and self-identity (Giddens 1991), and medical and behavioural science literature on steroids, violence, and muscle dysmorphia. This ethnography also informs recent efforts to cautiously "bring in" the biological to sociological debate (Williams *et al.* 2003). For example, although patriarchal ideology seeks to naturalize male power through an appeal to sex hormones, bodybuilders I interviewed viewed steroid behavioural effects through a social lens that challenged biological reductionism without writing out biology (Monaghan 2003). Like the modifiable bodybuilder's body, such research has the ability to help change the appearance of sociology as a body relevant discipline as it actively engages with myriad areas of embodied social life. And, it does this while remaining indebted to classic social thought such as Schutzian phenomenology and symbolic interactionism.

Opportunity, Pleasure, and Heterosexual Risk

We are in the third decade of HIV/AIDS. The threat posed by this disease has rendered social research on sexualities highly relevant, though the social paradigm to risk has been under-utilized compared to more individually oriented perspectives (Rhodes 1997). In the developed world, ethnographic research on workers in the nighttime leisure economy provides insights into the sociology of sexual opportunity, pleasure, and risk. Such research also helps empirically ground abstract discussion and re-animate and embody classic interpretive sociology. Again, and similar to Bloor (1995) who draws from Schutz (1970) when offering a phenomenological approach to sexual risk, my research draws from classic interpretive sociology. This research also seeks to embody such theorizing and conjoin dichotomies such as mind and body, reason and emotion.

Embodying more cognitive oriented approaches to sexual risk is therefore not simply an abstract, theoretical undertaking. It is grounded in ethnographic research on "bouncers" or "door supervisors" as they call themselves. Fieldwork among these predominantly male workers in British city centre nightclubs, bars, and pubs provided me with detailed understandings of their occupational culture. This study yielded thick descriptions and insights into various aspects of their life-worlds, and sustained methodological reflection on the emotional vicissitudes of assuming an "active membership role" (Adler and Adler 1987). That is, a role where I actually worked as a door supervisor and, for all practical purposes, was treated as a fellow worker who would lend his body if there was trouble. Ethnographic understandings, generated with my contacts over several years, were many and varied. Sexualities constituted one important theme and I will elaborate upon this below. However, other themes included: occupationally legitimated violence, worker solidarity and hierarchical relations, physical risk, legal risk, embodying competence and plural workplace masculinities. Following the above reference to Coffey (1999) on the body as a resource in ethnography, these understandings also informed methodological reflection on risky fieldwork as a form of embodied/emotional/edgework (Monaghan 2006). Again, this ethnography explicitly draws from, and is compatible with, symbolic interactionist writings. These include Athens (1997) on (near) violence and Lyng's (1990) Median/Marxist informed research on voluntary risk-taking.

Of course, and as exemplified in relation to sexualities, discourses of risk should not obfuscate pleasure. My research also considered urban male heterosexualities, the carnal pleasures and opportunities afforded through doorwork, in addition to social risks that could amplify or minimize the conditions of possibility of HIV transmission (Monaghan 2002b). For many doormen, who work long monotonous hours, flattering attention from female customers is viewed as a "perk of the job" (such attention sometimes brought a smile to my face). Convergent with a growing symbolic interactionist interest in the body, this ethnography offers an empirical study in the phenomenology of "erotic reality" (Davis 1983). Lessons for health promoters are also presented vis-à-vis the meanings of sexual risk-taking, the sense of which may largely appear indeterminable from a cold, disembodied stance. Namely, health threats must be interpreted in terms of cultural contexts embodied and enjoyed by actual flesh and blood bodies. In doing the work of a door supervisor over a prolonged period, I learnt firsthand that these men respond to life in ways that make sense even when their actions clash with middle-class or everyday expectations. Such sense-making is not only cognitive but embodied, visceral, and emotional. These men of honour and respect do what they think and feel is right at the time, albeit not necessarily under conditions of their own choosing.

In outlining the conditions under which doormen's heterosexual relations may be defined as risky from a member's perspective, this research explored various relevances. These extended beyond (un)protected sex to include: the normalization of non-exclusive or adventurous male heterosexuality, working in sexualized urban nightspots where (attractive) women do receptive/flirtations heterosexuality, and exploring multiple sexual opportunities in a society wherein monogamous heterosexuality is institutionalized. Ethnographic description and analysis of shifting social situations was facilitated using a typology of urban male heterosexualities. The typology included ideal types such as unsuccessful, indifferent, monogamous, flirtatious, and non-exclusive. Types of sexual risk, which include, extend beyond, and are possibly implicated in disease transmission, were also described, namely: risking existing intimate relationships and "ontological security" (Giddens 1992), violence, and embarrassment. These risks, and others, such as insolvency, were more-or-less associated with non-exclusive heterosexuality.

Given these multiple risks, questions emerge concerning the soundness of pursuing workplace sexual opportunities, especially for men in existing partnerships. Such questioning is taken-for-granted within everyday reality characterized by disembodied (calculative) rationality but less so within urban nightspots and erotic reality wherein corporeality, playfulness, and spontaneity are central. And, in contrast to models that portray social actors as deliberative economic agents, risk-taking within routinized socio-erotic contexts may largely remain taken-for-granted. During such processes the possibility of harm exists on the "horizon" of consciousness rather than becoming "thematic" or "topically relevant" (Schutz 1970). And, when exploring the situated rationality or sensuality of potentially "risky" heterosex there are identifiable attractions for doormen who may otherwise be discursively aware of sexual risks. Indeed, and especially in carnivalesque nightspots where gendered bodies are often adorned (adored) and displayed, socially constructed pleasures may be more motivationally relevant than possible danger. As a phenomenological study, this ethnography stressed how sexually related risks may become routinized as normal over time. Alternatively, from a calculative or "polythetic" (Schutz 1970) stance, incentives to risk-taking may outweigh the more distant gratification of abstention. All of this, of course, depends upon processes of symbolic interaction where bodies are potential vehicles of pleasure and pain. The organization and construction of "risky" sexualities in the nighttime economy is totally dependent upon interpretations, definitions, and meanings rather than unmediated organic feelings (Blumer 1966) and supposedly innate, natural, monolithic sexualities. Social paradigms, including sociological phenomenology, are therefore invaluable when researching and theorising such bodily or carnal matters.

Male Embodiment and the Obesity Debate

Historically and cross-culturally, degrees of fatness have been and continue to be adored not disdained. However, within contemporary Anglophone cultures, such meanings are discredited: fatness equals sickness and badness according to Western biomedical and aestheticized definitions. The orthodox view and associated "bodily sensibility" are increasingly taken-for-granted. For instance, the World Health Organization buttress the unacceptability of fatness when claiming there is a global obesity epidemic (WHO 1998). While the Western fight against fat exerts an unbearable weight on many women (Bordo 1993), men are also being sucked into dominant constructions of fatness as an expansive and expanding problem. Using rationalized calculations of weight-for-height, or BMI as an inexpensive proxy for adiposity, the National Audit Office claim almost two thirds of men in England are "overweight" or "obese" (NAO 2001). (According to BMI, lean bodybuilders would also fall into these categories as well as other athletes such sprinters.)

My current research critically engages the obesity debate, or, more accurately, "lack of debate" (Aphramor, personal communication; also, see Campos 2004). This research explores masculinities and weight-related issues while also questioning the "epidemic psychology" (Strong 1990) surrounding bodies that putatively "fail" to "fit in." Epidemic psychology is a Schutzian informed model for understanding the fragile social world. It was first proposed by Strong (1990) when making sense of the highly emotive and hysterical reactions to AIDS in the 1980s. Obesity epidemic psychology is comparable, at a time when mundane ways of gearing into the everyday world are apparently threatened by unusual but persistent trends. This epidemic brands literally millions of people as "at risk," "unhealthy" or "diseased" *because of their weight*. That, however, is a simplified and efficient yet irrational account. It comprises unjustified fear, moralizing action, and intense forms of social stigmatization (Monaghan 2005a). It is a case of pariah mongering that elides sociological knowledge of how material structures impact upon differentially endowed biological and social bodies. Aphramor (2005) describes it as "an epidemic of truncated theorizing."

Similarly dissatisfied with the dominant obesity discourse, Rich and Evans (2005) argue that this topic demands an ethical and politically informed analysis. I would add that it also warrants a gendered, micro-interactionist analysis. To be sure, important feminist work is available (see, for example, Gard and Wright 2005:153-67). And, as indicated in Sobal and Maurer's (1999a, b) edited collections, this topic lends itself well to symbolic interactionist readings. However, interactionist studies on masculinities and modalities of "fat male embodiment" or "bodily bigness" are scant. Existing literature also does not explicitly advance the case for an embodied sociology which re-reads classic social thought, such as Schutzian phenomenology, in a corporeal light (Monaghan 2005b). Yet, as discussed in this chapter, such an approach makes sense when exploring embodied life-worlds that are co-constituted by interacting body-subjects (including social actors largely defined in terms of their discredited corporeality rather than embodied sociality).

Again, my research explicitly draws from and embodies interpretive sociology while also remaining mindful of larger fields of power and material determinants of health. For example, I offer a revised application of the accounts framework (Scott and Lyman 1968) when exploring how people bridge the gap between what Stearns (1997) calls "bulky realities" and "slim ideals" (Monaghan 2006, forthcoming). Grounded in qualitative data (e.g. depth interviews, a slimming club ethnography), the research also explores the possible irrationalities of rationalizing bodies and the rationalization of resistance; i.e. embodied challenges to McDonaldized (Ritzer 2004), or streamlining, processes. Possible irrationalities include dissatisfaction with slimming (e.g. the predictability of failure) while resistances include the rejection of the BMI, even by slimming club consultants.

Another emergent theme may be termed "body-eclipsing" and "shining." Employing an astral metaphor, I argue that lived human bodies, similar to the sun, have the potential to radiate warmth and energy as they move within various social universes or provinces of meaning. However, given the negativity of fatness in Anglophone culture, and the tying of social selves to the physicality of the body, those (self-)typified as fat may be cast in the shadows or eclipsed by physical stigma. Even so, people denigrated for their weight always have the *potential* to shine, or at least align their bodies in socially accepted ways. For some this means intentionally trying to lose weight and keep it off. Yet there are alternative practices and vocabularies of the credited or creditable male body. For example, humour, intelligence, and meticulous grooming may enable some men to display embodied social fitness without necessarily having to cut their own bodies down in size. Of course, ambivalence and felt stigma are always possible. However, some "big" men project acceptability through a cultivated persona that is bigger than their flesh. Arguably, accommodating a larger body and eclipsing physical stigmata is a gendered social process that is generally easier for men than women. As Witz (2000) explains, men are often accorded the capacity to transcend their immediate corporeal selves while women are traditionally defined in terms of their (flawed) physicality.

I will finish this section by outlining understandings emerging from my online research on size acceptance/admiration (SA) groups (Monaghan 2005b). I initially stumbled across these during the early stages of my research. I typed keywords such as "men" and "fat" into internet search engines with the naïve expectation that men, who were reluctant to go to female dominated slimming clubs, would be sharing weight-loss tips online. That, of course, said more about my embodied habitus which was coterminous with dominant definitions of fatness. I was wrong. There is a whole world out there where fatness, or, more ambiguously and positively, "bigness," is accepted and admired. And, as I would later learn, some of these groups also have an offline presence, providing opportunities for people to meet face-to-face. For example, in some of Britain's larger cities there are popular gay clubs that cater to "big" gay men and their admirers. This may be especially important for older gay men who do not conform to the narrow gay ideal of a slim or waiflike male body, as displayed by the young "twink."

Cyberspace may be flat compared to situations of bodily co-presence. Nonetheless, it is a repository of positive meanings in an age when fat does not fit in with the favoured view. Primarily although by no means exclusively based in the USA, online SA groups foreground "bigness" or "fatness" and present positive typifications in response to the stigma of obesity. These body framings, comprising "face work" (Goffman 1967), or screen work, and advocated codes of self-body relatedness, include more flattering representations for those self-typifying as Big Handsome Men, Bears, and others (e.g. Chubbies, Gainers, Feedees, Foodies, and Gluttons). These online constructions of "fat male embodiment" are "virtual" given their digital expression (Hine 2000) and their relation to "actual" identities (Goffman 1968). In contrast to "degradation ceremonies" (Garfinkel 1956), or deflation ceremonies that discredit corpulent bodies, the flatness of cyberspace provides suitable conditions for esteem-enhancing inflation ceremonies. Online, participants in heterosexual, gay, and food-oriented space actively challenge the pathology of obesity (also, see LeBesco 2004) according to prevailing systems of relevance and typification (Schutz 1962). Here types of corpulent male body-subject and/or supportive others (e.g. Female Fat Admirers, Chubby Chasers, Feeders) virtually construct acceptable, admirable, and resistant masculinities. Participants appeal to "real" or "natural" masculinity, they admire and eroticize men's expansive/expanding bodies, they advocate corporeal transgression, fun, and the carnivalesque, and they discuss the gendered pragmatics and politics of fat male embodiment. This largely, although by no means always, occurs in spaces characterized by acceptance and solidarity. In online SA groups, corpulent men are virtually acceptable or admirable; they are correct bodies rather than correctable bodies. Of course, in everyday life, obesity entrepreneurs and profitable corporate interests reproduce typifications of fatness that are incompatible with notions of physical and social fitness. This degradation persists despite highly questionable and uncertain science (Gard and Wright 2005, Monaghan 2005a). In such a context, resisting the stigma of obesity online could be viewed as a healthful antidote to obesity epidemic psychology.

Conclusions

Drawing from my own body-relevant research, this chapter hopefully highlights the usefulness of embodied, interpretive sociology when making sense of the social. Discussion explicitly focused upon substantive issues, but more general and formal arguments emerge from these ethnographic studies in embodied sociology. These relate to the inescapable corporeality of social life and the broader relevance of an embodied sociology that remains indebted to, while seeking to expand, the sociological tradition. This tradition includes interactionist sociology: a rich body of work that is often forgotten in contemporary sociology (Atkinson and Housley 2003). Similarly, phenomenology (Schutz 1962), or everyday life sociology more generally (Adler *et al.* 1987), has value for social studies of bodies and embodiment. These are cognate and mutually reinforcing approaches that warrant a corporeal re-reading if sociologists wish to make sense of "somatic society" (Turner 1996).

Drawing from such literature, subjecting it to an embodied reading, and undertaking ethnography, leads me to the following conclusion. The brute materiality of physical bodies, their status as objects in the "natural" world, can never be divorced from shifting interpretations and definitions. Physical bodies are always from the outset social bodies (the product of relational bodies even prior to conception), the meanings and experiences of which are mutable and dependent upon processes of symbolic interaction, systems of typification, and relevance (Schutz 1962, 1970). Corporeality has no intrinsic meaning. Yet, corporeal indeterminacy provides openness for body-subjects (embodied selves) to collectively construct canopies that provide at least some shared warmth in an otherwise meaningless and potentially alienating world (Berger and Luckmann 1967). Here people forge definitions of individual and collective bodies within finite provinces of meaning, while also embodying such meanings. The task of embodied, interpretive sociology is to enter and engage with these meaningful realities (the body is a primary research tool) wherein bodies are hierarchically graded, inflated, pleasured, deflated, and stigmatized. These domains are where bodies live and die, in a physical and social sense. And, the micro-politics of these processes should be recognized. Throughout the larger social body there are myriad vested interests and structured concerns that ultimately relate to the organization, division, and regulation of bodies in ways that benefit some at the expense of many. Embodied, interpretive sociology should therefore also foster a critical attitude that questions the claims and practices of those seeking to strip embodied selves of sociality and render them imperfect, material bodies. Bodies matter, but the corporeal "matter" of fleshy bodies cannot be divorced from the social even if such matter is finite and labelled inadequate during processes of symbolic interaction.

Acknowledgements

The UK's Economic and Social Research Council (ESRC) supported two of the studies discussed in this chapter; namely, the projects on steroids and violence (L210252008) and the obesity debate (RES-000-22-0784). I would also like to acknowledge my indebtedness to Michael Bloor and Greg Smith for their teaching and ongoing support over the years. Finally, I am grateful to my ethnographic contacts for directly or indirectly helping me with my research.

References

Adler, Patricia and Adler, Peter. 1987. *Membership Roles in Field Research*. London: Sage.

Adler, Patricia, Adler, Peter and Fontana, Andrea. 1987. "Everyday Life Sociology." *Annual Review of Sociology*, 13:217–35.

Aphramor, Lucy. 2005. "Is a Weight-Centred Health Framework Salutogenic? Some Thoughts on Unhinging Certain Dietary Ideologies." *Social Theory & Health*, 3 (4): 315–340.

Athens, Lonnie. 1997. *Violent Criminal Acts and Actors Revisited*. Chicago: University of Illinois Press.

Atkinson, Paul and Housley, William. 2003. *Interactionism: An Essay in Sociological Amnesia*. London: Sage.

Becker, Howard. 1963. *Outsiders: Studies in the Sociology of Deviance*. New York: Free Press.

_____. 1967. "History, Culture and Subjective Experience: An Exploration of the Social Bases of Drug-Induced Experiences." *The Journal of Health and Social Behavior*, 8:163–76.

Berger, Peter and Luckmann, Thomas. 1967. *The Social Construction of Reality: A Treatise in the Sociology of Knowledge*. London: Penguin.

Bloor, Michael. 1995. *The Sociology of HIV Transmission*. London: Sage.

Blumer, Herbert. 1966. Sociological Implications of the Thought of George Herbert Mead. *The American Journal of Sociology*, 71 (5):535–44.

Bordo, Susan. 1993. *Unbearable Weight: Feminism, Western Culture and the Body*. Berkeley, CA: University of California Press.

Bourdieu, Pierre, Darbel, Alain and Schnapper, Dominique. 1991. *The Love of Art: European Art Museums and their Public*. Oxford: Polity.

Brain, Robert. 1979. *The Decorated Body*. New York: Harper and Row.

Campos, Paul. 2004. *The Obesity Myth: Why America's Obsession with Weight is Hazardous to your Health*. New York: Gotham Books.

Coffey, Amanda. 1999. *The Ethnographic Self: Fieldwork and the Representation of Identity*. London: Sage.

Davis, Murray. 1983. *Smut: Erotic Reality/Obscene Ideology*. Chicago: University of Chicago Press.

Dobash, Russell, Monaghan, Lee, Dobash, Rebecca and Bloor, Michael. 1999. "Bodybuilding, Steroids and Violence: Is There a Connection?" in Pat Carlen and Rod Morgan (eds) *Crime Unlimited: Questions for the 21st Century*. London: Macmillan.

Gard, Michael and Wright, Jan. 2005. *The Obesity Epidemic*. London: Routledge.

Garfinkel, Harold. 1956. "Conditions of Successful Degradation Ceremonies." *The American Journal of Sociology*, 61:420–4.

Giddens, Anthony. 1991. *Modernity and Self-Identity: Self and Society in the Late Modern Age*. Cambridge: Polity Press.

_____. 1992. *The Transformation of Intimacy: Love, Sexuality and Eroticism in Modern Societies*. Cambridge: Polity Press.

Goffman, Erving. 1963. *Behavior in Public Places: Notes on the Social Organization of Gatherings*. New York: The Free Press.

_____. 1967. *Interaction Ritual: Essays on Face-to-Face Behavior*. New York: Doubleday Anchor.

_____. 1968. *Stigma: Notes on the Management of Spoiled Identity*. Middlesex: Penguin Books.

_____. 1989. "On Fieldwork." *Journal of Contemporary Ethnography*, 18 (2):123–32. (Transcribed and edited by Lynne Lofland.)

Hine, Christine. 2000. *Virtual Ethnography*. London: Sage.

Klein, Alan. 1993. *Little Big Men: Bodybuilding Subculture and Gender Construction*. Albany, New York: State University of New York Press.

LeBesco, Kathleen. 2004. *Revolting Bodies? The Struggle to Redefine Fat Identity*. Boston: University of Massachusetts Press.

Lyng, Stephen. 1990. "Edgework: A Social Psychological Analysis of Voluntary Risk-Taking." *American Journal of Sociology*, 95:851–66.

Matza, David. 1969. *Becoming Deviant*. New Jersey: Prentice-Hall.

Monaghan, Lee. 2001a. "The Bodybuilding Ethnophysiology Thesis." in N. Watson (ed.) *Reframing the Body*. Hampshire: Palgrave.

_____. 2001b. *Bodybuilding, Drugs and Risk*. London: Routledge.

_____. 2001c. "Looking Good, Feeling Good: The Embodied Pleasures of Vibrant Physicality." *Sociology of Health & Illness*, 23 (3):330–356.

_____. 2002a. "Vocabularies of Motive for Illicit Steroid Use Among Bodybuilders." *Social Science & Medicine*, 55 (5):695–708.

_____. 2002b. "Opportunity, Pleasure, and Risk: An Ethnography of Urban Male Heterosexualities." *Journal of Contemporary Ethnography*, 31 (4):440–477.

_____. 2003. "Hormonal Bodies, Civilised Bodies: Incorporating the Biological into the Sociology of Health." in Simon Williams, Gillian Bendelow and Lynda Birke (eds) *Debating Biology: Sociological Reflections on Health, Medicine and Society*. London: Routledge.

_____. 2005a. "Discussion Piece: A Critical Take on the Obesity Debate." *Social Theory & Health*, 3, 4: 302–314.

_____. 2005b. "Big Handsome Men, Bears and Others: Virtual Constructions of 'Fat Male Embodiment.'" *Body & Society*, 11 (2):81–111.

_____. 2006. "Fieldwork and the Body: Reflections on an Embodied Ethnography." in Dick Hobbs and Richard Wright (eds) *Sage Handbook of Fieldwork*. London: Sage.

_____. 2006 (forthcoming) "Weighty Words: Expanding and Embodying the Sociology of Accounts." *Social Theory & Health*.

National Audit Office. 2001. *Tackling Obesity in England*. London: The Stationery Office.

Nettleton, Sarah and Watson, Jonathan (eds). 1998. *The Body In Everyday Life*. London: Routledge.

Pope, Harrison and Katz, David. 1990. "Homicide and Near Homicide by Anabolic Steroid Users." *Journal of Clinical Psychiatry*, 51 (1):28–31.

Pope, Harrison, Phillips, Katherine and Olivardia, Roberto. 2000. *The Adonis Complex: The Secret Crisis of Male Body Obsession*. New York: Free Press.

Rhodes, Tim. 1997. "Risk Theory in Epidemic Times: Sex, Drugs and the Social Organisation of 'Risk Behaviour.'" *The Sociology of Health & Illness*, 19 (2):208–27.

Rich, Emma and Evans, John. 2005. "'Fat Ethics': The Obesity Discourse and Body Politics." *Social Theory & Health*, 3 (4): 341–358.

Ritzer, George. 2004. *The McDonaldization of Society: Revised New Century Edition*. London: Sage.

Schutz, Alfred. 1962. *Collected Papers I: The Problem of Social Reality*. The Hague: Martinus Nijhoff.

_____. 1970. *Reflections on the Problem of Relevance*. New Haven: Yale University Press.

Scott, Marvin and Lyman, Stanford. 1968. "Accounts." *American Sociological Review*, 33 (1):46–62.

Shilling, Chris. 2003. *The Body and Social Theory*. (Second edition.) London: Sage.

Sobal, Jeff and Maurer, Donna (eds). 1999a. *Interpreting Weight: The Social Management of Fatness and Thinness*. New York: Aldine De Gruyter.

_____. 1999b. *Weighty Issues: Fatness and Thinness as Social Problems*. New York: Aldine De Gruyter.

Stearns, Peter. 1997. *Fat History: Bodies and Beauty in the Modern West*. New York: New York University Press.

Strong, Philip. 1990. "Epidemic Psychology: A Model." *Sociology of Health & Illness*, 12 (3):249–59.

Turner, Bryan. 1996. *The Body and Society*. (Second edition.) London: Sage.

Williams, Simon. 2003. "Beyond Meaning, Discourse and the Empirical World: Critical Realist Reflections on Health." *Social Theory & Health*, 1 (1):42–71.

Williams, Simon and Bendelow, Gillian. 1998. *The Lived Body: Sociological Themes, Embodied Issues*. London: Routledge.

Williams, Simon, Bendelow, Gillian and Birke, Lynda (eds.). 2003. *Debating Biology: Sociological Reflections on Health, Medicine and Society*. London: Routledge.

Witz, Anne. 2000. "Whose Body Matters? Feminist Sociology and the Corporeal Turn in Sociology and Feminism." *Body & Society*, 6 (2):1–24.

World Health Organization. 1998. *Obesity: Preventing and Managing the Global Epidemic*. Geneva: World Health Organization.

Chapter 10

Intelligent Bodies: Embodied Subjectivity Human-Horse Communication

Keri Brandt

Symbolic interaction is by its very nature limited. Symbols are only one of the many vehicles of communication that human and animal species may utilize in order to communicate. Because symbols depend on abstract associations between signifiers and signifieds, their operation is at times uncertain, controversial, or even impractical, as it is often the case when human species attempt to interact with animal species. As Keri Brandt points out in this chapter, humans and animals – in this instance female riders and horses – in fact recur to a type of communication that can be defined as iconic. Icons, such as the various somatic forms of tactile contact between horsewomen and horses, embody what they represent. Meaning, therefore, can be understood as residing within the experience of somatic perception of the symbolic presence of the other. On one hand, this observation points to the pre-reflexive carnality of communication. On the other hand, it highlights the symbolism upon which the co-existence of conscious bodies depends. Horsewomen and horses, and more generally, humans and animals, thus seem to be united in a moment of ekstasis (see Vannini and Waskul this volume) that Brandt understands to be inevitably gendered and specied.

Because interaction between humans and horses entails a high level of body-to-body contact, human-horse communication offers a unique lens through which to understand embodied interaction. In earlier research (Brandt 2004) I argued that the body is a basis for interaction and called for rethinking of the primacy of verbal language as a basis for symbolic interaction (also see Rochberg-Halton 1982). Here, I explore another element of the embodied language system shared between humans and horses and I challenge the predominance of the mind in theories of subjectivity. The relationship between embodiment and subjectivity remains vastly under-researched, and the mind and spoken language continue to occupy privileged status of subjectivity in much research and theory. Further, within symbolic interaction, the body as a basis for meaningful communication and self-understanding is regrettably underdeveloped (for a recent exception see Halton 2004).[1]

---

1   While the body as a basis for symbolic interaction has received little sociological attention, scholars from a variety of disciplines have investigated the body as a mode for

I explore how horsewomen use somatic sensations as a form of communication with horses. I bring women's experiences of embodiment to the foreground for a phenomenological analysis of embodiment as a lived process and argue that embodiment lies at the basis of subjectivity. Though horsewomen rely on a well-developed language system (Brandt 2004) they also draw from the experience of pre-linguistic somatic sensations as a resource to guide their interactions with horses. In this context, horsewomen rely on their bodies as a site for transacting information, ideas, emotions, and knowledge (see Dewey 1934). It is the women's embodiment – their lived and felt corporeality – that generates subjectivity. Simply put, bodies are intelligent.

Methods and Data

Over a two year period I conducted 25 in-depth interviews and observed women and horses working together in various horse barn settings. I strictly interviewed women because men's relationships to horses in the form of the cowboy, the ranch hand, the North American "Indian" warrior have been amply investigated. Consistent with feminist research principles, this research is an effort to bring women's relationships with others (horses, in this case) to the centre of empirical attention and to seriously regard women's unique ways of communicating with those others (Haraway 1996; Harding 1987; Mies 1991; Skeggs 2000).

My research was conducted in a large city in the American West. Within this landscape, the three chief areas of English style equestrian sports are hunter/jumper, dressage, and eventing. I focused mainly on participants in the hunter/jumper discipline of equestrian riding. Many of the women I interviewed also were interested in utilizing the philosophy and techniques of "natural horsemanship"[2] as a training method.

I was a known observer and full participant in this setting. As a horse owner[3] and rider I was a complete member and I added a research role to my existing membership role (Adler and Adler 1987). My role as a full participant helped grant entry and provided invaluable insider knowledge. Researchers like Bekoff (2002) and Sanders and Arluke (1993) assert that the unique endeavour of human-animal research requires that the researcher, to some extent, comes to the see the world through the eyes of the animals. This obvious challenge to traditional notions of

---

linguistic expression in sign languages (e.g. Davis 1995; Groce 1985; Liddell 2003; Schein and Stewart 1995; Taub 2001).

2   Natural horsemanship is a style of working with horses that is based on the premise that humans must understand the horse's thought process and way of being in the world and structure their interactions with horses based on this premise. As a training philosophy it endorses humane, non-forceful, and compassionate interactions between humans and horses.

3   The term "owner" reflects the language of the community and participants in this research. Individuals who have purchased a horse and pay for the horse's keeping do not use the terms "keeper," "caretaker," or "guardian."

objectivity, which is supported by reflexive feminist methodology, requires "that the investigator be intimately involved with the animal-other and the researcher's disciplined attention to his or her emotional experience can serve as an invaluable source of understanding" (Sanders and Arluke 1993: 378). My life experiences with horses provided me with the familiarity and knowledge of horse behaviour and their unique ways of relating in the world.

My interview format was designed to generate general descriptions of the women's history with horses, and also more detailed descriptions of their relationships with particular horses and the processes by which the two species communicated. I analyzed the data following a grounded theory approach (Emerson, Fretz, and Shaw 1995; Glaser and Strauss 1967).

Mind/Body Dualism

Dualisms such as mind/body, man/woman, subject/object, emotion/reason are central to the structure of Western thought (see Vannini and Waskul in this volume). As Derrida (1967) has pointed out, within dualist ideologies one term is always privileged over the "other." The latter remains the subjugated and subordinated counterpart. With mind/body dualism, the mind is valued over the body and the two entities are positioned in opposition. Since the diffusion of Cartesian philosophy, the mind has been theorized as the predominant force in shaping human subjectivity. At the core of the mind's elevated status over the body is its construction as the privileged medium for intelligence, knowledge production, and culture. In contrast, the body is the mundane and "merely physical" aspect of the human experience. In this view flesh is functional but not meaningful.

Within symbolic interactionism and pragmatism the philosophy and social theory of John Dewey (e.g. 1925, 1934) constitutes an advanced attempt to surpass dualism. Dewey's idea of transaction points to the reciprocal emergence of embodied self and world in organic interaction. As Vannini and Waskul remark in their chapter, for Dewey meanings are "had" before they are reflexively and consciously "known." For meanings to be had, they must be *sensed*. The embodied work of sensation consists of *sensing* (as in perceiving) and *making sense of* something (as in interpreting) (see Vannini and Waskul, this volume). Sensation works at the purely embodied, pre-linguistic level because it operates primarily at the level of qualitative immediacy (Dewey 1934; but also see Rochberg-Halton 1982 and Vannini and Waskul, this volume). Thus, sensing and making sense of are two interrelated activities by which beings – such as humans and horses – negotiate meaning. Because this negotiation occurs at the iconic level – mostly the level of tactile interaction – I posit that embodied communication between human and non-human animals is also a matter of iconic interaction, or transaction, rather than one of exclusively *symbolic* interaction as privileged in the literature. Symbols, in fact, are signs whose meaning depend on abstract conventions, such as words.

More recently, the deconstruction of the mind/body opposition has been particularly important for feminist and queer theorists. Elizabeth Grosz (1994) argues that mind/body dualism is at the heart of women's subjugation to men. Men claim the realm of the mind while women are perpetually situated (or confined) within the domain of the body. Men and the mind are synonymous with intelligence and knowledge production, whereas women and the body represent the lack thereof. Women are constructed as determined and essential beings who are tied to bodies that block their full actualization. Men, however, are granted full subjectivity with mental faculties that free them from the body that constrains women. Grosz (1994: 22) writes, "women can no longer take on the function of being the body for men while men are left free to soar to the heights of theoretical reflection and cultural production." Thus, an effort to displace the mind/body opposition is also a challenge to man/woman dualism. Not only does the collapsing of mind/body dualism allow for a rethinking embodiment and its relationship to subjectivity, but of women's subjectivity as well.

Because of women's troubled history with the body and reductionism, many feminist and queer theorists have turned away from examining the lived experience of embodiment. Embodiment is often associated with essentialism and, therefore, raises fears of oppressive biological determinism. In contrast, I believe it is important to carefully engage the relationship between embodiment and subjectivity as not to risk terminating the possibility of any understanding derived from the body.

Bodily materiality, sensation, and the way "we inhabit our skin" all have a meaningful impact on our intersubjective sense of the world around us. The skin is the immediate sensory organ that informs our experience of the world (Anzieu 1989). For all living creatures the body is our mode of being-in-the-world (Merleau-Ponty 1962). As Margrit Shildrick (1997: 178) writes, "the flesh and blood givenness of the physical body is not a passive surface, but a site of sensation." She argues that we cannot focus solely on a body conceived on purely discursive terms. An examination of the lived experience of the body and its interactions with textual practices is necessary for a more complete understanding of the fully embodied subject.

More recent work by transsexual theorists and others has argued for a deeper interrogation of the relationship between embodiment and subjectivity (Ahmed and Stacey 2001; Bailey 2001; Namaste 2000; Prosser 1998; Shildrick 1997; Tauchert 2002). This collection of work argues that the body is not simply an effect of language as many radical constructionists have argued. This attempt to investigate everyday embodiment and its relationship to subjectivity understands embodiment as a lived process that has a meaningful impact on how individuals understand themselves and others.

Informed by these literatures, I look to women who work with horses and reflect on the relationship between embodiment and subjectivity – a space where embodiment informs understanding. As I will illustrate, horsewomen speak of a subjectivity that is realized only though embodied pre-linguistic sensation and signification.

Having a "Good Feel"

While working with horses women have a heightened awareness of their bodies as a mechanism for communication. Because humans and horses do not have a shared symbolic language, they must both use their bodies as a basis for iconic transaction. Through a co-created embodied (iconic) system of cues, shared meaning is possible in the absence of spoken verbal language. However, beyond using a variety of bodily cues for communication, horsewomen spoke of a keen awareness of their bodily sensations – the experience of sensation, or what horsepeople refer to as "feel" – as a source of information to guide their interactions with horses.

There is an important difference between feeling, sensation, and emotion. Peirce's phenomenology – or phrenology – showed that feeling and sensation (the two will be used interchangeably in this chapter) are elements of Firstness, the qualitative immediacy of experience (see Rochberg-Halton 1982). Emotion, instead, stands higher in the continuum of reflexivity because it demands "inference" (Rochberg-Halton 1982: 164). Sensation is an essential part of communication, whether riding a horse or working with a horse from the ground. Horsepeople often speak of having a "good feel of the horse" or how much the horse "feels off" the person. This concept of "feel" is based in part on the idea that horses pick up on sensations through the body to body connection with humans. Because sense is pre-reflexive and purely embodied, it is a difficult concept to explain linguistically. Indeed, it must be acknowledged that some meaning will be lost in "translation" when putting into words a phenomenon that is non-linguistic. Sensation is partly tactile in the sense of touch, and it is also the experience of internal embodied processes. It is a hybrid concept. It is directly tactile in contact with the horse and at the same time "inner." For example, when I asked Lois, who has been a recreational horsewoman most of her life, if she thought the way humans and horses communicated was unique, she responded: "I'm trying to think of another animal that humans communicate with strictly by touch and feel." What is notable about Lois's response is that she distinguished between kinaesthetic touch and an internal sensation, understanding them as two distinct but inextricably interrelated parts of communication.

Through the corporeal experience of sensations and emotions horse and rider share meanings. Empathy – the embodied sensation of another's emotions – is employed in the service of communication. Empathy is not used only for the sake of *feeling for* the other, but rather it is used as a resource to *sense and make sense of* the other. This difference between feeling for the horse and sensing and making sense of the horse is an important distinction in the human-horse context. To *feel for* the horse is to use the experience of embodied empathy for the purposes of compassion and understanding. To *sense and to make sense of* the horse is to use empathy at the level of embodied sensation for the purpose of organic interaction. Emotional empathy, in the traditional sense, is a loss of self in the experience the other. It is a forgetting of the self to understand the feeling experience of the other. In the human-horse interaction, however, there is no loss or forgetting of the self. Empathy is more ecstatic (see Vannini and Waskul, this volume) as it is the medium through which communication can happen. The embodied experience of human-horse communication relies in part on what Kenneth Shapiro (1990: 192) calls "kinaesthetic empathy:" "empathetic experience involves appropriating a second body that then becomes my auxiliary focus. Through my lived body, I accompany yours as it attends an object." Thus, sensing and making sense of the other allows for a somatic and ecstatic transaction between humans and horses.

As said, horses' understanding is not mediated by formal language. I asked Sara if she could explain what she means by "horsemanship through feel." She responded:

> that would be their [horses] understanding of what they think you mean by what you're doing before you touch them. The way you move, the speed at which you move, the mood you're in when you approach them. If you're upset about your mortgage, your spouse or your job, it's not a time to be around a horse because they can feel that. Those sorts of stressful irrelevant energies have no place around a horse.

Using sensation to communicate with horses takes advantage of horses' acute sensitivity to emotions. Horses have a unique ability to pick up emotions and sensations via their somatic sensitivity. Jane Smiley (2004:198) writes that "if humans have smarter brains, horses have smarter bodies." Horses, in general, have highly sensitive bodies because their bodies are their medium of communication. Similarly, Vicki Hearne (1982:108) explains that when riding horses humans need to be aware of the horse's acute sensitivity because "every muscle twitch of the rider will be a loud symphony to the horse." Dewey himself (1934:19) finds that "the live animal is fully present, all there, in all of its actions: in its wary glances, its sharp sniffings, its abrupt cocking of ears. All senses are equally on the *qui vive*." And as my informant – Becky – said "when you're on them, you're connected to them. So any feeling you have in your body, then they can feel that." With the knowledge that horses can feel of the human, horsewomen work to develop their ability to sense and make sense of the horse as well. Thus, because both species are sensing and making sense of each other, sensation must be understood as a mode of communication and as the very ground of transaction (Dewey 1934).

Moria, a vet student and professional horse trainer, explained to me how the exchange of sensations is an important part of her horse-riding experiences:

> The most interesting thing I have found, more recently, is how much they feel off of me. Because if I ... you know, I'll just be riding, and if I feel tense about a jump at all, I can definitely sense the horse all of a sudden change his personality and, you know, kind of balk off of it or not go forward as much.... And I think I just make a lot of assumptions, too, without even seeing the signals, and my assumptions have been, so far, pretty correct.... I think it's a lot ... it's just my body, and just, you know, I get that feeling.

Moria explained how horses are sensitive to her emotional states, but she also acknowledged how she is sensitive to horses' emotions. These sensations are not based on "seeing signals," rather, she just "gets that feeling." For Moria and other riders, feeling sensations is a valuable resource in their interactions with horses.

Ultimately, the desired outcome for both horses and humans is to have a "good feel of each other" and to borrow from both Dewey and Merleau-Ponty (see Kestenbaum 1977), to acquire a "habitual" mode of relating to one another. Horsepeople talk about having a good feel of a horse or the horse having a good feel of the human. When a human has a good feel of the horse it means that she is keenly aware of the exchange of sensations between herself and the horse and is able to effectively communicate meanings to the horse through this mode of sensation. When a horse has a good feel of their rider it means that through the exchange of sensations the horse has a clear understanding of the rider's intent and literally feels good about working with that specific rider. Having a good feel of each other allows humans and horses to work in harmony, rather than in conflict.

A particularly illustrative example of a horse and rider having a good feel of each other is from Jane who reminisced about her relationship with a horse named "Shammy." Jane and Shammy competed successfully at the grand prix level in show jumping – the highest level of competition – and were a well known horse-rider combination in the region. At grand prix level competition horse and rider must navigate a set route over twelve to fourteen jumps that range between five and five and a half feet in height, with spreads up to six feet across. The goal is to make it over all the jumps (in a predetermined order) in a set amount of time without any penalties. The horse and rider team is penalized if the horse knocks down any part of the jump or refuses to clear a jump on the first try.

I: Why was your career with Shammy so successful?

R: Every once in a while, you just run into a soul mate. And he was considered a stopper. And he never, in his entire life, stopped with me, ever. Never even thought about it. But I never thought he would. And it was just … we just got along … they're very sensitive. I think they know if you like them. And I liked everything about him. He could have jumped a little better form, but he jumped his heart out.

I: What was he picking up? How was he sensing that you liked him?

R: Oh, just the way I touched him, and spent a lot of time with him. Never was rough with him. I always … when we'd go in the ring, before we'd start our course, I'd always reach up and just tug a little bit on his left ear. He loved that. [Laughs] It was just a habit – I'd just reach up and just hold his ear. I didn't pull it hard, but I just let it slide through my fingers … then we were ready to go. I never questioned him. And he wasn't easy. But I didn't try to change him too much; I tried to ride what I had…. And I got him because the guy who owned him, the person that was riding him before, he wouldn't jump for her. Just wouldn't. And there was nothing wrong with him. He just didn't like her. And she was a good rider. But I've seen that happen more times than not.

Jane considered Shammy her soul mate and "she liked everything about him," which most horsepeople would argue imparted a positive feeling to him. She had a good sense of him and "never questioned him," which enabled this notoriously difficult horse to perform at the top of his potential. Jane explained how he did not like his previous rider (did not have a good feel of her) and therefore did not want to make any effort for her. Jane's comment that she has seen horses not having a good feel of their rider "more times than not" also demonstrates that having a good feel is not always a given or even automatic. Good feel between horses and humans, as all habits do, often takes time and conscious skilful effort to develop. Still, sometimes, for whatever reason, horse and rider combinations never develop a good feel of the other.

For both Dewey and Merleau-Ponty "habits are not…experienced by the organism as cognitive or even conscious phenomena. Habits operate on a level of experience which precedes any sort of deliberate, critical, positing of distinct objects of reflection or consciousness" (Kestenbaum 1977:4). Habits, therefore, structure the knowledge that horse and horsewoman have of each other, at the pre-objective and pre-reflexive, as well as the pre-linguistic level. It is precisely at this level that organic transaction is primarily lived for Dewey.

It is important to note that although I have interviewed only horsewomen, horsemen talk of the same experience of feel with horses. Sensation is an approach to working with horses – a form of communication – that is found across all the riding disciplines and transgresses gender. Beyond technical and physical dexterity of both horses and riders, part of what makes horse and rider combinations successful is their ability to communicate through sensations and the habitual structures that sensations create. Therefore, horsemen, as well as horsewomen, must skilfully hone this mode of communication. I mention this because I recognize that this discussion of horsewomen's experiences of sensation may serve to further solidify the cultural construction of women as feeling/emotional and men as logical/unemotional. However, horses do not have the social construction of gender to contend with, and if a man or woman wants to achieve successful partnerships with horses this sense-based form of habitual communication is a skill they will have to develop.

As I stated earlier, iconic sense is difficult to explain in part because the only access to understanding this non-linguistic embodied experience (next to actually riding horses) is through words. Horsewomen are talking about an experience that is resistant to language. Their words are a representation of the experience and a representation is always limited in its ability to convey the qualitative immediacy of the experience. Moreover, because of the privileging of the mind and spoken language we have yet to create language-like tools that more accurately represent embodied sensations.

Embodied Subjectivity

Expressing subjectivity through words and spoken language that have shared meaning is not an option between horse and rider. The primary way a horse can know a human is through sensing and making sense of their body communication. Like horses, horsewomen's bodies have the task of sensing and making sense of horses' communication. By suggesting this I am directly challenging the notion that the body is a mere vessel of the mind and of cognitive knowledge, a view that for so long has left subjectivity within the domain of the mind. Horsewomen's experiences indeed reveal a self-understanding that is grounded in their embodiment, making the separation between embodiment and subjectivity problematic, if not false. Moria explained:

> I don't know, I definitely stress the fact that they feel so much more than we think they do. And it took me a lot of time, really, to realize that.... I think that ... what you learn about how much you're really able to feel on a horse is just an amazing lesson.... So yeah, I feel like it's definitely developed my being sensitive to touch. [Laughs] You know, like really raised my awareness in what I actually do feel.

Because Western culture has privileged a linguistic way of being-in-the-world, many scholars have failed to truly understand how we live through our bodies without necessarily involving language. Becky articulated this point when she said:

> I really do think that we just don't have enough respect for how much our bodies are capable of translating and expressing, human beings have gotten so wrapped up in verbal communication and visual communication I don't think we really think about the kinaesthetic side of things. I know that I don't really think about it unless I'm riding, that that's really when I'm aware of it.

As long as the mind and spoken language continue to have a stronghold on "intelligence" and subjectivity, the intellect of the body will remain undervalued, if even recognized at all. Exploring communication through sensation allows us to understand the fully embodied subject as well as embodied transaction.

Expert horsewomen talked about how they could strategically use their sensations to present different ideas to the horse. For example, Moria explained, "I kind of get the same kind of feeling, you know? If they're confident, I feel their confidence and I'm more confident. If they're scared, then I can definitely tell, and I try to overpower that by being confident." Moria senses the horse's emotional state and uses that sensation as information. If she senses confidence from the horse, her feeling of confidence is boosted. However, if she senses that the horse is scared, she actively manipulates that in order to communicate a different subjectivity to the horses. Habit and harmony between horse and rider is then at times created out of conflict. This embodied transaction is but a "contrast of lack and fullness, of struggle and achievement, of adjustment after consummated irregularity [that] form the drama in which action, feeling, and meaning are one" (Dewey 1934:16).

Becky spoke of a similar process where she consciously controls her emotions – that is, the embodied experience of emotionality – to communicate a feeling to her horse that she knows will help keep him stay calm and secure. She further explained how she tried to offer her horse support through her body when he is afraid or unsure. I asked what she meant by "support" and she responded:

> A lot of it, I would say, is just through my feeling that I have inside. Like when I'm nervous and I'm on his back, he can feel [it] ... in my body ... he feeds off of it ... we [Becky and her horse] have this happen all the time. If we're riding up to the water tank

and I'm nervous about it, because ten times before we've ridden up there and he shies and jumps around and is afraid, and if I'm thinking about that, if I've got that sick feeling in my stomach, that nervous feeling, he reacts. But if I just go – I just kind of have to bluff myself – if I just go, "come on, let's go," and I just ride him up there like we're just going to go get a drink of water, no big deal, then he doesn't get afraid, or if he does get afraid, it's a little bit, and then he kind of goes, "are you sure we don't need to be afraid of this?" I mean it's just a feeling. It's not really actions.

When the women talk about overriding a feeling they are talking about shifting their subjectivity by way of letting go of a feeling and by replacing it with another. Noting how women can shift their subjectivity in terms of their sensations – particularly the sensation of fear – is important because women historically are constructed as fearful while men are brave. Men are constructed as either not fearful and, therefore, brave, or they have a unique ability to use their minds to overcome their fear to have a different experience. However, the horsewomen's experiences challenge the sociocultural construction of women as fearful. Moreover, fear does not lead to paralysis; the body does not "take over" the mind. Not only are they not "overpowered" by their feelings of fear, instead they feel the sensation of fear and overpower it with a new feeling. Emotionality (femininity) is constructed as a lack of self-control, as "losing it." However, the women have tremendous emotional literacy that they draw on to quickly shift their subjective view from moment to moment. Here, the women are actors and express an agency that is counter-hegemonic to dominant notions of helpless emotional femininity.

Conclusions

An examination of the relationship between embodiment and subjectivity through the unique lens of human-horse communication offers insights reaching far beyond the world of horses and riders, as all human and non-human animals live in the world through their bodies. As Kenneth Shapiro (1990:192) writes, "our bodies do not encase us; rather, we are our bodies." Therefore, rather than "disembodying" theories of subjectivity, we must examine how different subjectivities are embodied to create a model of the fully embodied subject. We must continue the challenge to the primacy of the mind in theories of subjectivity to further our knowledge of the role of embodiment in self-understanding and meaning-making.

Phenomenological research that explores everyday lived experiences of the body and its relationship to selfhood allows for a more holistic understanding of the human and non-human animal experience. A phenomenological understanding of iconic, sensation-based interaction provides new pathways to a richer understanding of the relevance of embodiment, from experiences as diverse as communication with infants to dance to sport performance.

Finally, research that focuses on women's subjective lived experiences of their own bodies is sorely needed. We live in a society that perpetually objectifies the female body by specifying what the normative experiences of their embodiment ought to be. The horsewomen's experiences speak of a body that has its own intelligence. In terms of women's status, their experiences are important to the process of social change by offering alternative accounts for re-imagining female corporeality in new, more affirmative ways.

References

Adler, Patricia A. and Peter Adler. 1987. *Membership Roles in Field Research.* Newbury Park, CA: Sage.

Ahmed, Sara and Jackie Stacey (eds). 2001. *Thinking Through the Skin.* London: Routledge.

Anzieu, Dider. 1989. *The Skin Ego: A Psychoanalytic Approach to the Self.* New Haven: Yale University Press.

Bailey, Lucy. 2001. "Gender Shows: First Time Mothers and Embodied Selves." *Gender and Society*, 15 (1):110–129.

Bekoff, Marc. 2002. *Minding Animals: Awareness, Emotions, and Heart.* New York: Oxford University Press.

Brandt, Keri J. 2004. "A Language of Their Own: An Interactionist Approach to Human-Horse Communication." *Society & Animals*, 12:4.

Derrida, Jacques. 1967. *Of Grammatology.* Baltimore: Johns Hopkins University Press.

Dewey, John. 1925. *Experience and Nature.* Chicago: University of Chicago Press.
_____. 1934. *Art as Experience.* New York: Minton.

Emerson, R.M. and Fretz, R.I. and Shaw, L. L. (1995). *Writing Ethnographic Fieldnotes.* Chicago: University of Chicago Press.

Glasser, Barney, and Anselm Strauss. 1967. *The Discovery of Grounded Theory.* Chicago: Aldine.

Grosz, Elizabeth. 1994. *Volatile Bodies: Toward a Corporeal Feminism.* Bloomington: Indiana University Press

Halton, Eugene. 2004. "The Living Gesture and the Signifying Moment." *Symbolic Interaction*, 27:89–114.

Haraway, Donna. 1996. "Situated Knowledges: The Science Question in Feminism and the Privilege of Partial Perspective." in E. F. Keller and H. E. Longino (eds), *Feminism and Science.* Oxford: Oxford University Press.

Harding, Sandra. 1987. "Is There a Feminist Method?" *Hypatia*, 2(3):19–35.

Hearne, Vicky. 1982. *Adam's Task: Calling Animals by Name.* New York: Vintage Books.

Kestenbaum, Victor. 1977. *The Phenominological Sense of John Dewey: Habit and Meaning.* New Jersey: Humanities Press.

Lupton, Deborah. 1998. *The Emotional Self.* London: Sage Publications.

Merleau-Ponty, Maurice. 1968. *The Phenomenology of Perception.* London: Routledge.

Body/Embodiment

Mies, M. 1991. "Women's Research or Feminist Research? The Debate Surrounding Feminist Science and Methodology." in M. M. Fonow and J. A. Cook (eds), *Beyond Methodology: Feminist Scholarship as Lived Research*. Bloomington: Indiana University Press. pp. 60–84.

Namaste, Vivian K. 2000. *Invisible Lives: The Erasure of Transsexual and Transgendered People*. Chicago: Chicago University Press.

Prosser, Jay. 1998. *Second Skins: The Body Narratives of Transsexuality*. New York: Columbia University Press.

Rochberg-Halton, Eugene. 1982. "Qualitative Immediacy and the Communicative Act." *Qualitative Sociology*, 5:162–181.

Sanders, Clinton and Arnold Arluke. 1993. "If Lions Could Speak: Investigation Animal-Human Relationships and the Perspectives of Nonhuman Others." *Sociological Quarterly*, 34:377–390.

Shapiro, Kenneth. J. 1990. "Understanding Dogs Through Kinesthetic Empathy, Social Construction, and History." *Anthrozoos*, 3:184–195.

Shildrick, Margrit. 1997. *Leaky Bodies and Boundaries: Feminism, Postmodernism and (Bio)Ethics*. London: Routledge.

Skeggs, Beverley. 2001. "Feminist Ethnography." in Paul Atkinson, Amanda Coffey, Sara Delamont, John Lofland and Lyn Lofland (eds), *Handbook of Ethnography* Thousand Oaks: Sage. pp. 426–442.

Smiley, Jane. 2004. *A Year at the Races: Reflections on Horses, Humans, Love, Money, and Luck*. New York: Alfred A. Knopf.

Tauchert, Ashley. 2002. "Fuzzy Gender: Between Female Embodiment and Intersex." *Journal of Gender Studies*, 11(1):29–38.

Chapter 11

Professional Female Football Players: Tackling Like a Girl?

Joseph Kotarba and Matt Held

Phenomenology, much like symbolic interactionism, is a diverse enterprise. In the following chapter Joseph Kotarba and Matt Held owe primarily to the existentialist tradition in their grounded analysis the deeply personal meanings and experiences of females who play American football. Female football players are by no means as popular as their male counterparts, and indeed the marginality – and one might even suggest the deviant character – of such practices turns out to be precisely the source of meaningfulness, uniqueness, and distinction for their sense of self-identity. As these women become accustomed to tackling "like women," the social world of American football becomes feminized while at the same time their playing bodies begin to assume new meanings: from stigma to pride, from exclusion to inclusion, and from lack of comfort within one's skin to embodied authenticity. Tackling "like women" thus turns out to be an exercise in the care of the gendered self. As Kotarba and Held explain, for women who play football, performance is all about authentic femininity, one violent hit at a time.

As an acceptable arena for violence and aggression, competitive sports like football have been a traditional means for boys and men to construct a masculine identity, whether as players or spectators. When media images of women athletes are made available, they are dominated by images of feminine grace and beauty. Women's bodies are sexualized, while men are portrayed as powerful – as is typically the case in Olympic television coverage (Boutilier and San Giovanni 1983).

But how do these cultural stereotypes and rules play out when women "invade" one of the most hypermasculine of all professional team sports: football? What happens, then, when women "invade" the traditional male turf of football? Do female football players become "man-like," in a stereotypical sense, or does football become feminized? What kinds of interactional work are needed to be a woman and a football player at the same time? Above all, how do biographical, cultural, situational, and physical factors intersect to create the identity of the female football player? In this chapter, we will address these questions in terms of insights gathered from an ongoing study of injury management among professional athletes (Kotarba

2005).[1] Football provides a dramatic illustration of women's identity work. The specific organization in question is The Houston Energy.

A Brief History of Women's Professional Football

There have been several, largely unsuccessful, efforts to establish professional women's football in the United States. In 1965, promoters assembled the Women's Professional Football League (WPFL) barnstorming tour of 1965. This tour consisted of two teams playing each other in a series of exhibition games. Several regional conferences have come and gone, perhaps most notable was the National Women's Football League and the famous Oklahoma City Dolls of the 1970s (WPFL 2005). There are currently three professional women's football leagues, of which the WPFL has the most national visibility. Established in 1998, the WPFL's objective has been to establish a national women's professional tackle football league using rules borrowed from the men's National Football League.

The Houston Energy is one of seventeen teams in the WPFL. The Energy have been successful on the field, having made the playoffs four of their first six years in existence. The team originally played home games at Rice University Stadium, but low attendance (approximately 300 fans a game) pushed the team to a high school stadium for 2005. The ten game season schedule is played in the spring and early summer.

The work of playing women's professional football is not a full-time, or even part-time, employment. All the women have other primary sources of income. Jobs range from truck driver and custodian to attorney and clinical psychologist. There are also a few housewives on the team. The typical player receives a $1 salary each season to qualify as a professional, but she is expected to raise approximately $4,000 to cover her own expenses (e.g. travel and equipment).

Playing football includes off-season training, try-outs, practicing twice a week, and game time. Off-season training is variable and, perhaps, inadequate; one player said that about ten percent of the team stays in great condition throughout the year. The other ninety percent maintain minimal to mediocre training during off-season. Women who tend to maintain their physical conditioning regime are those who have day jobs related to athletics, such as trainer or physical therapist.

---

1   A grant from the National Institute on Occupational Safety and Health/Southwest Centre for Occupational and Environmental Health provided support for the writing of this chapter. The Houston Energy phase of the study was accomplished during the 2004 season. Jana Zacek served as research assistant for the Energy project. We began the study with an executive interview with the team owner, who also plays linebacker on the team. We then conducted conversational interviews with approximately twenty players, two coaches, and six members of the medical staff. We talked informally with numerous fans and family members, and conducted observations of five games, two try-out sessions, two press conferences, and so forth.

The Female Athletic Body and the Self

Popular and academic discourses on sports and women (such as those with which we introduced this chapter) are a good beginning to understanding the identity of the professional female football player, yet they are ethnographically simplistic and theoretically – from an interactionist perspective – wanting. Existential thought, both phenomenological and sociological, posits everyday life experience as embodied (Douglas and Johnson 1977). How we experience our bodies, however, is neither constrained nor explained solely by the body itself.

Borrowing heavily from the work of Merleau-Ponty (1962), Young (1990) suggests that the *situation* in which the body exists shapes a woman's experience of that body. The woman's bodily comportment, physical engagement with things, ways of using the body in performing tasks, and bodily existential self image are marked by three modalities of feminine motility: *ambiguous bodily transcendence*, *inhibited intentionality*, and *discontinuous unity with its surroundings*. She may not trust her body's ability to engage in physical activity. She may believe that her body can perform well, yet place unnecessary limits on the level at which her body can perform. She may direct one part of her body to perform, but leave the remainder of her body inactive.

Young's phenomenology adds a woman's perception of her body and its capacities to earlier physiological explanation for why girls throw baseballs "like girls" and why – in terms of the present analysis – girls should not be expected to tackle "like boys." Women treat their bodies as objects of action in such situations as opposed to the originators of action (Young 2000:150). If, as we will see, women use their bodies to play professional football much like male players do – tackling hard, engaging the whole body in a play, and ignoring the risk of injury when engaged in a violent play – then Young's analysis is left wanting. We need a model of the body that posits it as the originator of unified embodied action.

The existential sociological concept of the self refers to "a person's unique experience of being within the context of contemporary social conditions, an experience most notably marked by an incessant sense of becoming and an active participation in social change" (Kotarba and Johnson 2002:8). The concept focuses on *agency* in terms of the many ways adults search for new and renewed meaning for self in our postmodern world, such as adult women taking up a new and violent sport such as football to fill in an otherwise boring or less-than-fulfilling lifestyle. Furthermore, the concept of the existential self stresses the fact that we are first and foremost *embodied* beings who both respond to affective situations and create affective situations. We use the body in everyday life both as a driver for crafting a sense of self as well as an anchor for ensuring the self fits and complements the world around it. Consequently, we would expect a woman to play football "like a man" if her body directs her to engage in the same experiences as a man's body dictates. In the remainder of this chapter, we will describe ethnographically some of the organizational, biographical, and situational factors underlying the essential embodied experience of tackle football shared by both men and women: the desire and drive to, and thrill and satisfaction of "hitting" and being known as or identified as "someone who loves to hit."

Trying Out for and Making the Team

Try-outs are held in January or February each year. The coaches and veteran players conduct the try-outs.[2] Approximately 200 women try out each year for the Energy. Some women who try out for the Energy are former NCAA Division I, II, III athletes who played soccer, basketball, fast pitch softball, lacrosse, hockey, and track and field. Some are club rugby and flag football players from leagues such the NWFFA and IWFFA. Some who try out previously participated in local flag football leagues, which have offered non-contact league play opportunities to women athletes for years. Few have any tackle football experience. There seems to be no shortage of women anxiously seeking the opportunity to play for the Energy. The women offer several multiple reasons for their dedication. Training and disciplining their bodies is one. Joining a community of women who play football is another. The simple desire for physical contact, "to hit," is yet another common reason. As one linebacker explained:

> Since they first taught me how to tackle, I love it. One of my nicknames is "Tacklin' Pune" because I love it so much. It's the best feeling in the world for me to run down full force, on a kick off, and just way-lay someone. And do it the right way so no one gets hurt too bad.

This particular player also mentioned the skill involved in the tackle. It was important to some players to highlight aggression as purposeful and within the confines of the game. A defensive back notes:

> The contact is just part of the game. It's like a chess game. There's a lot of strategy involved, there's mental aspects to the game other than hitting each other. You have to be smart. The more you play and develop your skills, you still have the contact, but you can handle it better. You know how to take contact in a more appropriate way to minimize the risk of injury.

She goes on to state that there is also a level of intensity in football that does not exist in other sports:

> It's like if you put on a uniform right now and you play against me, I get to hit... and to see who gets up – that's the ultimate. And you wanna line up with as many people as many times as you can and see how many people won't get up, that you can knock down without them getting up, or to have to have somebody come and help them off the field, or to call a time-out because you knocked the wind out of them. That's a rush!

---

2   The coaches, incidentally, are all men whose day jobs are as high school boys' football coaches.

A defensive lineperson points to a level of aggressiveness that is found only in football:

> Because of contact. It's just knowing that the whole purpose of playing football is for somebody to knock you out. Period. To try to. It's not to make you fall, it's to knock you out, for you not to get back up for the rest of the game, really, it's not to hurt you, but to make you think you're hurt. To hit you so hard, you just want to take off your uniform and turn in all your stuff right there on the field and go home and not even worry about it no more.

On the field, women tackle with the same intensity and style as men. The team trainer has been with the team for four years and says that "they've really been tackling hard the last couple of years." This is beneficial to the players' own physical health because "less hesitancy means fewer injuries." A tight end bragged proudly that her "WPFL dream is to just hit someone."

While playing football is what these women do in their spare time, they certainly identify highly with their team and enjoy their status as football players. One of the linebackers even has a tattoo of the Houston Energy logo on her calf. A defensive end voices the common wish "to achieve a status that allows the games to be televised and gain enough support to allow everyone involved to make money at playing football." The players take football seriously and many profess to an ultimate goal of making it their full-time job.

Try-outs are broken down into new player try-outs and veteran try-outs. Turnover is a chronic problem among the Houston Energy and other teams. The team only retains about half its players from year to year. The other half leave because of competing priorities, or simply because they have proved to themselves and others that they could do it. The fact that none of these women has had prior experience with tackle football is evident when they were instructed to begin throwing the football to each other. Most threw it as if it were a softball. Their arm moved across their body rather than straight through. Many of the women probably grew up playing softball so they equated the football with a softball. The coach had to show the women how to throw and, once explained, the throwing style changed quickly and dramatically, contrary to Strauss' (1966) claim that the difference in throwing styles is innate. It is not that women cannot throw a football – most simply have had little experience doing it.

The women who perform best in try-outs are large and athletic. Those two words are normally not associated with women's sports, but ideal for football (regardless of gender). While a veteran did say that they had hoped for "more big girls," there were a few that really stood out. Their agility and speed often matched and occasionally beat the smaller and leaner players.

Players only practice twice a week. This is another hindrance. The team, while strong, has certainly not reached its optimal level of performance for basic logistical reasons. The inability to practice daily or concentrate on football, because it offers no source of income, keeps the team, and the league, in general, from operating at peak performance.

Football is a third shift for many of the players. A high level of commitment is required. The women are forced to balance family, school, work, and football. They understand the glaring differences between the quality of work among NFL players and themselves, as a place kicker notes:

> Exactly... it's their job. They have time. They wake up and they're like oh, I gotta go to the gym, and then they go do some sprint workouts, and then they're like I'm going to the gym again. Plus they have the facilities to do it. We have to find our own places.

Fan support is invaluable because it reinforces the identity of professional football player. As a result of an informal survey of fans in attendance at one game at Rice University Stadium, most fans are players' family members, co-workers, and friends. The players routinely mingle with fans in the stands during halftime. Fans can even be seen on the sidelines during games, along with volunteer nurses, trainers, emergency medical technicians, and hangers-on.

The Football Body

For Pierre Bourdieu (2001), the body is an unfinished entity that develops in conjunction with various social forces. Acts of labour are required to turn bodies into social entities and these acts influence the way people feel about and present themselves. These acts of labour are not innate, but rather highly skilled and developed throughout life. The labour of body management is important to self, body image, and status. Such labour is also central to the exercise of power and the reproduction of social inequalities. Consequently, there is a tendency for those with the resources to treat the body as a life-long project.

Bourdieu's insights apply directly to women's professional football. Our culture has commodified the body through mass-mediated marketing of "thin is beautiful." As Turner (1969:47) notes: "the growing emphasis on the aesthetic quality of the body in relation to consumerism has emphasized the virtues of thin-ness and self-regulation in the interests of looking good." Women can resist this cultural hegemony. The Women's Professional Football League offers one arena for such resistance: a wide range of ways to see, celebrate, experience and transform the female body into various social identities.

Case Study: "Big Sue"

Sue is a 41 year-old married mother of three children and a four year football veteran. She is a leader and an integral part of the team. Football takes a central place in her life, since her supportive husband is the main breadwinner. Sue's involvement with the Energy feminizes football – she changes her sense of being a woman while changing the gendered meaning of the sport itself:

I just have a job more so I have something to do during the day.... Football is for entertainment and for the whole family. Actually my kids and mom and sister and uncle and aunts, they all come to my games. I have a big crowd. My whole family is involved. One son is a water boy and the other helps getting stuff ready for games and whatever anybody needs him to do. That's why I really tried out for football. It was to bring the family together.... Our whole family just loves football.... So when I heard about Houston Energy I thought that was a way for me to bring something back into this family so that we can all become a family again and go to the games together and cheer.

For Sue and most Energy players, football is indeed a family affair. Sue's husband spoke of how he was initially sceptical and did not think she would make the team when she tried out. Now, he is completely supportive. He said that if it was co-ed football, he would feel differently, but since it is women playing against women he could accept it:

It's just like, well, something else women do together. Back when I was young, my mother would always get together with the ladies and cook or sew or somethin'. These gals, today, I'll tell ya, they got different way of having fun.

Sue's embodied self-identity has also improved since she began playing football. She is a large woman, 5'11" and 305 lbs, who feels stigmatized in a society that highly values slimness. She has found a place where big is not only acceptable, but highly valued. Her size is an asset, and not only for her team. When her husband calls her "Big Sue," a smile appears across her face. She notes that if her husband had called her "Big Sue" ten years ago, she would have tackled him to the ground. Now she can save it for the football field. Playing football provides Sue a means of accomplishment and, because her athleticism was prematurely interrupted, it also grants closure:

It's something that I wanted to do for myself personally too. I got pregnant at 17 in high school. I was playing basketball, I was the starter on the varsity team and I had U of H looking at me, and some of the other colleges looking at me. Then I kinda ended up getting pregnant so I kinda dropped out of school and let my life go. I ended up having him and stayed at home and raised my kids.

Sue loves her family and considers herself a mother and a wife first and foremost. Nevertheless, she still felt like she lost – and regained – a piece of her self:

So I stayed home and took care of my family. I've been married for 22 years so when I heard about the Houston Energy and football, it was like, oh my God, it'll be like a second chance to do something that I've always wanted to do. My first thought was, am I too old?, but you have to try or you'll never know. When I first got out there I was like how can I stand out. For one, I have my size because you saw a lot of average girls out there. Then I found out who was the offensive line coach and I got right in their face, and he was like so you think you can play football and I was like just stand back and watch me.

There is certainly a need for large, athletic women on the team. There are not enough veterans or women trying out that fit this body type. Veterans often have to recruit large athletic players from their personal social networks. One player said that she scouts big athletic girls on her college campus. Likewise, Sue works at Wal-Mart and approaches customers that fit this ideal type. These recruiting methods are only partially successful. Due to prevailing cultural values on the body many large women do not view themselves as athletic. Professional football encourages women to stay large, but insists on training and conditioning, so large women are also good athletes – a previously unheard of possibility for Sue:

> When you grow up as a kid people judge you on the outside by the way you look. I got judged my whole life because I'm a big girl and I come from a big family. You saw my mom, my sister, and my dad was 6'4". He's a big guy too. I could do the splits. I could do back flips. I could do anything, but I wasn't a cheerleader because my body wasn't a cheerleader. I represent the big girls that are coming up. It's like on the team, you have small girls, big girls, and they don't look at you as any different. They need big girls on the offensive line. For the first time, somebody needs a big girl to play the sport. They don't judge me, they appreciate who I am and how big I am because without me they can't make a hold, they can't get a ball off.

Although Sue is a large woman and an aggressive player on the field, her persona off the field is much different. As Zurcher (1977) has argued, a successful person today must maintain a "mutable self" – the ability to be different persons in different settings and under different social conditions. Similarly, Sue is a modest and reserved person on the sidelines. On the field, she has the persona of a determined and aggressive athlete:

> I usually fight one time a year on the field. The very first year I got into a fight and I found out she was a professional boxer. She was 10 and 0, I lost the fight. I protect my quarterback, that's what the offensive line does. Another time a player came back and clipped my quarterback in the throat. That's just a cheap shot to me. She was walking back and I was gonna let her know that next time she needed to back up. I was gonna get her. And so I just shoved her up in the shoulder a little.

Sue has always had two personas. Like most women, she has had to learn to balance the two – being as female and being a female (fill-in-the-blank):

> Well, it's a job to do on the field, and at home it's a different job. And it's a blast on the field, you just put your game face on, you're not mom, you're Big Sue the football player. I love being aggressive on the field. You can take all your anger and frustrations on the field. If you've had a rough time, you can take it out on somebody. In elementary school I used to fight the boys.

Playing football has provided Sue with the relationships needed to create a comfortable yet secure sense of self:

People look at me and think what is she doing? Does she sit at the house and on the couch all day long? At work, some of the customers come in and give me the attitude of, I don't want to talk to you because you're just some fat person, and I'll either flash them my ring or say, hey how would you like to come to the Houston Energy football game or play for the Houston Energy, and you can see in their minds, attitude, and eyes that it's been changed. They're like, oh you play football, you don't just sit around the house. No, I don't sit around the house and eat bon bons, I get up and I work and I kick butt on the field. To me it's like I am who I am. Accept me or don't accept me. And being my size has added to that. And yeah I do want to be a size 12, but who knows. I don't know if I do. This is who I am. I don't think I could do the things that I do now if I was smaller. I can move furniture. I can get out there and mow. I take my life in my own hands. I think people are created for different things. I know I was created for football. That's God's way of telling me it's ok you messed up, you didn't play basketball, you decided to raise your family for 22 years and this is the way I'm going to repay you, I'm going to let you play women's professional football, and give you three rings for each of your kids. Exactly what I wanted to do I did. I have a ring for each one of my kids, and if I was small and petite they wouldn't have even looked at me for football, but they did. They were like big girl, hey. Because we're hard to find, somebody that's big and agile and mobile. And according to my doctor I'm in good shape. He says, I don't know why you're here you're in such great shape. So football has been good for my health and kept me in good shape.

As we can see, the body and self exist in a tightly reciprocal relationship. As Waskul (2002) notes, the presence of the body implies a self. Therefore, compliments given to the body reflect upon the self. In Sue's case, compliments on her body's performance level directly impact her sense of self. These comments are seemingly directly to the performance aspects of her body, not necessarily the aesthetic aspects as dictated by American culture. Thus, football provides rules for self-identity that allow Sue and other large women to win the battle of the self.

Other Football Bodies

As Bordo (1993:196) argues, "the desire for a more masculine body appeals to some women because it symbolizes power in the public arena and a revolt against maternity and restrictive definitions of femininity. Mainstream American culture idealizes women who are both supermen in their muscles and superwomen in their breasts." WPFL players compare and comment on their bodies to each other. These perceptions are ambiguous because of the ambiguity in their identity as women and football players. The women typically frame these comments in humour to protect themselves and each other from embarrassment:

We laugh at each other. We pick at them and they pick at us. They pick at me because the way my pants fit. Some people got some funny walks. The primpy girls, they still trying to swish, it's like, man, this is football – you better put a pimp in your step.

Being petite in football is the exception and rather undesirable, which is ironically the opposite of our general cultural view of women's bodies. A quarterback felt that she constantly had to prove herself because of her 5'3", 120 lb. frame:

> In football, it's been kind of a roller coaster. I come out to play football and I'm seen as small and puny. If I had a dollar for every time somebody said "you're too small to play quarterback, you're too short to be playing football," if I had a dollar, I wouldn't need a salary. There's a part of me that sometimes wants to scream, like, excuse me I am playing quarterback so just shut up about me being too small.

Another player, a defensive back, felt that her small stature was an asset. She noted that it helped her and she made her body type of 5' work to her advantage. "Sometimes the quarterbacks don't see me behind the receivers and they will throw it at them and I'm there to catch intercept." She also felt that whenever she did perform on the field, her team was more laudatory than they would be for a taller player:

> You get a good hit and it's like yeah, and they come around me especially because I'm so small and so like any hit, they're like "hell yeah!" Because these girls are huge and then there's little itty bitty me.

Athletic women need to eat for energy and endurance. In football they need size and strength to tackle and, consequently, the meaning of weight is renegotiated:

> I try to put on a little more weight when it comes to the season because I'm so small and I figure the bigger I am the more chance I have of making the tackle. I guess the lighter I've gotten, the harder it is to tackle. If I gain weight then I don't care. If it's in the middle of the season and it's what I need, then I don't care.

Football is different from other sports because of the uniqueness of each playing position. Because a different body type is ideal for various playing positions, the sport opens the door to the wide range of body sizes and types of female athletes:

> When you look at the offensive line, you see your bigger girls. Your defensive line also has your bigger girls. Your receivers are thinner, shorter, and taller, faster girls. So you kinda have a body type. Just scrolling through, you're not gonna see a body type, but when you put us into the positions we play, you'll find a body type. Maybe it's not as distinctive as the guys are, but there is a body type.

Although it may appear ironic, football may in fact provide the most democratic and open athletic experience of all sports for women. Whereas a woman needs her body to play effectively, she can escape many of the cultural constraints placed on women's bodies by experiencing it as a *subject* as well as an *object* (Merleau-Ponty 1962:1223).

Conclusions

We have provided some observations on self-identity work among professional female football players that illustrates the complexity of the body in that experience. Overall, the body drives the women's essential desire to "hit." Our key argument has been that these women can succeed in this violent sport by moving away from the constraints of traditionally experiencing their bodies as objects and moving towards the liberating experience as subjects. The latter approach is not only needed to play football, but is also valuable in constructing a self-identity that transcends all the roles the women must simultaneously juggle.

These women must learn how to make sense of and organizationally manage these new embodied experiences as adults, quickly and efficiently. The inner self of one who desires to hit, however, may have been with them throughout life under the guise of a different identity, such as that of *tomboy*. We occasionally heard respondents mention that they either felt like tomboys or were labelled tomboys as youths. As Martin (2002) notes in her stories about girls, while tomboys are tolerated and even enjoyed as children, once girls reach adolescence they are naturally expected to transform into feminine bodies, and to actualize this transition easily, and to continue to do so through womanhood. Girls who throw a ball "like a girl" may be those who try to imbed their embodiment into a hypermasculine culture. Future sociological research should focus on the emergence of self-identity of those girls – a few of whom may turn up as football players later in life – who hit "like a boy" on *their own terms*.

References

Bordo, Susan. 1993. *Unbearable Weight: Feminism, Western Culture, and the Body*. Berkeley: University of California Press.

Bourdieu, Pierre. 2001. *Male Domination*. New York: Polity Press.

Boutilier, Mary A. and Lucinda San Giovanni. 1983. *The Sporting Woman*. Champaign, IL: Human Kinetics Publishers.

Douglas, Jack D. and John M. Johnson (eds). 1977. *Existential Sociology*. New York: Cambridge University Press.

Janofsky, Michael. 1992. "Yamaguchi has the Delicate and Golden Touch". *The New York Times*, 22 February, p. 31.

Kotarba, Joseph A. 2005. "Professional Athletes' Injuries: From Existential to Organizational Analyses." in Kevin Young (ed.), *Sporting Bodies, Damaged Selves: Sociological Studies of Sports-Related Injury*. Boston: Elsevier. pp. 99–116.

Kotarba, Joseph A. and John M. Johnson (ed). 2002. *Postmodern Existential Sociology*. Walnut Creek, CA: Alta Mira Press.

Martin, Jessica. 2002. *Lizzy's Do's and Don't's*. New York: HarperCollins.

Merleau-Ponty, Maurice. 1962. *The Phenomenology of Perception*. (trans. Colin Smith.) New York: Humanities Press.

Straus, Erwin W. 1966. *Phenomenological Psychology*. New York: Basic Books.

Turner, Bryan. 1991. "Recent Developments in the Theory of the Body." in Mike Featherstone, Mike Hepworth and Bryan Turner (eds), *The Body: Social Process and Cultural Theory*, London: Sage. pp. 1–35.

Waskul, Dennis. 2002. "The Naked Self: Being a Body in Televideo Cybersex." *Symbolic Interaction*, 25, 2:199–227.

WPFL (http://www.womensprofootball.com/history.htm)

Young, Iris Marion. 1990. *Throwing Like a Girl and other Essays in Feminist Philosophy and Social Theory*. Bloomington: Indiana U Press.

Zurcher, Louis. 1977. *The Mutable Self.* Beverly Hills, CA: Sage.

Chapter 12

The Addict's Body: Embodiment, Drug Use, and Representation

Richard Huggins

How do we understand other people? How do we make sense of who they are and what they stand for? What do we know about others and how do we accumulate such knowledge? As Shutz argued, it is primarily through embodied presence and visual interpretation of the symbolic meanings associated with bodies that we come to have a sense of the other. Understanding these signifying cues is part of a complex hermeneutic process that is informed by the dialectical relation between bodies and the contexts in which embodiment takes place. For Richard Huggins such process takes on disconcerting twists when the other is the subject of fear, disgust, moral condemnation, and aesthetic stigma, as is the case with drug addicts. The body of the drug addict – through popular representations – becomes a spectacle of the grotesque, in virtue of embodying decay, decadence, physical weakness, and perhaps the moral panic of a sober, silencing majority, rather than an individual's self.

> Everyone knows what a junkie is supposed to look like: hollow cheeks, panda eyes, a haunted expression, wasted, decadent desperate. And yet, narcotic addiction, as a physiological or psychological condition is invisible. It offers no infallibly visible markers of its presence.
>
> Hickman (2002:1475)

This chapter has developed out of my interest in general and diffuse issues of crime and disorder as a social and practical problem. Over the last ten years I have spent considerable time working with those charged with bringing "order" to communities and individuals. At the same time I have also developed a significant interest in the cultural significance of crime and disorder and its representation in popular media and public discourses. Much of this focus has been on issues of drug use and, in particular, "heavy-end" drug use often associated with notions of addiction, for example, heroin and "crack" cocaine. Furthermore, such interest is also informed by a deep involvement in the practical issues of service delivery to drug users in the form of my involvement with three community drug agencies and close working with a range of statutory agencies.[1]

---

1   I am a Director and Trustee of the Substance Misuse Arrest Referral Scheme (SMART CJS) Ltd, Community, Action, Development Ltd and OUT, a pioneering user advocacy service.

Clearly the significance of drug use has a long, diverse and interesting history and many scholars have focused on the politics, significance and effects of drug control and drugs policies (Carnwarth and Smith 2002; Courtwright 2001; Gossop, 2000; Manderson 2005). This chapter is an attempt to get to grips with the "problem" of drugs but not as a problem of drugs and crime (Bean 2004; Seddon 2000) or drugs as a public health issue, instead I examine the cultural significance of drug use and the representation of drug use – addiction and associated issues – through discourses and images of the addict's body in popular media (also see Ferrell and Sanders 1995; Ferrell and Hamm 1998; Ferrell and Websdale 1999; Presdee 2000; Lalander 2003). In particular the chapter explores how representations of drug use and addiction work to construct the user as outsider and marginal subject to mainstream society through a focus on particular images and metaphors which tend to stress the abject body, bodily decay, and embodied "Otherness." This chapter analyses the ways in which representation of the addict's body contributes to both production of the idea and popular understandings of addiction, drug use, and contributes to a culture of control that can be said to characterize late modernity (Garland 2001; Reith 2004).

I offer here a hermeneutic analysis of images and discourses of drug use and drug addicted bodies contextualized in terms of historical, socio-cultural and political perspectives. The idea of addiction and the social practices and behaviours that accompany it are heavily reliant on particular themes that recur through and in the representation of drug use and the "addict." In this sense I am working from a tradition that regards the idea and meaning of addiction as socially constructed. Furthermore, as I will emphasize, the body of the addict plays a significant role in these representations and discourses and to some degree, this focus on the body and body parts accounts for the power of many representations of drug use. However, I also argue that representations and images of drug use in different popular cultural forms (for example, in public policy campaigns, literature, film and photography) reveal several themes that are central to the social construction of both addiction and of the addict's body. The body, body parts, and actions of the addict (such as injecting) are central to such representations. Furthermore, the addict's body acts as a kind of map for the (perceived) social significance of drug use and addiction. Indeed one maps onto the other and back again as the centrality of symbolic and representational form both enhances and is enhanced by the socially marginal location of the addict (Fraser 1996; Hunt and Derricott 2001; Meyers, 2004).

Reading Drug Use and the Everyday

One can identify a number of relatively consistent and persistent characteristics of drug use and addiction in popular cultural representations of drug use. First, the central focus of discourses about drug use tends to concentrate on the decaying body and, in particular, on the effects of drug use on the body's physical and psychological integrity and, as such, drug use is measured through its effects on the body. Second, the addict is represented as occupying the margins of society in both social and geographical terms. Third, the notion of the drug addict and user is often represented as an "Other," a consistent feature of cultural representation of addiction and drug use throughout the last two centuries (Kohn 1997). Fourth, representations of the addict focus on the body in ways that reflect both the perceived social otherness and marginality of the addict.

One approach to fears about and responses to drug use has been to stress the role played by moral panic in relation to the specific issue of illicit drug use and the more general issue of the prevalence of crime in society (Cohen 1972; Goode and Ben-Yehuda 1994; Hunt 1997). In such panics certain events, individuals or groups of individuals (such as youth gangs) are defined as a threat to societal values and interests (Cohen 1972). In these panic discourses specific and central roles are given to the mass media, and central political, social, and moral actors through which the "threat" is averted, diffused, or contained. There are some clear parallels; the social construction of drug use as a problem resulting in moral panics as reflected by specific fears about particular drugs and their use at specific times or, indeed, users themselves. Such examples could include the outbreak of "Reefer Madness" in the 1930s in the US (Sloman 1979; Goode and Ben-Yehuda 1994), crack panics in the 1980s (Reinarman and Levine 1997) or random drug violence (Brownstein 1995). Jenkins (1999) catalogues a range of "synthetic" panics across a range of man-made substances across the twentieth-century arguing that the role of symbolic politics is critical to understanding representations of drug use.

However, this model is limited in that it really only focuses on one aspect of the "drug problem" and tends to explain numerous and often diverse social phenomena in the same or similar ways – as panic responses either elite engineered or self-generated by an ignorant or inherently "conservative" general public. Although clearly linked to issues raised in this chapter, the moral panic explanation does not sufficiently explain the power and durability of representational images of drug use and addiction which characterize much popular media. It is important to recognize that representations of drug use are complex, often contradictory and ambiguous. On the one hand we all *know* what addiction is and what an addict looks like – but in reality very few of us actually do and as Hickman (2002) notes it is this very process of trying to make what is invisible visible that is significant.

It is clear that the penetration of drug-related images and drug discourses is now manifest and examples are numerous. For example, in November 2004 the *Buffalo ArtVoice*[2] ran an advertisement for Feel Rite: Fresh Markets informing the reader that their turkeys "don't do drugs". Simultaneously playing on a multiplicity of discourses from Reagan era "Just Say No" campaigns, to the humour (real or perceived) in actually doing drugs, especially in this case turkeys that, in lieu of Thanksgiving and Christmas, might well need some respite. Whilst all along, in actuality, the advertisement reassures us that Feel Rite turkeys are "pure, safe and organic". The Feel Rite campaign is reflective of a wide variety of representations of

---

2   This is a free paper available in Buffalo, NY, USA.

drugs and drug users in popular culture – including movies, television dramas and sitcoms, and music.

Importantly, such an example demonstrates not only the mainstreaming of certain images of drug use but also the fact that analysis of the representation of drug use in popular culture can not simply reflect one or other particular interpretation. It is a complex, ambiguous, and multi-levelled phenomena which lends to multiple readings. Drug use is increasingly located within the highly consumerist cultures of contemporary society, societies in which the body, itself, has become a "principal vehicle for ... consumerist desire" (Turner 1996:6). South (1999) argues that in recent years the whole issue of drug use in contemporary society has become more complex to analyze and understand due to changes in both the organization of everyday life and drug use as substance use has apparently become "normalized" (Parker *et al.* 1998; Shiner and Newburn 1997). For South (1999:3) drug use has ceased to be located at the margins of social experience and society and has, instead, become part of the "paramount reality of everyday life."

Against such a backdrop the significance of the cultural and political representation of drug use as a social and political issue with powerful and important impacts on the lives of individuals and social groups is manifest. There exists a potent relationship between the symbolic, metaphoric, emotional and representational that impacts directly on individuals and on our understanding of drug use and addiction. For Manderson (1995:799) the war on drugs is a war about emotional imagery and contested symbols, and in particular about the idea of the boundary "a matter crucial to the metaphysics and social organization of Western society" and if we are to fully understand discourses around drug use we must first "appreciate the aesthetic forces which influence attitudes to this question, and the symbolic meaning which is attached to the imagery of drugs." Indeed, it is the failure to recognize that we are dealing with the symbolic which "bedevils" both drugs users and legislative policy. Likewise for Campbell (2000:38) the significance of narratives and representations of drug use is clear:

> The narratives of drug discourse do not proceed as simple discussions of "fact," but instead assess the moral and symbolic value of particular paths and patterns of risk and blame. These stories must achieve the rhetorical effect of realism – "facts" must not overshadow the values and images they inflect.

The importance of the representation of addiction is amplified precisely because this is not a new development. Lindesmith's (1940) paper, "The Drug Addict as a Psychopath," aimed to discredit what he called the dominant theory of addiction at that time which suggested that before becoming addicts individuals were distinguished by physical or mental abnormality. Lindesmith provided sustained criticism of a number of studies which claimed to demonstrate the link between "abnormality" and drug use. In addition he challenged the strong association of illness with addiction, criticizing Sando Rado's notion of "pharmacothymia," a term referring to a kind of disease which consisted of the desire to ingest drugs in any form. Lindesmith hinted at the close relationship between professional, clinical, political discourses and how they map onto public accounts of the addict as weak. As Lindesmith (1940:919) noted, "Addicts, to a greater or lesser extent, have always been a pariah class which has not been in a position to refute any charges levelled against it."

Nearly 70 years later the war on drugs can still be characterized as the routinization of caricature which promotes worst case scenarios as the norm and sensationalizes drug use in the media (Reinarman and Duskin 1999). Representations of illegal drug use are often moralistic, fuelled by race, class and gender concerns (Beyerstein and Hadaway 1990) and media representations of drug users and traffickers continue to stress that those who are perceived as the "dangerous classes" such as racial minorities and as "Other" threaten the world order of white, middle-class protestant morality (Boyd 2002:387; Kohn 1997). In these ways representations and images of drug use and addiction can play a significant role in identifying and defining social problems and those seen as responsible for them. In the next section I will briefly discuss some of the recent developments in social and sociological theory which underlie this approach and examine the idea of the social construction of the both the body and drug use.

Understanding the Addict's Body

Drawing upon a structural-hermeneutic and phenomenological approach my analysis focuses on the ways by which we understand the "Other's" (the addict's) body through popular representations of addiction. In departing from transcendental phenomenology Schutz (1962) attempted to understand the alter ego by analyzing the ways in which the ego could make sense of fellow human beings without being able to directly access their consciousness. For Schutz (1962) the alter ego can only be understood in a "signitive" way, or in other words through signs and significations. Existing contextual and biographical knowledge about others is therefore put into intentional practice in the act of making sense of the alter ego, in this case the addicted body's mediated presence. Knowledge of the "Other" is always fragmentary and is characterized by multiple qualities of experience and even contradictions, because the process of interpreting the meanings of the "Other" through his/her signitive presence is, hermeneutically speaking, a dialectics of approximation dependent on the proximity of textual and contextual cues.

For Luckman (1983, and see also Berger and Luckman 1966:97–146) human social practice is inevitably interpretive practice; a practice which leads us to communicating with embodied others by way of "decoding" the signs of their embodied realities. But in order to come to terms with everyday life meanings we often rely on embodied habits of interpretation and perceptions. These habits tend to form the basis of our understanding of the "other". In this way, understanding of the "other" is never entirely new as, hermeneutically, the signitive presence of the "other's" body is always given meaning to in relation to the working of a historical context which forms the basis of interpretation. Thus, understanding the alter ego is a questionable act as the meanings given to the alter ego's body may or may not overlap with the alter ego's conscious experience of his/her being-in-the-world. Our (existential) desire to understand the alter ego's embodied presence is thus a matter of routine, but surprise as well, as our interpretations of the alter ego's motives for action alternate between the taken for granted and the novel, as the historical context for our interpretations of the alter ego's body as text, and signitive bodies change over time.

Metaphors and other heuristic tools aide the ego in understanding the alter ego. Turner's idea of the "somatic society" (Turner 1984, 1992, 1996, 2003) in which "our present political problems and social anxieties are frequently transferred to the body" (1992:1) is of particular significance in relation to the analysis of representations of drug use and addiction. As such the body can be seen to act as a metaphorical map of social problems and community, public space and in particular the margins (of the body and society) and the marginalized (bodies and social groups). The case of addiction is even more complex as – for many – drug use *is* an actual social problem and not simply a metaphorical one. But I maintain that the close relationship between representations, social meanings and actual practices conflate around notions of the addict in mutually reinforcing ways.

For Turner (2003:1) the body is a key site for social metaphors: "dominant concerns and anxieties of society tend to be translated into disturbed images of the body." Furthermore, body metaphors can illustrate the fact that the body provides a convenient and accessible metaphor for moral and political problems of society (Turner 2003). For Turner such a process has a long and detailed history traceable in the dark symbolism of the *danse macabre* as a response to the devastation of the social order caused by the Black Death, the paintings of Hieronymous Bosch in which the torments of the fifteenth century are expressed through "a series of images of bodily defecation in which the sinful beings of this world are finally expelled in the form of faeces, vomit and spew" (Turner 2003:3).

Thus, the body "offers a profound and rich source of metaphors, similes and modes of conceptualization of the crisis, hazards, dangers and paradoxes of individual collective existence" (Turner 1996:8). In such discourses the body and the fluids it contains and expels, or in the case of addiction ingest through consumption and injection, frequently act as metaphors and signifiers of order, disorder, orderliness, safety, danger and threat. If we extend such analysis we can identify a range of metaphors of drug use, including disease, demonization, weakness, flaw, and decay. Such metaphors and representations often reveal significant assumptions about normal (and "abnormal") behaviour. In this way the addict's body may be understood as an example of how the body can be understood as a set of maps and metaphors for the wider social body: the ravaged body of the addict is depicted in ways that aim to discipline and to promote anti-drug messages.

The significance of the work of Mary Douglas (1966) is central to much contemporary commentary on the body. For Douglas the relationship between the body and social order is critical and to some extent she sees the individual body as embodying the social body (also see Brook 1999). For Douglas understanding the significance of the human body is about understanding issues of boundaries and transgression of phenomenological bodily processes and fluids such as blood, semen, saliva and tears. In this analysis the human body is prone to leakages of bodily fluids which cross from inside to outside and permeate the fragile boundaries of social, cultural, moral, and corporeal order. As such leaky bodies signify transgression and disorder. As an offence against order, social ritual and behaviour is organized around containing or re-ordering.

Similarly, drug use can be seen as an offence against order and Douglas's approach helps explain the depth of the response to injecting drug users, the fascination with images of injecting use, and the concern with containment and contamination that often accompany representations of drug use. Now, whilst Douglas' work is clearly focused on the meaning of public ritual and taboo, it still seems relevant to reflect on the importance of the relationship between bodily order and social order and the significance of the addict's body in contemporary culture.

Douglas's central theme that disorganized bodies express social disorganization (see Turner 1996) is particularly relevant to a discussion of addicts and addiction who are officially represented as "problem" or "chaotic" users and as such are discursively constituted as dangerously disorganized in both drug use and lifestyle. Furthermore the transgression of boundaries by body fluids is a central feature of injecting drug use as blood issues from the hypodermic penetration of the skin and, interestingly, the transgression of the bodies' external boundaries is further achieved by the injection of a fluid *into* the body of the user. As Fitzgerald (2002:381) notes:

> At the level of the individual, the wounds are health-related; at the level of the community the images show a community in turmoil; at the level of the sovereign state, they show the political wounds that supposedly can be remedied by western democracy and global capitalism. The making visible makes the individual, the community and the state amenable for intervention.

Such analysis emphasizes the ways in which the larger social group, be it local or national community comes to be symbolized by the body and how discourses about the body can signify a number of tensions within the political and social order at any given moment. At this level the social or political body is a way of imagining the wider social or political area in anthropomorphic terms (Waldby 1996).

Katovich (1998:277) notes that although the focus of the "war on drugs" periodically changes, the images rarely do and he argues that the "reality of illegal drugs as social objects has always been dependent on how people agreed to define such objects" and the substantial meaning of illegal drugs emerges in the process of creating responses to them. For Hickman (2002:122) such strategies of envisioning addiction, of "rendering the invisible visible" do not emerge from a void. They have a long history which reflects a range of social and historical processes. For Hickman the representation of drug use can be charted through four distinct phases: from *definition* in the years 1870–1920 in which the "problem" of addiction emerges, through *demonization* during the 1920–1950s, the emergence of a *counter-discourse* in the 1950s and then a phase of *commercialization* or "heroin-chic" in the 1990s. Throughout these phases presentation of the drug user as "Other" is critical in representations of drug use and cultural products frequently demonstrate the composite effect of representations that place the war on drug outside of US or Western borders, construct the drug user and dealer as depraved and deranged and avoid engagement in the social, political and legal factors that shape drug use (Boyd 2002; Kohn 1997).

Representing Addiction: Order, Chaos and Community

In 2004 an anti-drugs campaign was launched across 17 London boroughs relying on billboards, public house beer mats, and flyers showing six pictures of American drug addict Roseanne Holland. The images were derived from police "mugshots" over an eight year period. These shots (Figure 12.1) map the physical effects and impacts of her drug use, her transformation from a "pretty blonde" to a "cadaver in a wig."[3] This Metropolitan Police campaign was directed at the capital's estimated 45,000 crack cocaine "addicts" with accompanying slogan "Don't let drug dealers change the face of your neighbourhood."[4]

This is a strong campaign, visually powerful and full of impact working on the basis that nothing can be worse for a woman than to lose her looks and prematurely age, but also importantly highlighting the metaphorical links between physical bodily damage

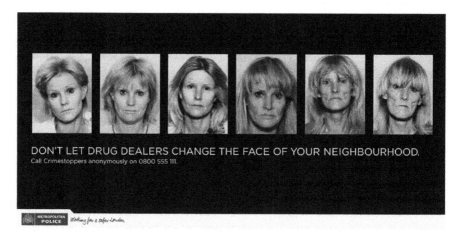

DON'T LET DRUG DEALERS CHANGE THE FACE OF YOUR NEIGHBOURHOOD.
Call Crimestoppers anonymously on 0800 555 111.

**Figure 12.1   Body Metaphor – Metropolitan Police Anti-Crack-Cocaine
            Campaign**
Copyright Metropolitan Police Authority 2004

---

3   See http://www.met.police.uk/drugs/advertising.htm.

4   The campaign also features two other American women: first, Melissa Collara from Florida, who was arrested 17 times between the ages of 18 and 21 for offences related to prostitution. Second, Penny Wood from Chicago charting her physical decline over a four year period. Interestingly Penny is reportedly a methamphetamine, not crack, user but let not detail stand in the way of a good metaphor. See http://www.met.police.uk/drugs/advertising.htm.

Special investigation

....

Chaos meets order – the result is tragedy

Figure 12.2 *Guardian Newspaper* **Headline Linking Drug Use, Tragedy and Chaos**
Copyright Guardian Newspapers Limited 2004

and community order and integrity. Furthermore, the campaign utilises a marketing strategy that draws on gender stereotypes emphasizing that drugs make individual women *look bad* rather than utilizing substances to enhance physical appearance. Such campaigns raise interesting issues about drug use and embodiment, bodily pleasures, and perceived risks. The campaign overtly links both bodily decay and community disorder through the representation of the (perceived) effects of individual drug use and the possibility of community decay and disintegration. Perhaps Cocteau (1990:62) was right when he argued that "Opium desocializes us and removes us from the community. Further the community takes its revenge. The persecution of opium addicts is an instinctive defence by society against an antisocial gesture."

Such use of representations of the female form is not new to anti-drug campaigns. In the 1940s the Federal Bureau of Narcotics also employed representations of women depicting the effects of addiction in very similar ways by utilizing forensic style photographs that depicted the passage of addiction from its start in 1937 through 1942 until the subjects' complete mental and physical breakdown in 1947. Hickman (2002), commenting on these FBI pictures, notes that if the physical marks are so obvious why do the FBI need to add the dramatic labels to tell us exactly how to read such pictures? He also notes that the image is deceptive: the model's skin around her eyes darkened to add further (though cosmetic) impression of wasting.

Such images are critical as they can be seen as categorising the drug user as someone who looks *like this*.[5] Fitzgerald (2002:380) argues that the particular faces produced in drug photography reproduce drug users as "strange, suffering and powerless victims," creating problems for drug users who may wish to deviate from the identity of suffering or mobilize new or different identities for political or other purposes and he notes that there is rarely a face "for an ordinary, living drug user, only a suffering or a monstrous, freakish, diseased Other."

As the front-page headline in Figure 12.2 and the image that accompanied it – of a ravaged, female addict staring at a half-filled syringe – from *The Guardian* newspaper[6] illustrates a key theme is how the image of the addict comes to represent

---

5   There is a long history of attempts to typify and categorize the "deviant" see, for example, Horn (2003), *The Criminal Body: Lombroso and the Anatomy Deviance*, New York: Routledge.

6   See *The Guardian*, Tuesday, 13th April 2004, page 1, guardian.co.uk.

a site of social order and chaos as reflected in bodily disorder and chaos. In what Fitzgerald (2002:369) calls "drug photography"[7] we can further explore the tensions, complexities, and problems of "making visible" a social problem (through, for example, social realism in film or documentary photography as well as the meanings of these representations, socially, politically, morally). As Fitzgerald (2002:374) argue, "There is a tendency in drug photography to attempt to make images of dark, seedy, secret worlds resulting in the 'Othering' of the individual and in the development of a range of pre-existing, citational images of drug use which then come to inform and define what might be called the landscape of authentic drug photography."

Figure 12.3 is one such image: the injecting drug user is portrayed as the ultimate symbol of both addiction as well as individual and collective moral, social, and political collapse. For Weimar (2003:268) the "symbols associated with addiction helped separate drug users from mainstream society. Arguably the most recognizable and powerful symbol of addiction is the hypodermic syringe, a symbol that denotes heroin addiction." The syringe is a potent symbol for a number of reasons, again in Weimar's (2003:268) words:

> First, the hypodermic needle violates the boundary between the body and the outside world. This violation is normal if an injection is related to a ... medical procedure. Yet, injection nullifies this normality because the voluntary introduction of an illegal substance into a person's bloodstream violates the "normal use" of a hypodermic needle. Moreover, instead of medication, an illegal pollutant is placed in the body. Thus, the ultimate boundary of the body plays a role in deciding what is normal and what is deviant because what one allows into the body contributes to identity formation.

Fitzgerald highlights images reflective of the work of Susan Watts (2002:376) who focuses on a day in the life of "Gloria," an injecting drug-using sex-worker whose body has become a "canvas of scabs, scars and disfigurations." Such images focus on bodily damage, depravation, blood and injection. As such, these images utilize dominant framing techniques and thus "rather than just depicting a technical method of drug administration, the images of the injecting scene has a number of functions" (2002:379). It can be a form of narrative disclosure, it can categorize, individualize or isolate a character. Importantly, the injection scene effectively distances the drug users from "normality." The power of the image of the injecting drug user is critical to establishing the absolute violation of self and the social. For many (Duterte *et al.* 2003; Manderson 1995; Vitellone, 2003) images of injecting drug use arouse immediate waves of discomfort and distaste as the syringe acts as the ultimate boundary violation, reinforcing Douglas's idea of pollution and taboo and as such delineate the boundary between social inclusion, exclusion and deviance.

---

7   For Fitzgerald this would include the work of John Ranard, Geoffrey Biddle, Larry Clark (1995), Nan Goldin (1989, 1993, 1996), Brenda Ann Keneally, Susan Meiselas, Eugene Richards (2000), Tyrone Turner and Susan Watts but could also be extended to include any photograph working in the documentary/social realist tradition with a focus on drug use such as 1998 Pulitzer (Photography) Prize winner Clarence J. Williams with his series of images entitled *Orphans of Addiction.*

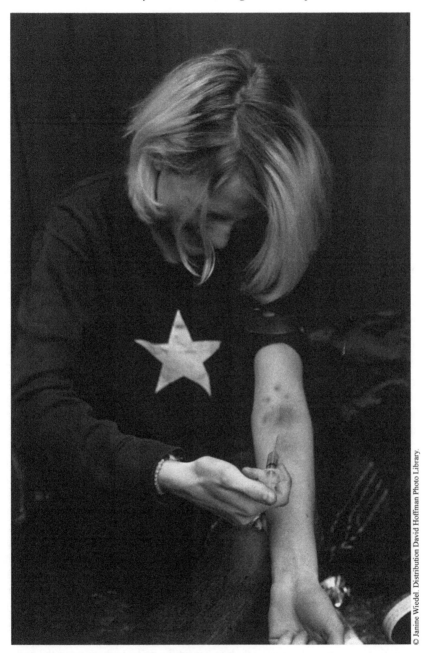

Figure 12.3 Symbolic Image of Drug Use

Conclusions

The representation of drug use and addiction, through the imagery and visual representation of the body is an important element of popular culture and public discourse. These representations have a variety of meanings which reflect ambiguous and sometimes contradictory views of drugs use and addiction and range from horror and abjection to celebration and fascination or, on rare occasions, apparent neutrality. It can be shown that certain popular representations map specific official, political, and moral discourses and agendas and importantly the addict's body can be seen to be utilized as a metaphor and symbol of social and moral decay and likewise social and moral decay is reflected in the marks left by drug use and addiction on the addict's body.

The textual representation of drug use and addiction through the imagery of the body is an important element of popular culture production and, as we have noted, such representations have a long and important history that is deeply contextual and situated within the growth of medical, political and moral discourses. In hermeneutic analytic fashion I have argued that such popular representations directly inform and are informed by particular social, moral and political agendas, not all of which are necessarily about drugs themselves – although drug use may become a signifier of other threats perceived to be embodied in certain social groups.

However, other representations are less directly clear. There appears to be some mileage in suggesting that the body is the central representational form or image, and the effects of drug use on the body's physical and psychological integrity. Furthermore, the addict is frequently represented as occupying the margins of society, including its social practices and groups – both social and geographical.[8] In some representations the addict's own self comes to occupy the margins of his or her own body. Representations of the addict as an "Other" are a consistent feature of both fictional and non-fictional representations and discourses of addiction throughout history (Boyd 2002; Kohn 1997; Reith 2004). Finally, representations of the addict focus on addiction, at the level of both the individual and collective body, and the physical and embodied experience of drug use.

In these ways "junky culture" and the image of the "junky", "crack-addict" and "smackhead" work as sets of multiple signifiers of multi-faceted deviance on to which all sorts of social discourses, anxieties and fears can be placed. Not just about drugs but about groups of people who are perceived as more threatening or, in this case, more likely to use, deal, or trade drugs. Whether we endorse, seek out, reject, or seek to control deviance, the notion of the junky, the user of needles, of spoons, of pipes, of "smack" or "crack" is instantly and readily understood as deviant. The addict is defined by, and with reference to certain substances in the body, the absence of will to resist, by the threat of disorder and lack of control – including the method of administration, and effects of such drug use on the body. In these ways the body of

---

8   For example Walsh's characters in *Trainspotting* (1993), Selby Jr's in *Requiem for a Dream (*1979), Burroughs' in *Junky* (1963) or Algren's, (2000), *The Man with the Golden Arm*, or more recently Elliot's *Happy Baby* (2005).

the addict, the activities of that body (real or imagined), and the marks on that body define or make real (or visible) the nature of "addiction" and the social implications of conventionally defined unruly behaviour. Furthermore, the accounts of the addict, fictional or non-fictional, rely on the body. More precisely they rely on gender differences and bodily metaphors for effectiveness. In order to communicate the story of addiction the narrator relies on the body to explain. But, equally, the social body of the community or nation is represented as threatened, through infection, corruption, disorder by the (injecting) drug user.

In the face of all the social anxieties and perceived threats located within and carried by the body, the regulation of drug use and availability is an issue that requires urgent control. The government of the body, similar to the processes outlined earlier by Turner (1996, 2003) have become increasingly crucial to notions of government and social order. Of course this does not occur at the level of national, regional, or even local government through the formal institutions of social order and control but more readily at the level of interaction and social construction by individuals and social groups – including the self – in the course of everyday life and communicative exchange. Indeed the quest for the well-regulated and "good" body is a critical element of the creation of body as a province of meaning (see Waskul and Vannini, this volume).

References

Algren, Nelson. 2000. *The Man with the Golden Arm*, Rebel Inc., Edinburgh.

Bean, Philip. 2004. *Drugs and Crime*, 2nd Edition, Cullompton, Willan Publishing.

Berger, Peter and Luckman, Thomas. 1966. *The Social Construction of Reality*, Garden City, New York: Anchor Books.

Beyerstein, Barry and Hadaway, Patricia. 1990. "On Avoiding Folly," *Journal of Drug Issues*, 20, 4:43–57.

Boyd, Susan. 2002. "Media Constructions of Illegal Drugs, Users and Sellers: A Closer Look at *Traffic*," *International Journal of Drug Policy*, 13:397–407.

Brook, Barbara. 1999. *Feminist Perspectives on the Body*, London: Longman.

Brownstein, Henry. 1995. "The Media and the Construction of Random Drug Violence," in Ferrell, Jeff and Sanders, Clinton (eds), *Cultural Criminology*, Boston: Northeastern University Press, pp. 45–65.

Burroughs, William. 1977. *Junky*, London: Penguin.

Campbell, Nancy. 2000. *Using Women: Gender, Drug Policy and Social Justice*, New York: Routledge.

Carnwarth, Tom and Smith, Ian. 2002. *Heroin Century*, London: Routledge.

Clark, Larry. 1995. *The Perfect Childhood* (ed. with Keller, W.), Zurich: Scalo.

Cocteau, Jean. 1990. *Opium: The Diary of His Cure*, London: Peter Owen.

Cohen, Stanley. 1972. *Folk Devils and Moral Panics : The Creation of the Mods and Rockers*, London: MacGibbon and Kee.

Courtwright, David. 2001. *Forces of Habit: Drugs and the Making of the Modern World*, Cambridge, Mass: Harvard University Press.

Douglas, Mary. 1996. *Purity and Danger*, London: Routledge.

Duterte, Micheline, Hemphill, Kristin, Murphy, Terrence and Murphy, Sheigla. 2003. "Tragic Beauties: Heroin Images and Heroin Users," *Contemporary Drug Problems*, 30:595–617.

Elliott, Stephen. 2005. *Happy Baby*, London: Picador.

Featherstone, Mike, Hepworth, Mike and Turner, Bryan. 1991. *The Body: Social Process and Cultural Theory*, London: Sage.

Ferrell, Jeff and Hamm, Mark (eds). 1998. *Ethnography at the Edge: Crime, Deviance and Field Research*, Boston: Northeastern University Press.

Ferrell, Jeff and Sanders, Clinton (eds). 1995. *Cultural Criminology*, Boston: Northeastern University Press.

Ferrell, Jeff and Websdale, Neil (eds). 1999. *Making Trouble: Cultural Constructions of Crime, Deviance and Control*, New York: Aldine De Gruyter.

Fitzgerald, John. 2002. "Drug Photography and Harm Reduction; Reading John Ranard," *International Journal of Drug Policy*, 13:369–385.

Fraser, Penny. 1996. "Social and Spatial Relationships and the 'Problem' Inner City: Moss-Side in Manchester," *Critical Social Policy*, 16:43–65.

Garland, David. 2001. *The Culture of Control: Crime and Social Order in Contemporary Society*, Oxford: Oxford University Press.

Goldin, Nan. 1989. *The Ballad of Sexual Dependency* (ed. with Heiferman, M., Holborn, M. and Fletcher, S.), London: Secker and Arburg.

_____. 1993. *The Other Side* (ed. with Armstrong, D. and Keller, W.), Manchester: Cornerhouse Publications in association with the D.A.A.D. Artists.

_____. 1996. *I'll be Your Mirror*, (curated by Sussman, E. and Armstrong, D.), New York: Whitney Museum of American Art; Scalo.

Goode, Erich and Ben-Yehuda, Nachman. 1994. *Moral Panics: The Social Construction of Deviance*, Oxford: Blackwell.

Gossop, Michael. 2000. *Living With Drugs*, 5th Edition, London: Ashgate.

Hickman, Timothy. 2002. "Heroin Chic: The Visual Culture of Narcotic Addiction," *Third Text*, 16:119–136.

Horn, David. 2003. *The Criminal Body: Lombroso and the Anatomy Deviance*, New York: Routledge.

Hunt, Arnold. 1997. "Moral Panic and Moral Language in the Media," *British Journal of Sociology*, 48, 4: 629–648.

Hunt, Neil and Derricott, Jon. 2001. "Smackheads, Crackheads and Other Junkies: Dimensions of the Stigma of Drug Use," in Mason, Tom, Carlisle, Caroline, Watkins, Caroline, and Whitehead, Elizabeth (eds), *Stigma and Social Exclusion in Healthcare*, London: Routledge, pp. 190–206.

Jenkins, Philip. 1999. *Synthetic Panics: The Symbolic Politics of Designer Drugs*, New York: New York University Press.

Katovich, Michael. 1998. "Media Technologies, Images of Drugs, and an Evocative Telepresence," *Qualitative Sociology*, 21, 3:277–297.

Kohn, Mark. 1997. "The Chemical Generation and its Ancestors: Dance Crazes and Drug Panics Across Eight Decades," *International Journal of Drug Policy*, 8, 3:137–42.

Lalander, Philip. 2003. *Hooked on Heroin: Drugs and Drifters in a Globalized World*, Oxford: Berg.

Lindesmith, Alfred. 1940. "The Drug Addict as Psychopath," *American Sociological Review*, 5, 6:914–920.

Luckman, T. 1983. *Life-World and Social Relations*, London: Heinemann.

Manderson, Desmond. 1995. "Metamorphoses: Clashing Symbols in the Social Construction of Drugs," *Journal of Drug Issues*, 25, 4:799–817.

Marez, Curtis. 2004. *Drug Wars: The Political Economy of Narcotics*, Minneapolis: University of Minnesota Press.

Meyers, Marian. 2004. "Crack Mothers in the News: A Narrative of Parternalistic Racism," *Journal of Communication Inquiry*, 28, 3:194–216.

Musto, David. 1991. "Opium, Cocaine and Marijuana in American History," *Scientific American*, 265, 1: 20–27.

Parker, Howard, Aldridge, J., and Measham, F. 1998. *Illegal Leisure: The Normalization of Adolescent Recreational Drug Use*, London: Routledge.

Presdee, Mike. 2000. *Cultural Criminology and the Carnival of Crime*, London: Routledge.

Reinarman, Craig and Duskin, Ceres. 1999. "Dominant Ideology and Drugs in the Media," in Ferrell, Jeff and Websdale, Neil (eds), *Making Trouble: Cultural Constructions of Crime, Deviance and Control*, New York: Aldine De Gruyter, pp. 73–90.

Reinarman, Craig and Levine, Harry (eds). 1997. *Crack in America: Demon Drugs and Social Justice*, Berkeley: University of California Press.

Reith, Gerda. 2004. "Consumption and Its Discontents: Addiction, Identity and the Problems of Freedom," *British Journal of Sociology*, 55, 2:283–300.

Richards, Eugene. 2000. "Crack Annie," *Aperture*, 160, Summer, p. 2.

Schutz, Alfred. 1962. *Collected Papers I: The Problem of Social Reality* (ed. Maurice Natanson), The Hague: Martinus Nijhoff.

Seddon, Toby. 2000. "Explaining the Drug-Crime Link: Theoretical, Policy and Research Issues," *Journal of Social Policy*, 29, 1:95–107.

Selby Jr., Hubert. 1996 [1978]. *Requiem for a Dream*, London: Marion Boyars.

Shiner, Michael and Newburn, Tim. 1997. "Definitely, Maybe Not? The Normalisation of Recreational Drug Use amongst Young People," *Sociology*, 31, 3:511–529.

Sloaman, Larry. 1979. *Reefer Madness: A History of Marijuana*, New York: St. Martin's Griffin.

South, Nigel. 1999. *Drugs: Cultures, Controls and Everyday Life*, London: Sage.

Turner, Bryan. 1984. *Body and Society*, Oxford: Blackwell.

_____. 1991. "Recent Developments in the Theory of the Body," in Featherstone, Mike, Hepworth, Mike and Turner, Bryan (eds), *The Body: Social Process and Cultural Theory*, London: Sage.

_____. 1992. *Regulating Bodies: Essays in Medical Sociology*, London: Routledge.

_____. 1996. *Body and Society*, 2nd Edition, London: Sage.

_____. 2003. "Social Fluids: Metaphors and Meanings," *Body and Society*, 9, 1:1–10.

Vitellone, Nicole. 2003. "The Syringe as Prosthetic," *Body and Society*, 9, 3:37–52.

Waldby, Catherine. 1996. *AIDS and the Body Politic: Biomedicine and Sexual Difference*, London: Routledge.

Weimar, Daniel. 2003. "Drugs-as-a-Disease: Heroin, Metaphors, and Identity in Nixon's Drug War," *Janus Head*, 6, 2:260–281.

Welsh, Irvine. 1999. *Trainspotting*, Vintage/Minerva: London.

PART 4
The Socio-Semiotic Body:
Body as Trace of Culture

Chapter 13

Body Ekstasis: Socio-Semiotic Reflections on Surpassing the Dualism of Body-Image

Phillip Vannini and Dennis D. Waskul

Psychological and social psychological literature on body image, as Phillip Vannini and Dennis Waskul argue, has been unaffected by the somatic turn in the social sciences. Despite its potential for applicability across analytical domains within the sociology of the body, the concept of body image continues to be affected by a variety of dualisms that subjugate it to a logic of Cartesian heritage. The solution is simple, Vannini and Waskul argue, sociologists of the body need a new concept that reflects the active role played by social agents in constituting representations of the body to the self and others. Drawing from Peircean semiotics and Dewey's pragmatist deconstruction the concept of body, "ekstasis" attempts to capture semiotic and social relations that transcend binary oppositions and forms of determinism.

Traditional psychological and social psychological approaches to the study of body-image are vitiated by a variety of serious problems. The concept of body-image – defined as "the picture of our own body which we form in our mind" (Slade 1994:497) – is made inadequate by scholars' reliance on a host of dualisms which permeate Western culture writ large. Such dualisms include the dichotomies of body and mind, of individual and society, and of materialism and idealism. In this chapter we suggest surpassing dualism by way of theoretical reflection and articulation of an alternative concept. After fleshing out our criticism we propose a new non-dualist understanding of body-image that draws from the pragmatist philosophy of John Dewey and the semiotics of Charles Sanders Peirce. Our goal is not only to produce a more robust conceptualization liable to generate more refined empirical insight, but also posit a more solid foundation for coherent cultural criticism.

Decomposing Body-Image: The Decay of Dualism

Dualism is an ideology as old as Western civilization itself (Synnott 1993). As Synnott reported, ideas, values, and meanings associated with the human body are particularly subject to dualist thinking. It is no accident that such ideology has been at the intellectual core of the genesis and historical development of Western medicine, psychology, religion, and many of the patriarchal discourses and institutions of our society that contribute to the regulation, control, and fabrication of bodies (Synnott 1993).

At its core, dualism is a semiotic accomplishment (Derrida 1967). The dualist assumption is a juxtaposition of dichotomous terms within a system of signification that manufactures difference, which is then presumed to create meaning. This ontological view of meaning is typical of theoretical perspectives founded upon the semiology of Saussure, such as the structuralist anthropology of Levi-Strauss as well as Parsonian structural-functionalism in sociology. Indeed, Saussure's semiology was instrumental in reifying dichotomization to the status of positive science (Hodge and Kress 1988).[1] As Derrida (1967) argued, the binary oppositions which structuralists presume to constitute the essence of culture are in actuality nothing but intellectual gambits operating upon the unquestioned assumptions of dualism and the metaphysics of presence. The foundational status of dualism, therefore, is but an illusion.

Semiotically speaking, body-image – as conceptualized within mainstream sociology, social psychology, and clinical psychology – is a signifier. Certainly, body-image signifies different referents for different groups of scholars. For clinical psychologists an individual's body-image has as its referent an ideal, generalized, normal or healthy body-image. For psychological social psychologists – much like for clinical psychologists – an individual's actual body-image is often the distorted representation of a real and undistorted body concept that an individual *should* have, on the basis of how s/he "really" is. Sociologists suggest that a person's body-image is understood as the incarnate representation of ideologies of beauty, gender, age, physical ability, and sexual preference. Nonetheless, in spite of a diversity of discourses, these various disciplinary arguments insist the same point: body-image – especially when it is distorted, unhealthy, or negative – is nothing but a reflection or representation of a reality existing outside the individual's mind and body. Let us take a closer look at some of these perspectives.

Body-image in Psychology

"Body-image" cannot be understood apart from the procedures used to measure it. Not only do these procedures highlight the epistemological underpinnings of how we can know the body but by specifying dimensions and indicators of body-image they also shed light on how the body and body-image are ontologically fashioned. Clinical and social psychology employ two measures of body-image: perceptual and subjective/attitudinal (see Thompson 1990, 1996).

---

1 For Saussure the most elementary unit of difference – which stood as the basic ontological genesis of all forms of difference – was the relation between a signified and a signifier. A signifier is a sound-image of a signified, that is, a mental concept invoked by a signifier. Within this idealist model the unity of signifier and signified – regardless of the materiality or lack thereof of the signified – constitutes a sign.

Perceptual assessments test an individual's ability to accurately gauge body size. Three main types of assessment are used: whole-image adjustment, body-site adjustment, and perceptual measurement with weight categories. In experiments conducted through whole-image assessments researchers produce a set of distorted photographs of a person's body, then ask a research participant to select amongst the distorted images which one more closely resembles his/her actual body. The more distant a subject's choice from the accurate photograph, the more distorted his/her body-image. In contrast, experimental psychologists who use body-site adjustment procedures ask participants to estimate the size of their body parts. Body-image is once again assessed in relation to the deviation of participants' estimates from objective measures. Finally, studies conducted by use of perceptual measurement with weight categories utilize weight categories (e.g. underweight, overweight, normal weight) as benchmarks for subjects' self-assessments. Individual assessments are contrasted with researchers' objective assessments and, once again, body-image is derived from the contrast between an external objective referent and an internal (i.e. cognitive) representation.

Perceptual assessments are more common in clinical research. Subjective assessments of body-image are frequent in social psychology – in both sociology and psychology. Subjective assessments assume a variety of methodological forms including scales, questionnaires, and somatomorphic matrices. The basic mechanism underlying these assessments is a reflexive, cognitive, and affective self-evaluation. Studies utilizing subjective assessments generally focus on body-image as a precursor of body dissatisfaction. Dissatisfaction with appearance is often studied in conjunction with behavioural investments in appearance, attitudinal judgements, and other somatic domains, including dimensions of health and fitness. Common amongst these studies, as well as studies utilizing perceptual assessments is a rigid distinction between procedures measuring emotional and cognitive indicators (Thompson and Altabe 1991; Thompson and Dolce 1989).

Psychological research has been pivotal in claims-making efforts aimed at elevating issues of body dissatisfaction – broadly defined – to wide acceptance amongst social scientists and the general public. Psychologists have been particularly adamant about stressing the psychiatric and psycho-somatic problems associated with a negative body-image, such as depression, self-harming behaviour, disordered eating and fasting, and so forth. Nevertheless, the conceptualization of body-image prevalent in psychology suffers from the shortcomings of a dualistic outlook of body and mind, as well as individual and social.

Hermeneutic approaches to science and epistemology have long argued that the intellectual development of academic disciplines and theoretical paradigms is inevitably shaped by socio-historical context (e.g. Foucault 1973). Psychology is no exception. Despite claims to value-neutrality, universality, and objectivity, modern psychology is deeply entrenched in a typically Western outlook on the relation between individual and society. Feminist critics, among others, have pointed out that psychology's main bias resides in the overly individualist characterization of subjectivity – an individualist bias that risks turning psychology into an oppressive tool rather than an emancipatory agent (see Wolszon 1998).

The philosophy of individualism runs deep throughout the history of Western civilization. Conflated with liberalism, individualism posits the original ontological and moral separation of individuals from one another and from the social. Such bifurcation of individual and society is then justified as the foundation of civic and human rights of self-determination. Individualism theorizes the subject as an autonomous terminal of free will – whose only restrictions must come at the intersecting point with other individuals' freedom. In individualist ideologies persons are motivated by self-interest, and action is understood as an instrumental repertoire of behaviours oriented toward maximization of pleasure.

Most psychological research and theory posits human development as a life-course quest toward autonomy, often understood as a healthy separation from the dysfunctional forces exercised by familial, sexual, or cultural constraints. Psychotherapy's goal is, by no accident, the liberation of the individual from oedipal struggles and the shackles of early, or even innate, tendencies toward dependence on others. Also typical of psychological research is the decontextualization of persons from one another and from the greater realms of the cultural and social (especially characteristic of experimental psychology), as well as the reification and dichotomization of constructs (affective vs. cognitive, behavioural vs. attitudinal levels of observation, etc.). Thus, on the surface, psychological research on body-image takes into account the strength of "social" forces (whether in the form of peer pressure, parental influence, media exposure, etc.), upon closer inspection these approaches implicitly hinge on individuals who (fail to) resist and reject these appeals. Despite the strength of culture and society as an "independent variable," and despite the individual's status as nothing but a dependent variable, much of psychology demands that we exert individual resistance – therefore effectively turning the person into the sole agent responsible for one's moral and physical health. As Wolszon (1998:546) insightfully asks: "how can we be so embedded in culture and yet so able to detach ourselves from it?"

The individualist bias of this type of psychology is further exacerbated by individuals' internalization of supposedly deleterious traits. For example, the dysfunctional effects of undue exposure to nefarious magazines, television, Hollywood imagery, and pop culture discourses may be magnified by individual susceptibility, inaccurate perception, or perhaps by the presence of certain personality traits and dispositions such as tendencies to perfectionism or irrational thought. Here it is the dualism of stimulus and response – which Dewey (1896) criticized in his paper on the reflex arc concept in psychology – that pre-empts a comprehensive and organic understanding of embodiment by reducing organic interaction to a "patchwork of disjointed parts [and] a mechanical conjunction of unallied processes" (Dewey 1882–1898, 5:97). Thus conceived, people are reduced to psycho-cultural dupes. Or to put it in semiotic terms, people turn into signifiers – lies, standing for something they are not.

Body-Image in Sociology

Within much of sociology the concept of body-image tends to lose the definitive boundaries typical of psychological constructs and becomes conflated with a loosely embodied version of the self-concept, as well as with body-imagery in general.[2] In other words, it tends to lose its external and internal validity. Not all sociologists partake in this form of intellectual poaching, whereby an operational measure endemic to one discipline is preyed upon by another, causing the purity of the original concept to be lost. For some researchers within social psychology, the experimental and paper-and-pencil measures typical of psychological research exert great appeal, and their scholarship can hardly be distinguished from the mainstream approaches in psychology. Yet, for the majority of sociologists interested in issues of body-image, feminist theory is the true beacon of light and the exact interest is not a precise measurement of body-image, but instead the broader issue of embodied inequality. There is, of course, an enormous variety of feminist approaches to the body (for a review see Howson 2005), but despite the sophistication of some of these, for many feminists body-image is still vitiated by a number of dualisms. Let us look for example at the theory of Susie Orbach (1988) and Kim Chernin (1983) whose works are quite influential in sociology.

For both Orbach and Chernin women's bodies are fundamentally different from men's. These natural differences provide the basis for the evolution of patriarchal systems, which in turn magnify the shaping of men's and women's bodies in differing and unequal ways. Orbach and Chernin not only suggest innate body differences between men and women, they also believe that bodies have natural sizes and shapes, which are then distorted by social forces. For example Orbach (1988) finds that some women engage in compulsive eating because their natural feeding patterns are disrupted by oppressive ideologies produced and distributed by the media and the beauty industry. Whereas becoming thin is a form of normative conduct, becoming fat for Orbach is a symbolic reaction against a phallocentric system which continuously distorts women's body-image. Not only is there an obvious form of gender dualism at work here, but also a significant dichotomization of culture and nature, body and mind, as well as individual and society (not to mention a gross homogenization of internal differences among men and women). As Shilling (2003: 59, emphasis in original) remarks "for Orbach, *thin* is natural, while fat is distortion." Hence, even though bodies are subject to change, such change always occurs in a dualist and causalistic pattern of unidirectional influences: society forces individuals to become adjusted (i.e. co-opted) or maladjusted, minds generate ideologies that mould bodies after their fantasies, and females are nothing but the passive victims of male desire.

---

2   Within much of sociology body-imagery refers to the circulation of images and discourses of and about the body in the mass media and public discourses and while it does not always get at an individual's introspective assessment of physical appearance, research on body-imagery uses a variety of indicators (some quantitative, some qualitative) to suggest that many people are dissatisfied with their body.

Equally concerned with body dissatisfaction is Kim Chernin (1983) who ponders how and why women become sufferers of a tyranny of slenderness which impairs their natural development and self-growth. Chernin shares many of the same themes of Orbach's position. Women, as opposed to men, fail to take pride in their bodies and become obsessed with weight loss and other forms of appearance management. Also similar to Orbach's (1988) analysis, women's negative body-image is nothing but the result of men's oppressive politics, this time emerging as a response to the threat represented by women's innate parental connection. Much like Orbach, Chernin's arguments are vitiated by essentialism; women's and men's bodies are naturally different from one another, and culture and society are seen as negative forces distorting biological realities and individual development. This is dualism at its clearest.

Chernin and Orbach are not the only influential theorists to deal with body-image, of course. Yet, their approach to the body is exemplary and symptomatic of the general preference amongst empirical sociologists to treat the body as an *object* of action. As we said earlier, from a semiotic perspective, body-image – as the name itself suggests – is but the signifier of a referent to which it is tightly coupled. Whereas many psychologists (including Chernin and Orbach) commit the mistake of seeing the individual as primordial, many sociologists incur in the opposite error of structural determinism, whereby issues as diverse as class standing (e.g. Bourdieu), discourse (e.g. Foucault), and social order (e.g. Turner 1984) literally *make* the body and body-image a social and semiotic by-product of joint action.

As our critique illustrates, across psychology and sociology the concept of body-image suffers from a variety of dualisms that do little justice to the body's polysemy and creative force. In the following section we suggest a socio-semiotic reformulation of body-image that treats the body not only as a sign vehicle, but as "sense," and how this approach can renovate interpretive sociological interest in this important concept.

Ekstasis and the Ecstatic Body

Body-image research traditionally fails to explain how body-image is constituted and why a negative body-image has increasingly become a "normative discontent" (Wolszon 1998:545). Such problems originate, in part, due to the psychological and sociological tendency to treat "body-image" as a definite concept, rather than a sensitizing one. A sensitizing concept "gives the user a general sense of reference and guidance in approaching empirical instances. Whereas definitive concepts provide prescriptions of what to see, sensitizing concepts merely suggest directions along which to look" (Blumer 1954:7).

Regarding body-image as a sensitizing concept ought to enable a broadening of conceptual and methodological horizons, and in turn allow us to better understand the social and semiotic processes by which body-image is constituted. A sensitizing conceptualization of body-image ought to help in rejecting conceptualizations and methods that are overly-individualistic, de-contextualized, and overly-cognitive. We are suggesting an abandonment of traditional methodological procedures of studying body-image, the rejection of body-image as a definitive concept, and an updating of our understandings – all in a framework that surpasses the various forms of dualistic thinking attached to it. As our previous critique illustrates, the concept of "body-image" fundamentally owes to problematic dualisms. We therefore propose a fresh concept, namely an *ecstatic* formulation of the body (from the ancient Greek *ekstasis*). An ecstatic formulation of the body emphasizes the active, interactive, and transactive state of ekstasis – being at once both inside and outside one's self, body, and society and in virtue of doing so annihilating those boundaries. Ekstasis entails *the qualitative evaluation of the aesthetic potential of one's body*.

Body ekstasis has several advantages over body-image. First, the concept of body-image does not adhere to its application. An image is most often an icon – in the classic Peircean differentiation among indexes, icons, and symbols (Peirce 1958; also see Rochberg-Halton 1982). Iconic signs are embodied representations of the object they represent. In other words, icons express something by referring to themselves, like musical notes or facsimiles. Despite this, traditional approaches to body-image patently disregard the iconic quality of body-imagery, and instead treat body-image as a symbol – which conveys meaning via a rule-based association with an object. Ekstasis, on the other hand, is not only perceived and interpreted, it is fundamentally somatic and aesthetic; the ecstatic body is fully amendable to symbolic, indexical, and iconic meaning.

Second, the word "image" clearly connotes a *visual* concept. Emphasis on the visual is problematic at a multitude of levels. The primacy of sight is clearly linked to cultural and historical biases in which sight reigns as the supreme sense (Synnott 1993). This is clearly observed in our folks sayings such as "seeing is believing," "I'll believe it when I see it" – each suggestive of sight as the ultimate empirical verification – thus lending merit to urge disbelievers to "see for yourself" (Synnott 1993:207). Indeed, in these ways and many more (see Synnott 1992) the privileged status of sight is directly linked with the most privileged of human faculties – knowledge and reason. Thus, for related reasons, the cultural supremacy of sight partially owes to the emergence of the modern world, and further represents a somatic consequence of a continued androcentric bias. In other words, to reduce the aesthetic evaluation of one's corporeality to the visual is a particularly male logic; the politics of the gaze are decidedly gendered: the gaze "is political surveillance, control, domination and power" (Synnott 1993:222). Furthermore, image, in this sense, connotes an overly-static mental *picture*. Sight is certainly important to the ecstatic body which, by virtue of a self, engages in body *imaging* – an active and reflexive rendering of the body as a visible object, materially *and* in one's mind. However, sight is but one sense that constitutes the ecstatic body.

Third, body-image smacks of Cartesian dualism: "I think about my body, therefore my body *is*." Or, alternatively, "I have a thought about my body, therefore I have a body." The problem with the concept of image is that traditional research regards the body as a sign-vehicle, or representation, of the object created in one's mind. As said, conceived this way body-image is nothing but the signifier of a mental concept. Not only is this a problem in terms of dualism, but it is also over-reliant on idealism and solipsism. Body-image connotes nothing but a ghost in the machine. In contrast, ekstasis is transactive and denotes obliteration of the alleged boundary between mind and body, self and body, and body and the bodies of others. Ekstasis is a fluid state of being and becoming. Moments of ekstasis may be beyond reason and self-control, a state of intense exaltation of emotionality and somatic sensitivity that alters mood, cognition, and action.[3]

In many cultures ekstasis is also a departure from the spatial limitations of one's body by way of embracing fusion with the divine or with other bodies. Without suggesting that ekstasis is necessarily a mystical experience we are positing here that the ecstatic body has the power to implode the artificial differences between body and mind, self and others, emotion and cognition, pre-reflexive and pre-linguistic sensation and linguistic reflexivity, as well as perception and action – perhaps even the boundary between this world and another. Let us examine some of the characteristics of the body-ekstasis.

Habit and Meaning: Ekstasis as Evaluation

Our first contention is that ekstasis is evaluative. The ecstatic body is a habitual body; old and new habits are the emergent outcomes of non-dualistic processes of transactive evaluation – the starting point of this argument is Dewey's idea of organic interaction, or transaction. For Dewey (1925, 1934) self and world, mind and body, and subject and object cannot be specified in isolation from one another. Transaction is the concept that Dewey employs to describe the relationship of codetermination of experiencing and experienced. For him such relationship "was a single structure, not two separate, discrete structures which somehow causally 'act' upon one another" (Kestenbaum 1977:1). Dewey recognized that consciousness was not something first existing in itself and only later entering into a relationship with something else. Indeed Dewey's (1929:294) belief that "the characteristic human need is for possession and appreciation of the meaning of things" led him to suggest that meanings are "had" before they can be known, or in other words they are sensed in qualitatively immediate ways that are distinct from, and preconditions of, reflexive knowledge.

People sense and evaluate the immediacy of meanings through the operation of habit (Dewey 1922; also see Kestenbaum 1977). The concept of habit allows

---

3   The concept of the ecstatic or ecstatic body is not a new one. Leder (1990:11–35) discusses at length how "as ecstatic, the body projects outside itself into the world" (1990:69). Significantly, Mead (1934:273–281) recognized the significance of ekstasis in remarkably similar terms, however without using the term. Ekstasis is implicit in moments of "fusion" of the "I" and the "me," which Mead described as "particularly precious" situations that lead to "intense emotional experiences" of a kind and quality that he likens to religious and patriotic exaltation: "This, we feel, is the meaning of life."

us to surpass the binary of freedom vs. determinism. As Crossley (2001:136–137) explains, habits are forms of embodied creative agency shaping meaningful and purposive conduct arising out of the "interaction between the organism or agent and the world." However, habits are also the "result of imitation" (Crossley 2001:137) and the crystallization of historical meaning and value. Habit plays a pivotal role in Dewey's philosophy of embodiment and selfhood. For Dewey (1922:40–41) "habit:"

> express[es] that kind of human activity which is influenced by prior activity and in that sense acquired; which contains within itself a certain ordering or systematization of minor elements of action; which is projective, dynamic in quality, ready for overt manifestation; and which is operative in some subdued form even when not obviously dominating activity.

Habits constitute the basic nature of the embodied self (Dewey 1922:25) and the basic nature of the body-mind unity, as well as the organic unity with bodies-minds of other people.

Body-ekstasis, we contend, is a form of habit. I am my own ecstatic body in that all I sense, feel, or think "emerges out of behaviours which follow a habituated pattern" (Crossley 2001:140). As a form of habit, body-ekstasis is nonetheless a form of motion; it is indeed the potential for both stasis (old habit) and movement beyond stasis (new habit). The ecstatic body indeed emerges by becoming committed to its future projects. Again, following Crossley (2001: 140), there are old habits and "'habit-busting' habits; habits which both equip and incline me to question and change the way in which I live my life." This is so because habits are reflexive, in that they enable us to turn to our embodied self as an object of reflection and action, when old habits get "busted" and replaced with new ones. This happens, for example, when the evaluative processes underlying ekstasis lead to the person's adopting and engaging in new forms of body maintenance and modification, or reflexive body techniques (Crossley 2005). Out of such ekstasis also emerges another stasis: as a habit of sensing the potential of one's body that remains temporarily stable until another movement of ekstasis gathers up speed. Such structure (stasis) and anti-structure (ekstasis) of experience is a continuous process of development "from a state of wholeness to a state of wholeness by way of an intervening phase of reconstruction" (Alexander 1987:127). Yet, this is not a simple or even a teleological progression from automatic routine to automatic routine via mechanical reintegration. Rather, such is the very temporal condition of experience "as a total field of action which has a complex structure at each and every moment and different degrees of focus, clarity, obscurity, and organization... by increasing articulation, illumination, meaning, and apprehension" (Alexander 1987:127). Ekstasis is temporally dynamic, yet ordered.

Habits are reflexive, but because they are impulsive they are also pre-objective and pre-reflexive (see Alexander 1987:136–137). Humans are sense-giving, sense-having beings who operate on a level of access to the world that is firstly immediate and meaningfully tacit. For Halton (2004:90) it is through the "breathing, palpitating, bodily awareness of the situation [that] the spontaneous soul is brought to bear on life." Through this organic interaction "the living gesture bodied forth in the signifying moment [connects] with the very conditions out of which the human body evolved into its present condition" (Halton 2004:90). It is at this pre-reflexive level that habits first operate – thus temporally preceding linguistic formulation, reflexive consciousness, and deliberate critical knowledge. Hence, it is at this level that ekstasis is originally constituted and *then* shaped throughout processes of linguistic reflection; the constitution of the ecstatic body is coterminous with the genesis of the embodied self. As the infant develops embodied habits, and therefore a rudimentary sense of self, s/he learns to sense the bodies of others and one's own. That sensing is of course pre-linguistic and only crypto-reflexive. Yet, it is creative by definition because it creates the conditions of existence of the ecstatic body by making sense of embodied self, others, and the world.

The infant's sensing habits are aesthetic in nature. Recall that the meaning of the word "aesthetic" is rooted in the Greek word for "sense" and "perception." This sensing is also evaluative. As infants sense their being-in-the-world they evaluate the immediate qualities of objects in relation to their potential for meaning and value. A parental face and touch, for example, is sensed and evaluated for the comfort it brings to the body. Recognition of others – following this argument – is therefore firstly aesthetic.

As the perception of one's body and others' becomes more and more reflexive something else happens. In addition to developing habitual and reflexive knowledge about the ecstatic body on the basis of the interpretation and internalization of others' evaluations of us (Cooley 1902; see Part One of this book), the embodied self also communicates his/her aesthetic evaluation of others' bodies to those others. This can be as simple as an infant crying in the presence of a stranger, or as complex as a group of friends organizing an intervention to persuade a dear one to lose weight or stop smoking. The process of constitution of ekstasis is thus parallel not only with the somatic constitution of body, self, and society, but also with the constitution of physical inequality, via differential evaluation of the unequal aesthetic potential of others' bodies. More on this later.

The Aesthetic and Qualitative Nature of the Ecstatic Body

Our second contention is that ekstasis is an aesthetic experience. In other words, in suggesting that the constitutive process of ekstasis relies on the immediacy of sense and therefore on qualitative immediacy we are arguing that the ecstatic body is aesthetic in nature. Dewey (1934) used the word "esthetic" or "aesthetic" to denote not art, but instead the consumption of the inherent quality of an act, situation, or object (see Rochberg-Halton 1982). In Dewey's anti-dualist thinking this conceptualization of aesthetics avoided any undue distinction between the object of aesthetic evaluation and the perceiving subject. In fact, in the case where the aesthetic quality of an object is believed to either "lie in the eye of the beholder" or in the object itself (on the basis of objective aesthetic standards or conventions), beauty is respectively thought as either a subjective or objective experience. But if we understand an aesthetic evaluation to emerge as a *transaction* between the unique and immediate qualities of an object and the unique ways of sensing that object, then aesthetic evaluation is a holistic experience and the ecstatic body is in therefore an emergent intersubjective accomplishment (see Joas 1983). Understood this way, the aesthetic quality underlying the constitution of the ecstatic body is not dependent on the opposition between object and subject on which the concept of body-image depends.

It is somewhat ironic that aesthetics is never mentioned in the psychological or social psychological literature on body-image. As Rochberg-Halton (1982:172) nicely puts it: "the lack of attention given to aesthetic quality is another of the effects of the Cartesian world in which we live. Social scientists tend to ignore aesthetic quality as if it were solely a matter of convention, or else physiology." Such is of course the case of mainstream discourse on body-image. When the body's ability to sense aesthetically is excluded, living bodies and their sensations become accidental byproducts of the mind alone and its projections. Instead, a pragmatist formulation of an ecstatic body sensitizes us to the existence of a living, feeling, communicative body – a *somatic* body that is oriented toward the immediate quality of sensing-and-being-in-the-world.

We also suggest that ekstasis is a qualitative experience. By qualitative we refer to the Deweyan (and Peircean) concept of qualitative immediacy and to the "mercurial essence that is the vital source of meaning" in Dewey's philosophy of quality (Rochberg-Halton 1982:162). Dewey (1925, 1934) argues that humans have the capacity of sensing and are able to "make sense" (Dewey 1925:258), or in other words that sensation differs from reflexive thinking in that the experience of sensing entails capturing the immediate qualities of existence. Thinking is somewhat more detached from embodied experience because it relies on symbols, whereas sensation is the interpretive experience of icons, and icons do not depend on the same rules of abstraction on which symbols depend.

Peirce (1958) argued that signs have differing qualities of firstness, secondness, and thirdness. Of course these are not separate and distinct experience, but rather contiguous aspects of experience understood as a continuum of reflexivity (Alexander 1987). Firstness refers to immediate consciousness of sensing – so immediate that the word "consciousness" may even be misleading (as we further discuss later). Sensation and firstness are not synonymous with emotionality, as emotionality requires a deeper level of reflexivity, knowledge, and interpretation. Sensation and firstness are instead correlates of quality, "… an instance of that sort of element which is all that it is positively, in itself, regardless of anything else" (Peirce 1958, 1:306). From this conceptualization, experiencing or sensing meaning is a purely embodied affair occurring in the present in relation to past experiences and future action:

Imagine, if you please, a consciousness in which there is no comparison, no relation, no recognized multiplicity (since parts would be other than the whole), no change, no imagination of any modification of what is positively there, no reflexion – nothing but a simple positive character.

Peirce (1958, 5:44)

The "material" of the ecstatic body – we suggest – consists of qualities. Whereas in the mainstream psychological conceptualization body image is a cognitive experience resulting in the formation of a set of symbols that stand for experiences that are never seriously experienced (they are more like reactions), our conceptualization treats ekstasis as immediately felt and part and parcel of an aesthetic process that only later becomes an integral process through intellectual reflection. In sum, ekstasis is dependent on reflexivity, but such reflexivity can only exist insofar as we keep in mind the origin of ekstasis in pre-reflexive sensation and the unity of aesthetics and reflection. In empirical research dualism occurs as categories such as cognition and perception are reified and thought to encompass experiences and objects that are essentially different from one another. Our formulation instead, while it respects such qualitative differences as those existing between aesthetic and intellectual experiences, posits that one cannot exist without the other; one is mutually constitutive of the other.

Ekstasis as Potential

For our argument, one of the most important aspects of qualitative immediacy is potentiality. "Potential" is an interesting word because it connotes *emergence* – a foundational concept in pragmatism and symbolic interactionism (see Mead 1934) – but also because in Peircean semiotics potentiality is not contrasted to actuality. Potentiality is meaning, because potentiality is sense, as Rochberg-Halton (1982:165) explained:

> ...potentiality is itself genuine.... [In] trying to delineate a mode of being concerned with potentiality, with what "might happen," Peirce tried to account for the importance of immediacy in experience, as well as showing how essential it is to novelty, uniqueness, to the creative aspect of human experience and the world at large.

Defining ekstasis as a form of potentiality, therefore, points to the possibility of developing an aesthetic evaluation of one's body that is not merely a passive internalization caused by way of exposure to the ideological codes produced by the "mechanical other" (Halton 2004:91). We do not deny that ideologies – in particular hegemonic discourses of gender, race, ethnicity, and sexuality – have a great role in the development of the ecstatic body, but by embracing a view of ekstasis grounded in potentiality and the immediacy of embodied sensation we suggest that the concept of the ecstatic body relies on an understanding of the body that is neither stuck in passivity, nor entrenched in dualism. Furthermore, potentiality indicates the processual constitution of the ecstatic body. Traditional research on body image, by necessity of operationalization and dimensionalization, instead treats body image as a structure – a structure of cognitive beliefs and dispositions *about* the body, rather than *of* the body, as potentiality implies.

By suggesting that ekstasis is about firstness, immediacy, and potentiality we are advancing the point that the development of the ecstatic body depends on the purely embodied sensation of one's body, self, objects, and others. When we say purely embodied sensation we mean that the development of ekstasis depends on firstness, that is, the pre-reflexive and even pre-conscious transaction between the person and the world.

Furthermore, by suggesting that ekstasis is dependent on qualitative immediacy we are positing that the body has and is comprised of immediate meaning, since not only does the body make sense, but the body also is the origin of sense. This is a difficult concept that requires careful explanation. The basic starting argument is that the ecstatic body is a sign. In Peircean semiotics a sign is "something which stands to somebody for something in some respect or capacity" (Peirce 1958, 2:228). A sign has creative power because by addressing somebody it creates another sign – which Peirce named interpretant. A sign also involves an object, or referent, and a sign vehicle used to represent said object. So, how is the body a sign? We know that obviously the body may work as a sign vehicle (when it represents something) or even as an object (when, for example, it is object of emulation; see Stephens and Delamont, this volume), but to complete the Peircean semiotic triad the body must also be sense and have the capacity of making sense.

The body *makes sense* of things for it connects with the qualitative immediacy of its world (indeed, recall that the firstness of qualitative immediacy is such that it can only be sensed and therefore its embodiment precedes its enselfment). Secondly, the body *is sense* in virtue of its being an icon. An iconic sign conveys information by embodying an object, in this case itself. Of course a body cannot be sense by itself for sense (i.e. the Peircean interpretant), which depends on an interpersonal communicative achievement; a body therefore is sense for somebody whom it addresses. The body or to be precise, *bodies*, therefore are meaning and meaning-full. By conceptualizing bodies as signs of firstness we have put in place the conditions for a pre-reflexive, pre-conscious, embodied agency. At the same time we have begun to erase the embodied individual-society dualism.

Understanding the body as sense does not preclude us from thinking of the body and ekstasis as thirdness. Ekstasis is also a form of thirdness because it entails introspective reflection and knowledge obtained through linguistic reflexivity and interpretation. But thirdness cannot exist without firstness. Such a formulation is extremely important in erasing the dualism of mind and body. Through this formulation the body is of the mind as the mind is of the body. The concept of ekstasis precisely captures this dialectic process. The relation between body as a sign, self as a triadic sign (Peirce 1958), and society as a triadic sign gives rise to sense, or an interpretant, which is a new sign, from which new semiotic and social relations emerge. What we have here is a post-dualistic vision of the constitution of body, self, and society.

The Ecstatic Body and Structures of Embodied Difference

As an evaluative process, the constitution of the ecstatic body is also the genesis of socio-semiotic structures of bodily differences. In fact, the ecstatic body is relational and comparative; its meanings and values emerge out of a reflexive looking-glass process whereby the qualitative potential of one's body is dependent on an evaluative contrast with others. I may feel deficient in muscular mass, for example, in comparison to my perception of your muscular mass. Or you may feel obese as you sense the thinness of my body build. The point is that the constitution of the ecstatic body is necessarily rooted in difference.

From our pragmatist perspective there is nothing morally improper with the existence of such differences. Difference is the condition of existential uniqueness. The absence of difference would mean that no tension exists in organic interaction, and the absence of tension would mean the lack of potential for existential growth. Without the tension emanating from structures of differences transaction would be empty and meaningless and aesthetic experience would be impossible (Dewey 1934). As Alexander (1987:124) puts it, for Dewey meaning arises in a world in which there is "structure and destruction; one in which action matters because it can effect a reconstruction; one in short, in which there are both stable and precarious features so that *growth* rather than static, bare existing is the mark of life."

A problem, therefore, occurs when the structure of embodied differences is reduced and stasis becomes the norm. This is not an uncommon occurrence. Many of the discourses on health, fitness, and appearance abundant in popular culture and everyday life (see Edgley, this volume) indeed prescribe that the bodies of the citizens of our polity resemble *this* body size rather than *those*, *this* shape rather than *that*, and *this* style, look, etc. rather than another (see M. Atkinson, this volume).

Embodied social inequality is therefore not the inevitable product of organic interaction, but instead the unfortunate byproduct of the discursive and practical solidification of ideologies. Such discursive and practical solidification results in the constitution of shared social habit (Crossley 2001). Such social habits have a direct consequence in the process of formation of the embodied self. The "Me," for instance, may feel the stigma associated with certain socially shared habits and feel a sense of deficiency and dissatisfaction toward one's ecstatic body. As Crossley (2001:150) puts it, all societies "involve basic systems of classification which are focused upon the body or particular 'markers' thereon. And these systems of classification both construct and enforce a particular definition of the me, creating significant forms of structural (vertical) differentiation." Needless to say, the embodied self is reflexive, and following Mead (1934) it would be an obvious mistake to reduce the self to the "Me." Then again, what may (and does) frequently happen is that the extent to which certain habits are commonly shared and regularly unchallenged results in the *stasis of habits of recognition*.

A clearer understanding of this can be achieved by way of distinction among types of habit. In *Art as Experience* Dewey (1934) differentiates between habits of *recognition* and *perception*. In recognition the meaning of an object is merely dependent on previous habits of interpretation, whereas in perception the meaning of an object comes to live through a novel sensation of its unique qualities. Many of our mundane transactions with the world are based on recognition rather than perception and herein lies the foundation for sociological and cultural criticism: *whenever vertical structures of differentiation become so habitual that they effectively reach a relatively enduring static hegemony people temporarily lose their capacity for novel and creative sensation.* This is what happens, for example, when we recognize beauty in always the same forms, shapes, sizes, colours, types, and tones prescribed by hegemonic social discourses. And this is what happens when we aspire to have and to be the body prescribed by ideologies of gendered beauty. When this happens ideologies become embodied in habits of recognition that end up shaping the ecstatic body of self and others in unjust and unequal ways; unjust and unequal because stasis recognition curbs the dynamic potential of ecstatic aesthetic evaluation. In other words, the potential of body-ekstasis is stymied; bodies are either appealing or not on the basis of discriminatory hegemonic prescriptions. In those cases, the reduction of potential difference generates in many people dissatisfaction with one's body, and dissatisfaction becomes therefore a normative discontent.

Conclusions

We have detailed the inherent dualism implied and evoked in the concept of body image. We have also crafted an alternative framework suggesting that aesthetic body assessments (poorly framed as "body image") are actively fashioned in the margins between stasis and ekstasis. We have further located those dynamics in classic pragmatist and socio-semiotic perspectives that are central to interactionist thought and practice. We conclude with brief commentary on body-stasis, body-ekstasis, and the *potential* of liminality.

As previously discussed *potential* is significant, not only to body-ekstasis but also to classic pragmatism and socio-semiotics as well as contemporary symbolic interaction as manifest in concepts such as emergence. Indeed, Blumer's (1969:18) "play and fate of meaning" owes to a legacy of potential and continues to characterize symbolic interaction. Our formulation of body-ekstasis is equally pregnant with potentiality, not only because it relates to the classic literatures we have already cited, but also because potentiality is ever-present in circumstances of liminality. Indeed, the potential of body-ekstasis is bred in the fertile dynamics of liminality.

Our characterization of body-ekstasis significantly owes to Victor Turner (1967, 1969). Akin to interactionist formulations (see Waskul 2005), Turner suggests that all social worlds are composed of two parallel, yet seemingly contrasting models. On one hand, there exists society as "a structure of jural, political, and economic positions, offices, statuses, and roles in which the individual is only ambiguously grasped behind the social persona." On the other hand there is "society as communitas," experienced in betwixt and between moments – at the interstices and edges of norm-governed and institutionalized social order – where "concrete idiosyncratic individuals... confront one another integrally, and not as 'segmentalized' into statuses and roles" (Turner 1969:177). One juxtaposes the other in a relationship that is mediated by moments of liminality, a condition that is "neither here nor there" but "betwixt and between the positions assigned and arrayed by law, custom, convention, and ceremonial" (Turner 1969:95). Turner's model magnifies how individuals are necessarily tied to the social world through institutionally grounded statuses and social roles, yet also experience with equal necessity moments of ekstasis where "men [and women] are released from structure... only to return to structure revitalized by their experience... what is certain is that no society can function adequately without this dialectic" (Turner 1969:129). The same dynamic is implied in our conceptualization of body-ekstasis.

Body-ekstasis is a liminal moment in which the qualitative and aesthetic potential of one's body is evaluated and re-evaluated. This liminal moment is necessarily active and is, indeed, an act – an act of what Dewey would call "perception" "in which an object's meaning includes its unique qualities as well as a person's culturally conditioned habits of interpretation" (Rochberg-Halton 1982:171). In this way, body-ekstasis juxtaposes body-stasis. In fact, body-stasis is fully situated in the exact opposite – what Dewey (1934) calls "recognition": "an object's meaning is solely dependent on previous [passive] habits of interpretation." Like Turner, we suggest that body-stasis and body-ekstasis juxtapose one another, but not as a dualism, instead as a relationship that is actively mediated by liminality: aesthetic experiences that stand over and against the experiences of merely *recognizing* the aesthetic potential of one's body and other people's body in everyday life; it is a kind of liminal *perceptual* experience where both the aesthetic potential of one's body and others' may be re-evaluated in a context of loosened temporal, physical, and normative constraints. The ecstatic-body transcends the static-body and, in that transcendence, potentiality is realized.

References

Alexander, Thomas M. 1987. *John Dewey's Theory of Art, Experience, and Nature.* Albany: SUNY Press.

Blumer, Herbert. 1954. "What is Wrong with Social Theory?" *American Sociological Review*, 18:3–10.

_____. 1969. *Symbolic Interactionism: Perspective and Method.* Berkeley: University of California Press.

Chernin, Kim. 1983. *Womansize: The Tyranny of Slenderness.* London: The Women's Press.

Cooley, Charles H. 1902. *Human Nature and the Social Order.* New York: Scribner's Sons.

Crossley, Nick. 2001. *The Social Body: Habit, Identity, and Desire.* London: Sage.

_____. 2005. "Mapping Reflexive Body Techniques: On Body Modification and Maintenance." *Body & Society*, 11:1–35.

Derrida, Jacques. 1967. *Of Grammatology.* Baltimore: Johns Hopkins University Press.

Dewey, John. 1882–1898. *The Collected Works of John Dewey: The Early Works 1882–1898. Volume 5.* Edited by Jo Ann Boydston. Carbondale: Southern Illinois University Press.

_____. 1896. "The Reflex Arc Concept in Psychology." *Psychological Review,* 3:357–370.

_____. 1922. *Human Nature and Conduct.* New York: The Modern Library

_____. 1925. *Experience and Nature.* Chicago: Open Court Publishing.

_____. 1929. *Experience and Nature.* Second Edition. Chicago: Open Court Publishing.

_____. 1934. *Art as Experience.* New York: Minton.

Foucault, Michel. 1973. *The Birth of the Clinic.* London: Tavistock.

Joas, Hans. 1983. "The Intersubjective Constitution of the Body-Image." *Human Studies,* 6:197–204.

Halton, Eugene. 2004. "The Living Gesture and the Signifying Moment." *Symbolic Interaction,* 27:89–113.

Hodge, Bob and Gunther Kress. 1988. *Social Semiotics.* Ithaca: Cornell University Press.

Howson, Alexandra. 2005. *Embodying Gender.* London: Sage.

Kestenbaum, Victor. 1977. *The Phenomenological Sense of John Dewey.* Atlantic Highlands, NJ: Humanities Press.

Leder, Drew. 1990. *The Absent Body.* Chicago: University of Chicago Press.

Mead, George H. 1934. *Mind, Self, and Society.* Chicago: University of Chicago Press.

Orbach, Susie. 1988. *Fat is a Feminist Issue.* London: Arrow Books.

Peirce, Charles S. 1958. *The Collected Papers of Charles Sanders Peirce.* Volumes 1–8. Cambridge, MA: Harvard University Press.

Rochberg-Halton, Eugene. 1982. "Qualitative Immediacy and the Communicative Act." *Qualitative Sociology,* 5:162–181.

Shilling, Chris. 2003. *The Body and Social Theory.* Second Edition. London: Sage.

Slade, Peter. 1994. "What is Body Image?" *Behaviour Research and Therapy,* 32:497–502.

Synnott, Anthony. 1993. *The Body Social: Symbolism, Self, and Society.* London: Routledge.

Thompson, J. Kevin. 1990. *Body Image Disturbance Assessment and Treatment.* New York: Pergamon Press.

_____. (ed.) 1996. *Body Image, Eating Disorders, and Obesity: An Integrative Guide for Assessment and Treatment.* Washington DC: American Psychological Association.

Thompson, J. Kevin and Manuel Altabe. 1991. "Psychometric Qualities of the Figure Rating Scale." *International Journal of Eating Disorders,* 10:615–619.

Thompson, J. Kevin and Joseph Dolce. 1989. "The Discrepancy Between Emotional vs. Rational Estimates of Body Size, and Ideal Body Ratings: Theoretical and Clinical Implications." *Journal of Clinical Psychology*, 45:473–483.

Turner, Victor. 1967. *The Forest of Symbols*. Ithaca, NY: Cornell University Press.

———. 1969. *The Ritual Process: Structure and Anti-Structure*. Ithaca, NY: Cornell University Press.

Waskul, Dennis. 2005. "Ekstasis and the Internet: Liminality and Computer-Mediated Communication." *New Media & Society*, 7:47–63.

Wolszon, Linda Ridge. 1998. "Women's Body Image Theory and Research." *The American Behavioral Scientist*, 41:542–557.

Chapter 14

Eating the Black Body: Interracial Desire, Food Metaphor and White Fear

Erica Owens and Bronwyn Beistle

Socio-semiotic and interactionist understandings of the body attempt to capture the inevitably social and political dynamics whereby definitions of signs, and the situations in which signs are meaningful, are negotiated. Meaning in other words is a form of power, and to make something mean is therefore an act of power shaping what an object represents and what others may make it represent. In this chapter Erica Owens and Bronwyn Beistle reflect on the power of the black body as represented within personal ads written by white men and women seeking sexual partners. Emerging out of these ads is a powerful food metaphor in which the black body is alluring, tantalizing, and mysteriously "exotic," while also a pollutant, contamination and gluttonous sin. No matter what connotation is prevalent, Owens and Beistle show that the meanings of the body emerge out of a semiotic process grounded in profound ideological roots.

> [Beloved] had two dreams: exploding and being swallowed.
>
> Toni Morrison, *Beloved* (1991: 164)

"SWM seeks SBF for chocolate vanilla swirl" (WM seeking BF). "Cup of cream looking for some dark coffee to warm up with" (WM seeking BF). "Vanilla looking for some brown sugar" (WF seeking BM). "White knight seeks chocolate kiss" (WM seeking BF). These are just a few Internet personal advertisements for white men and women seeking black partners for romantic and sexual relationships (data from Owens 1999, 2004). In each of these the use of food metaphors is striking – likening the black body to an object for consumption – this chapter unpacks the discursive eating of the black body.

Few studies link racism and racist expression back to the theoretical underpinnings beneath the distaste or fear felt by many of those in the dominant culture. This chapter will take a critical view of one particular form of distasteful racist expression – the representation of black bodies as food in personals ads – and expose the socio-semiotic and sociocultural factors involved in the use of this ideological construction. We draw from theoretical literature in several areas, including socio-semiotics, symbolic interactionism, and critical race theory and Marxist theory, to accomplish this goal.

The central argument advanced in this chapter is that the black body, as represented within the personal ads we examine, stands in a uniquely liminal socio-semiotic space. First, the black body has meaning as pollutant, as framed by the racist ideological discursive formation that we call the "pollution discourse." The pollution discourse re-casts the language of "miscengenation" such that the concept of contamination and taint is present but no longer overt in these imaginings of interracial pairings. But on the other hand the black body is compelling, even fascinating to these racist ad writers. The black body seduces them, titillating them and enchanting them into seeking the very "pollution" and "contamination" feared by the authors. We identify this discursive thread as the "seduction discourse." The two discursive formations, with their competing but yet complementary meanings, and the semiosic processes whereby the black body assumes these situated meanings within the structure of the personals ad, are both framed within the larger structure of "cannibal talk" (Obeyesekere 2005), which encompasses fascination, exaggeration, horror, and taboo.

The Pollution Discourse

For our purposes it is critical to establish the link between interracial sexual contact and the psychosocial basis of the ideological discursive formation of white racism. Disapproval of interracial sexual contact represents a bottom-line taboo for many white persons, including those who consider themselves nonracist (Feagin and Sykes 1994). A possible reason for this disapproval, according to Frankenberg (1993:103), is an essentialist form of racism: "hostility toward interracial relationships hing[es] on constructions of racial and cultural differences as absolute and of families and communities as monoracial and monocultural." Sexual contact between persons of different race creates a fault line in the perceived "monoracial and monocultural" identity. The belief in a racially "pure" identity leads the rejection of the possibility of incorporating a racial "other" into one's family group. Frankenberg (1993:104) sees the act of "disowning" a child because of interracial sexual contact as a primary example of defending against a breach in racial identity:

> Beyond its economic aspect, the act of disowning makes the statement that "you are no longer my child," a symbolic severance of genealogical ties to a family member who has, in the parents' eyes, joined the "wrong" genealogical group.

The rejection of interracial sexual activity is related to a fear that one's own identity, perceived as biologically homogeneous, could be "tainted" by an implicitly inferior "other:" a fear of miscegenation. Because the fear of miscegenation presupposes heterosexual partners of different races, we limit our arguments to heterosexual contact, although we recognize that it is not the literal biological "mixing" of two parents of different races in offspring that is the source of hostility toward interracial sexual contact. If it were, the lack of intent to conceive, the use of contraception, or the sterility of a partner would nullify hostility. As it is, intimate contact between persons of different race itself conjures the spectre of racial mixing, as if intimacy causes a "mixing" of otherwise "pure" identities regardless of whether that intimacy produces a child, the concrete symbol of such admixture. So strong is the taboo in this instance, that the *desire* for such contact is cast as unacceptable. Control extends beyond action to emotion and intent. One should not *wish* to cross this racial divide; to do otherwise is, the discourse implies, an act of ethno-treason against one's "white" origins.

Whites and black sexual contact, more than any other, is a cultural trigger of which otherwise latent racism becomes overt. For many white people, the possibility of a racial "mixing" which involves sexual intimacy with a black person is an unthinkable breach of white identity. This premise is supported by the groundbreaking work of Kovel (1970), who analyzes how white persons conceptualize blackness along a continuum of dirt, filth, stink, and danger. Kovel asserts that many white people have the irrational fear that "blackness," represented by dark skin, can somehow rub off and sully whites who come into contact with it. Much like the smell of something rotten, which permeates other objects in an enclosed space, whites fear that close contact with blackness will similarly "taint" and result in a sudden, and perhaps permanent, invasion their own being.

The Seduction Discourse

One might think, then, that the desire for interracial sexual contact represents a sign of acceptance of persons of another race. Simply put, if racist discourses prohibit sexual contact between members of different racial groups, then discourses that support interracial sexual contact ought to be anti-racist. However, previous research shows that some white persons who desire a partner of another race base their desire in a wish for the exotic or wild "other" who is more a sexualized object than an equal partner (see Hsia 1997; Vigoya 2002; but see Yancey 2003 for a contrasting viewpoint). An entire industry of "sex tourism" has grown around the desire to penetrate the "ethnosexual frontiers" that are present when two or more races, ethnicities, and national origins are present in a potential pairing (Nagel 2000). Often, appreciation for the "differences" of a potential partner of another race is a mirror image of racist discourse, and comprised of cultural appropriation or stereotypical objectification (Owens 1999). Therefore, desire for this racialized "other" is potentially problematic: how do whites looking for black sexual partners represent blacks as objects of desire?

Previous research has shown a tendency for white persons to use food metaphors when seeking black partners through personals ads (Owens 2004). Although these metaphors are not prevalent, they occur in sufficient frequency to warrant further investigation. We propose that formulating the black-and-white liaison generally, and the black body especially, as food implies consumption and thus an assimilation of the black body. We argue that white-on-black desire cannot be simply read as anti-racist, but rather, must be analyzed in relation to a long history of discursive tension between essentialist racism and an ideology of assimilation. Descriptions of the black body as food discursively resolve the tension between the reality of racism and the idea of America as a body which devours and assimilates all difference.

Clearly, we do not suggest that there is not (or cannot) be love and respect between white and black partners. Nor are we asserting that our data are typical of interracial dating discourse, experience, or sexual expression. We were first intrigued by the use of food metaphor when analyzing Internet dating pages, and we recognize that the medium of personals advertisements may encourage mere sexual contact rather than emotional closeness. However, we also found that few whites categorize non-black persons by use of a similar food metaphor. This indicates that there is something about the food metaphor that extends beyond the objectification of the singles ad scene. The food metaphor is used not to declare "consuming" passions in general, but is linked specifically to white-black relations. By extending this metaphor and considering its implications in light of other critical work in the field of race and race relations, we have taken the use of food metaphor well beyond the realm of dating. It is our contention that expressions of sexual desire are only one nuance of the food metaphor used; the underlying root, whether used in a sexual or nonsexual context, is the protection of whites' sense of identity.

The Discourse of Digestion

As we mentioned earlier, sexual desire for the black other implies the threat of losing whiteness by having a nonwhite child. The perceived social danger of sexual contact with a racial "other" is implicit in the "one drop rule," which declares "black" any person with one drop of "black blood" regardless of appearance (see Feagin, 1989). Thus, white desire for the black other potentially signifies and evokes this threat of a loss of whiteness. Such fear of "darkening" propels an ever-more urgent desire on the part of some whites to assimilate the threatening black body, to incorporate and render it harmless or inert. The fear of loss of whiteness may be partly contained or mitigated by making the black other into an object designed for consumption or use – sexually through copulation, and figuratively as food – rather than an individual worthy of a committed longer-term pairing.

The use of food metaphors is especially revealing when considered as a tactic used to enact this distancing. Feminist theorist bell hooks (1992:36) notes that food metaphor is often used to denote the enforcement of power imbalance: "what racism, imperialism, and sexist domination prevail by courageous consumption. It is by eating the Other ... that one asserts power and privilege." This "assertion of power and privilege" arises metaphorically from food's unique ability to "become" the body which consumes it, as well as its function as fuel for the consuming body. Further, once the body digests a food product, the remaining material is expelled as waste. Neither the waste nor the useful product is recognizable as the original product; the body destroys the uniqueness of different foods and converts all into itself. Similarly, hooks (1992:36) notes that "the commodification of difference promotes paradigms of consumption wherein whatever difference the Other inhabits is eradicated, via exchange, by a consumer cannibalism that not only displaces the Other but denies the significance of the Other's history through a process of decontextualization."

The production of waste from food is central. If we trace the full meaning of food metaphor through to completion it is possible to deconstruct meanings inherent in this discursive form. Judith Butler (1990, in Witt 1998) has addressed this process of "othering" through analysis of the body boundary symbolized by the digestive tract and intestines. Butler argues that it is through the digestive tract that the self-other dichotomy can be transcended for a time; the digestive process stands as a metaphoric model for determining what is "self" and what is other – and "other" is, by extension, worthless. Although Butler delves further into the nature of food metaphor, she does not specifically address the tensions inherent in white discourse regarding contact with the black body. Butler's analysis has not fully captured the dichotomy of hunger and revulsion betrayed by this linguistic form. Eating never fills for long. The state of hunger begins again as soon as consumption is completed. The white body, having only momentarily sated its hunger, will remain empty and therefore still vulnerable to the semiotic seductive power of the black body.

Also, as Weiss (1998) notes, the act of eating, absorbing, incorporating, and then expelling exemplify both love *and* hate. Food by its very nature is designed to be consumed. Consumption by a human implies that a food product is deemed wholesome or flavourful enough to eat, barring extreme circumstances of hunger which may remove the element of choice. As the consumed object is chosen for consumption it is tacitly granted value. However, if it is not consumed, it will rot in its original form and serve no useful purpose; it only becomes fully itself (food as opposed to garbage) if it is eaten. It is also an object of a transitory nature. Once a piece of food enters the human body its chemical makeup changes and it is recognized immediately as no longer being "food" or worthy of eating. Milk in the glass is a beverage, milk held in the mouth for two seconds and spit back into the glass is waste. Thus, food only becomes fully itself by becoming fully other. Its only option other than co-optation is to become waste. In this manner, food misused becomes "dirt" by virtue of being out-of-place (see Douglas 2002/1966). The food metaphor, with the implied co-optation and reduction to faeces, therefore speaks also to the notion of "place" in relation to race and belonging. Black persons, in the estimation of many whites (see Feagin and Sykes 1994; Kovel 1970) do not "belong" in relationships with whites. When a black body is in bed next to a white one, it is out of place and the desire that brought the pair together stands as potential contaminant.

When whites use a racialized food metaphor to construct a black object of desire, then, they are representing the black body as having no separate selfhood – in fact, a black body which has a separate existence from the consumer is rendered a waste product. This requires us to dig further than Hooks' "decontextualization." Eating the black body is not only deconstructive but of active spoilage and obliteration.

The following examples represent the imagined or desired black partner as food, and the white writer of the advertisement as a consuming subject, an eater (Owens 2004:227):

> White knight seeks chocolate kiss. (WM seeking BF)
> White Brotha lookin for that sweet redbone. (WM seeking BF)
> I love dark meat unless you are serving chicken or turkey. (WF seeking BM)

In order to ensure that earlier research did not contain an unusual grouping of examples due to time constraints or choice of sites, three new searches were performed over the period of several weeks using a new site. Identifying information and contact numbers have been removed from these examples to preserve the privacy of the advertiser. A common theme that has emerged is the description of "meat" (Owens 2004:227):

> I am looking for black studs I am a real nasty kinky nympho for black meat. (WF seeking BM)

Interestingly, most of the advertisements which exclusively represent the other as food, rather than also using food metaphors to describe the self, use "meat" as their food metaphor rather than the chocolate, coffee, brown sugar, cream and vanilla most often used by those who describe both self and other as food. This identification of the black body with "meat" evokes a very old stereotype, which Henry Louis Gates, among others, has identified: that Africans, and, later, African-Americans, are closer to the animal than to the human (Gates 1993: in Rice 1998:43–69). Like a non-human animal, the black body is represented as a source of meat. One of these advertisements (see above) even compares "dark meat" to chicken and turkey, accentuating the idea that blacks, like chickens and turkeys, are a different species, a species which is not only lower on the food chain, but also domesticated and raised for consumption. Another advertisement uses a much more prevalent form of the same stereotype; a white woman who states her desire for "black meat" in the same advertisement says "I am looking for black studs," emphasizing the sense of the black body as a domesticated animal, used both for breeding and meat.

Cannibal Talk and Iconic Power

The discourse of "black meat," a subset of the construction of the black body as food, has intimate ties to the eighteenth- and nineteenth-century European discourses of Africans and indigenous peoples as cannibals. Alan Rice (1998:110) states: "The European view of cannibalism [was] buttressed by the pseudoscientific writings of the leaders of the Enlightenment, such as Thomas Jefferson and David Hume, who compared Africans to animals and denied their ability to think rationally, implying a bestiality that was directly linked with cannibalism." In the aforementioned personals advertisements it is the white subject, not the black object, who is presented as a cannibal. Rice (1998:115–116) cites pro-slavery tracts from the nineteenth century which elucidate the connection between nineteenth-century ideologies of race and twenty-first century interracial sexual desire:

> All markers of the bestial are habits that civilized Europeans see as taboo, as vices that differentiate the civilized from the primitive. The triangle of vices includes "idolatry, cannibalism, and sexual excess" (Mason 63). All three vices are alluded to in the discourse around slavery. It appears in writings by pro-slavery apologists such as William Gilmore Simms, the South Carolina novelist, who in a lecture entitled "The Morals of Slavery" (1837) stated that "the Negro comes from a continent where he was a cannibal destined to eat his fellow or be eaten by him."

The cannibal must either eat the other or be eaten by him or her. In the previous examples, it is clear that the writers of the advertisement intend to be at the top of the food chain, as they do not admit the possibility of being consumed themselves. Therefore, since a cannibal exists either to eat or be eaten, the only remaining possibility is for the imagined black object of desire to become meat. Interestingly, the comparison between the black body and farm animals represses the fact of this "white cannibalism," so that the writer can imaginatively engage their own taboos, projected onto the bestialized other, but at the same time avoid them; all they are really doing is consuming what is meant to be consumed, raised to be eaten. Still, the white consumer does not escape becoming "food" him or herself. In eating or desiring to eat, one becomes consumed by one's own hunger. The relative power enacted in this "apparatus of culture" (see Denzin 1992:98) is held by the iconic fetishized image of the black Other. If communication is, as Denzin argues, "an ensemble of sexual practices, social forms, social relationships, and technologies of representation which construct definitions of reality," then these ads betray the vulnerability of the white consumer in the face of his or her own desire and fascination.

This tendency is present in Obeyesekere's (2005) work on "cannibal talk," where reports of the dark-skinned Other as cannibal arises in part from early British childhood socialization through nursery rhymes where the "naughty" or "bad" person is eaten by an ogre, witch, or giant. Nursery rhyme cannibalism is a way to make difficult persons disappear. Thus, when British explorers reported cannibalism among native persons, they designated the native as 1) problematic, 2) less than human, and 3) capable of base action. In a little-mentioned aspect of the cannibal-settler dynamic, some researchers have noted that native persons and kidnapped slaves viewed their oppressors as likely cannibals as well. Rice (1998) cites accounts of Middle Passage voyages where slaves, who were being force-fed to prevent resistance through starvation, assumed that they were being fattened up as food for their white kidnappers. Obeyesekere (2005:29) states that when the Cook voyage encountered native Hawaiians, both groups considered the other through "paranoid lenses," and thought that the *other* would surely attack and eat them. Cannibalism is always more than eating or hunger. Cannibalism is domination, fear, absorption, revulsion, and dehumanization. The threat of being eaten, not just killed but devoured and obliterated, forms an effective deterrent to resistance by subordinates (Petrinovich 2000).

The eighteenth- and nineteenth-century association of cannibalism and sexual excess with a bestialized black other persists in these twenty-first century advertisements. The following advertisement deserves particular attention as it demonstrates the connections between racialized sexual desire, slavery, and bestialized images of the black body (in Owens 1999):

> Looking for a couple of heterosexual males aged 20–40 to help my 37 year old wife bring in the new millennium. Would prefer one of the males to be African American as I want to watch her being aggressively plowed by dark meat. (WM for BM)

The image of a black man plowing a field while a white man oversees the labour literally evokes cultural memories of slavery. At the same time, since the black body here is figured as "dark meat" which is also "plow[ing]," the black man is clearly imagined as a farm animal: a source of both labour and "meat." Finally, the fact that the advertiser wants to see his wife "aggressively plowed" shows that he wishes to see a particular scene enacted: he wishes to see a black man aggressively overpowering a white woman in sex. This scene, once enacted, would violate both the most intense form of the taboo against interracial sexual activity, and also, more importantly, would confirm, for the white male observer, the idea that black men desire to rape white women (see Frankenberg 1993). Again, we return to the notion of the black body as a site of power which is both coveted and feared. In these personals ads, we see a black body that has seductive power over the white consumer. It is this power that threatens the hegemonic, supremacist control wielded by the white author. In these narratives of eating and hungering, co-optation and incorporation of sexual desires cannot be finalized. Hunger cannot be fully satiated, and in the end the potential for sexual competition or violation has not been quelled.

Food Metaphor and Assimilationist Discourse

While whites do not generally characterize persons of Latino or Asian descent as food, some white advertisers describe their own bodies as food. These advertisements (taken from Owens (1999)) which rarely make use of the "meat" metaphor are, on the surface, much less vicious:

> SWM seeks SBF for chocolate vanilla swirl. (WM seeking BF)
> Cup of cream looking for some dark coffee to warm up with. (WM seeking BF)
> Vanilla looking for some brown sugar. (WF seeking BM)
> Light to Dark chocolates' delicious! Try me as your Yummy Vanilla! (WM seeking BF)

Interestingly, we have only found evidence of the white self being described in terms of food in cases of imagined sexual contact involving a black person. In these advertisements, white and black bodies alike become consumable at the moment that sexual contact between them is imagined. It is almost as if, being juxtaposed with the "dark coffee" or "chocolate" or "brown sugar," suggests to the white advertisers that their bodies are also food of a complimentary and opposite type to the black partners they desire: cream to coffee, vanilla to chocolate or brown sugar.

In most of these examples, as both the advertiser and the desired partner are represented as food, the consumer, the eating self, disappears. The very fact that the advertisers describe themselves or their desired liaisons as food, whether a "chocolate vanilla swirl" or a cup of coffee with cream, implies that consumption is expected. Unlike in the "dark meat" advertisements, the agent of that consumption is obscure. What replaces the relationship of eater to eaten is the combination of foods with each other.

In fact, what characterizes these advertisements is an emphasis on tasting rather than on eating. The light and dark chocolates are described as "delicious;" vanilla, brown sugar, and even cream are all foods used as flavourings. Thus, the idea of race that underlies these metaphors differs in some ways from that underlying the metaphor of black body as meat. Where the "meat" metaphor partakes of a tradition of brutally essentialist racism, advertisements that describe both the black and white bodies as food borrow from an assimilationist tradition Frankenberg (1993:156) calls power evasion:

> If the sharp edge of color evasion resides in its denial of the differences that race makes in people's lives power evasion involves a selective attention to difference, allowing into conscious scrutiny – even conscious embrace – those differences that make the speaker feel good, but continuing to evade by means of partial description, euphemism, and self-contradiction those that make the speaker feel bad.

Upon further analysis, however, the binary opposition between power evasion and essentialist racism collapses. Essentialist notions of race underlie even assimilationist positions. The interviews Frankenberg (1993:144–5) conducts with her respondents reveal that they oscillate between denial of racial difference (or at least of the aspects of racial difference that make them feel bad) and speech which reveals an actual, though denied, hyper-awareness of racial difference:

> RF: "So you think that's the best way to be-color-blind?"
> Joan: "Yes. Don't just look at them and immediately say, 'Oh, I shouldn't like them.' I really don't think I even thought I was different from them. I just took it in stride – like a bunch of kittens – all of them are different colors.'"

As Frankenberg notes, this respondent's initial assertion of colour-blind unawareness of race crumbles beneath her statement "I just took it in stride," which indicates that race is a social obstacle she must negotiate, or step around. It is also quite telling that even in this example of purported *unawareness* of race, persons of colour are characterized as small, defenceless animals, a characterization the speaker does not extend to herself when she employs the distancing pronoun 'they'. As Denzin (2000:172) notes, an easy answer to racial difficulties is not available but it is deeply wished for nonetheless. When images of assimilation and integration are presented, they are understood as being controlled by whites:

> In the end, it all comes back to black and white bodies that matter; to race and sex and gender; to love, intimacy, and family; to male and female bonding; to taboos surrounding miscegenation and to male desire.

> And here it gets complicated. In every scene in the [*Lethal Weapon* movie] cycle where homoerotic banter occurs, it is the white man, Riggs, who utters the words of desire to the black man, Murtaugh.

Of course, none of the advertisers we study purport to be colour-blind. But the same oscillation between essentialist notions that race is immutable and assimilationist notions that race is infinitely deconstructable that Frankenberg finds in her respondents' attitudes occurs in these personal advertisements as well. The tension present in these narratives does not allow a resolution where both parties in a potential pairing – whether for one evening or for a longer-lasting relationship – are allowed full and unique personhood. The use of food metaphor by white partners maintains active personhood for oneself, while denying active participation to the black partner.

We must note again that not all whites who seek black partners take this tack in characterizing the desired partner. The use of food metaphor is common enough to be considered a pattern within white online dating narratives, but we do not claim that all white persons seeking black partners are attempting to consume and thereby own the sexuality of an objectified other. It should also be noted that online dating advertisements represent a growing, but still self-selecting, pool of courtship. It is impossible for us to reliably tease out all of those posters who are seeking only (or predominantly) sex, rather than long-term committed relationships. Even among those who state that they want more than a casual encounter may be stating this in an effort to widen their pool of interested partners. We cannot impute motive that is not stated, but we must take into account that posters are crafting online personae to present a given public self.

Conclusions

The black body is an emotionally and politically laden discursive field. There is a seductive semiotic power to the black body as fetishized through white desire. This iconic body, inherently sexual and exotic, compels the white consumer to hunger for what is forbidden yet tantalizing. But white hunger for the black other can never be satisfied. Just as bodily hunger is only ever temporarily quelled, and hunger begins at the moment that eating stops, so sexual contact with the black partner does not "solve" the struggle over pollution, desire, and hegemony expressed in these personals advertisements.

White authors' choice of food metaphor does more than play off of the sexual notion of oral play. These authors employ the language of consumption, implying both absorption and the potential for pollution through unclean or inappropriate sustenance. At the same time, the semiotic power of the black body is seductive, and exerts a compelling draw over the white consumer. The cannibalistic eating involved in this discourse is generative, perpetuating the cycle of hunger and attraction rather than resolving the attraction.

References

Asante, Molefi Kete. 1993. "Racism, Consciousness, and Afrocentricity." In Gerald Early (ed.), *Lure and Loathing: Essays on Race, Identity, and the Ambivalence of Assimilation.* New York: Viking Penguin.

Butler, Judith. 1990. Cited in Witt, Doris (1998) "Soul food: Where the Chetterling Hits the (Primal) Pan." In Scapp, Ron and Seitz, Brian (eds) *Eating Culture.* New York: State University of New York Press.

Denzin, Norman K. 1992. *Symbolic Interactionism and Cultural Studies: The Politics of Interpretation.* Oxford UK, Cambridge MA: Blackwell.

_____. 2002. *Reading Race: Hollywood and the Cinema of Racial Violence.* Thousand Oaks, CA: Sage.

Douglas, Mary. 2002/1966. *Purity and Danger: An Analysis of Concept of Pollution and Taboo.* London, New York: Routledge.

Feagin, Joe R. 1989. *Racial and Ethnic Relations* (3rd edition). Englewood Cliffs, NJ: Prentice Hall.

Feagin, Joe R., and Sikes, Melvin P. 1994. *Living With Racism: The Black Middle-Class Experience.* Boston: Beacon Press.

Frankenberg, Ruth. 1993. *White Women, Race Matters: The Social Construction of Whiteness.* Minneapolis: University of Minnesota Press.

Gates, Henry Louis. 1993. "Loose Canons: Notes on the Culture Wars." Cited in Rice, Alan (1998). "'Who's Eating Whom': The Discourse of Cannibalism in the Literature of the Black Atlantic from Equiano's Travels to Toni Morrison's *Beloved.*" *Research in African Literatures*, 107 (winter).

Goux, Jean-Joseph. 1990. *Symbolic Economies: After Marx and Freud.* Ithaca NY: Cornell University Press.

hooks, bell. 1992. "Eating the Other." In bell hooks, *Black Looks: Race and Representation.* Boston: South End Press.

Hsia, Hsiao-Chuan. 1997. *Selfing and Othering in the "Foreign Bride" Phenomenon: A Study of Class, Gender, and Ethnicity in the Transnational Marriages Between Taiwanese Men and Indonesian Women.* Unpublished doctoral dissertation.

Kovel, Joel. 1970. *White Racism: A Psychohistory.* New York: Pantheon Books.

Lingiss, Alphonso. 1998. "Appetite." In Scapp, Ron and Seitz, Brian (eds) *Eating Culture.* New York: State University of New York Press.

Mason, Peter. 1990. *Deconstructing America: Representations of the Other.* London: Routledge.

Morrison, Toni. 1991/1987. *Beloved.* New York: Signet/Penguin Books.

Nagel, Joane. 2000. "States of Arousal/Fantasy Islands: Race, Sex and Romance in the Global Economy of Desire." *American Studies*, 41 (2/3):159.

Obeyesekere, Gananath. 2005. *Cannibal Talk: The Man-Eating Myth and Human Sacrifice in the South Seas.* Berkeley: University of California Press.

Owens, Erica (n.d.). "Whiteness as Currency." Unpublished manuscript.

_____. 1999. "Racial Dimensions of Perceived Sexual Attractiveness and the White Self." Paper presented at the annual meeting of the Southern Sociological Society, Nashville, Tennessee.

_____. 2004. "Race, Sexual Attractiveness, and Internet Personal Advertisements." In Waskul, Dennis (ed.) *net.seXXX: Readings on Sex, Pornography, and the Internet.* New York: Peter Lang.

Petrinovich, Lewis. 2000. *The Cannibal Within.* New York: Aldine de Gruyter.

Rice, Alan. 1998. "'Who's Eating Whom': The Discourse of Cannibalism in the Literature of the Black Atlantic from Equiano's Travels to Toni Morrison's Beloved." *Research in African Literatures*, 29(4):106–121.

Roediger, David R. 1991. *The Wages of Whiteness: Race and the Making of the American Working Class.* New York: Verso.

Vigoya, Mara Viveros. 2002. "Dionysian Blacks: Sexuality, Body, and Racial Order in Columbia." *Latin American Perspectives*, 29(2):60–77.

Weiss, Allen S. 1998. "Edible Architecture, Cannibal Architecture." In Scapp, Ron and Seitz, Brian (eds) *Eating Culture.* New York: State University of New York Press.

Yancey, George. 2003. "A Preliminary Investigation of Differential Sexual Attitudes Among Individuals Involved in Interracial Relationships: Testing 'Jungle Fever'". *Social Science Journal*, 40(1):153.

Chapter 15

Claiming the Bodies of Exotic Dancers: The Problematic Discourse of Commodification

Carol Rambo, Sara Renée Presley and
Don Mynatt

Much like the meanings of black bodies examined in Chapter Fourteen, which are framed within existent ideological discursive formations forged under unequal and unjust social circumstances, the meanings of female exotic dancers' bodies are equally subject to a colonizing gaze that originates in misunderstanding and the desire to foster theoretical agendas rather than give voice to subjects of research. In this chapter Carol Rambo, Sara Renée Presley, and Don Mynatt show how academic researchers frame strippers and stripping according to the competing logic of victimization and deviantization. A thorough review of the sociological literature demonstrates how the body of an exotic dancer is very much a contested socio-semiotic field, and yet – as interviews with dancers show – one that is reclaimed by the women themselves. Rambo, Presley and Mynatt thus provide us with the quintessential socio-semiotic-interactionist strategy: the uncovering and the exposition of ideological meaning by social agents themselves.

Upon hearing the words "stripper" or "exotic dancer" many possible images come to mind: a beautiful woman unapologetically using her sexual prowess to stimulate and excite her audience for money; a scared young girl with little education forced to strip in order to survive; a woman with poor character, to be dismissed as immoral or deviant; someone with a diagnosable mental illness or drug addiction; or perhaps just someone doing a job. Less frequently, we might consider a male in the role such as a Chippendale dancer or a man who dances in gay clubs for other men.

The first author has researched various aspects of "stripping" or "exotic dancing" since 1984 as a participant observer (Rambo Ronai 1999; 1998; 1994; 1992a; Rambo Ronai and Ellis 1989) and as an interviewer (Rambo Ronai 1994; 1992b; Rambo Ronai and Cross 1998; Rambo Ronai and Ellis 1989). Over the years she has heard differing opinions of what being a stripper "really" means from her students and other audiences, but the debate does not stop there. The three authors of this chapter assert that the bodies and selves of exotic dancers are contested and claimed by researchers. This is carried out through the application of specialized technical discourses (Foucault 1977) in the framing of research projects and descriptions of dancers.

When sex, or the idea of sex, is exchanged for currency in the marketplace, sex and the body become commodified and a discourse is generated which structures much of how we as a culture "look" or "gaze" at exotic dancers. Through this particular expression of discursive order, the definition of dancers' bodies and selves are both gendered and politicized in everyday parlance and the research literature. With this in mind, we examine what we "know" about dancers according to the social science literature and what dancers have to say about it.

Through a content analysis of 87 abstracts found online in Sociological Abstracts on striptease dancers, we make the case that striptease dancers are characterized by researchers as either deviant, exploited, liberated, or both exploited and liberated. These characterizations or exemplars are not applied in an egalitarian manner and each serves to discursively constrain (Cordell and Rambo Ronai 1999; Rambo Ronai 1997; 1994; Rambo Ronai and Cross 1998) the narrative possibilities for the construction of a dancer's self. Furthermore, from life history interviews with female dancers currently being collected by the second author, we will show how dancers are now "talking back" to feminists and other researchers by resisting (Ronai and Cross 1998) the discursive constraint that is conferred upon their bodies and identities through the application of deviance/pathology and exploitation/liberation exemplars. From an analysis of the abstracts and the interviews, we hope to engage in a socio-semiotic, interpretive and *reflexive* sociology, which neither colonizes the lifeworld of its research participants, nor romanticizes their practices.

Methods

For the first part of this study, we gathered and coded 87 abstracts – eight dissertation abstracts, 12 conference papers, 61 articles and six book chapters. We retrieved these abstracts by typing in the search terms stripper, striptease, exotic dancers, and sex workers. We were aware of articles on the topic of striptease which were not listed in Sociological Abstracts, including some authored by the first author. Some of the articles did not have abstracts while others were not obtainable. We decided to use materials from Sociological Abstracts so that the data set would be consistent and available for anyone who wanted to replicate this part of our study.

There was an overlap of authorship between dissertations, conference papers, and articles. We decided to treat each abstract as an individual case rather than eliminating overlap because each represented a site where discourse was produced and potentially transmitted to others. One oddity we noted was an article by Graves Enck and Jim Preston (1988) published in *Deviant Behavior*, which was published again, verbatim, in 1995 by an author named Philip O. Sijuwade (1995) in *Social Behavior and Personality*, and again, word for word in the *International Journal of Sociology of the Family* (Sijuwade 1996). After some inquiry and thought, we decided to include all three abstracts because, again, each is a site where discourse can be disseminated.

We examined the abstracts and coded them for the following: deviance exemplars, exploitation exemplars, liberation exemplars, exploitation and liberation exemplars, and those which did not make use of any of these exemplars. In the many cases where it was discernable, we also coded for the gender of the strippers, and the gender of the customers. We made note when the article focused on the identity of the dancer, stigma, or the concept that deception was somehow involved in the relationship between customers and strippers. In addition, we coded for it when an article focused on the laws and ordinances surrounding the occupation or when some other role in the strip club setting was the focus of the article.

The Discourse of Commodification and Striptease Dancing

Dancers use "the sensual exhibition of one's body for financial remuneration" (Boles and Garbin 1974:114). They show no inhibitions or shyness about the body or about sex. For these reasons it has been noted by Marilyn Salutin (1971:19) that strippers were viewed as "bad:"

> because they strip away all social decorum with their clothes. The privacy of the sex act disappears as does its personal quality. In the strip bars the sex act is made a packaged commercial deal.

When sex is sold it becomes simultaneously a commodity and an object of discourse, "invested with symbolic meanings and symbolic value – use-value, sign-value, exchange-value, and sign exchange value – through the functioning of a *discursive order*," (Waskul and Vannini 2006, introduction to this volume). The discourse of "commodification of the body" is a vocabulary that, within the cultural contexts surrounding sex, suggests that either something shameful or exploitative occurs when sex becomes a commodity. If a woman sells sexuality and the concomitant use/sign values in an exchange, she is considered either criminal, mentally ill, or an exploited victim. As reflected in everyday parlance, stripping becomes pathologized or problematized.

When the commodification of the body is viewed as deriving from something abnormal, researchers frame their scholarship in terms of "deviance/pathology exemplars." When the commodification of the body is viewed as potentially exploitative, researchers frame their projects in terms of "exploitation/liberation exemplars." When scholars employ these frames, they become agents who produce specialized knowledge (Foucault 1977) regarding strippers. In scholarship, strippers are socially constructed, defined at the same time they are described. Through language, researchers work through the institution of the academy to affect stripper's lives, thus establishing and reinforcing power relations between strippers and society. In scholarly framing practices investigators claim the selves and the bodies of exotic dancers. The contest between researchers regarding the character of those selves and bodies, harnesses the language of commodification of the body through frames such as deviance/pathology, and exploitation/liberation. These frames reproduce gendered and politicized mainstream cultural understandings of exotic dancers.

Deviance/Pathology Exemplars

Deviance/pathology exemplars were found within the context of criminology, law, and medicine. They occur when the researcher characterizes striptease as something abnormal or pathological. For example many authors examined "contingencies" which led to the occupational choice of stripping, stressing factors such as coming from a broken home or being sexually abused at an early age. Some discussed how the occupation facilitated lesbian behaviour. A few projects explored various aspects of the law or the medical hazards associated with the occupation. Others characterized the occupation as some form of deception or counterfeit intimacy, whereby dancing is equated with a confidence game in which emotional closeness is manufactured with the customer in order to make money. Many focused on the stigma associated with the occupation. Often the "problematic identity" or "self" of the dancer was the central topic. A few examples from the abstracts illustrate this:

> Modalities of subjectivity are "leaky" for both customers and dancers and … it is difficult to keep the selves they occupy in the club separate and distinct from their other "selves" outside the clubs.
>
> Egan (2000)

> [To] increase cash reward, dancers may allow their body boundaries to be "fluid," deciding on a customer-by-customer basis how they will interact physically. These body compromises can lead to a variety of identity problems for the women.
>
> Wesley (2003)

> [Dancers] relied heavily on cognitive & emotive dissonance to reduce the emotional strain of the work & to alternately embrace their role as dancer & distance themselves from it as the situation seemed to dictate.
>
> Thompson, Harred, and Burks (2003)

And likewise for male dancers:

> Ultimately the alienation of the dancer from this virtual self may result in behaviors and encounters that violate the normative and moral expectations of the dancer's actual self.
>
> Boden (2002)

Deviance/pathology exemplars reinforce a societal norm and assume that striptease is a form of individual pathology or "wrong doing" which has negative consequences that must be managed. A "we" and a "they" dualism is wrought and marginalization is manufactured (see Vannini and Waskul in this volume).

Exploitation/Liberation Exemplars

The bodies and selves of exotic dancers are also claimed in exploitation/liberation exemplars. These appear in three forms: exploitation, liberation or, a more complex synthesis, exploited *and* liberated. Each of these frames pose an answer to the question: Are exotic dancers' oppressed by the experience of exotic dancing or are they exercising new found sexual and financial liberation, and/or engaging in resistance to mainstream male domination? Again, dualistic answers abound in the literature, thus effectively representing the stripper's body as a sign-vehicle of this or that academic discourse of choice (see Vannini and Waskul, this volume).

Exploitation

In some radical feminist discourses exotic dancers are passive sex objects who lack agency and unwittingly reinforce traditional patriarchal values with their participation in striptease dancing. They are characterized as exploited and oppressed, perpetuating societal norms of "a culture in which sex is defined in terms of dominance and submission" (Kitinger 1994:209).

If a dancer claims she is not exploited or oppressed, if she expresses job satisfaction or enjoyment, resists oppression, or feels like an exploiter or powerful herself, then she is characterized as a victim of false consciousness – a passive agent and cultural dupe who has internalized her oppression. In such cases she cannot, because she is a victim, provide valid descriptions of her lived experience in a "conscious" manner. One abstract excerpt sums up the exploitation frame well:

> These exchanges occur in a context in which interactions are structured by the collective dominance of male patrons and male workers and a social organization of the work that devalues and demeans strippers. While strippers use a variety of coping mechanisms and resistance tactics an examination of these techniques shows the majority of women are overwhelmingly unsuccessful in resolving the troubles of stripping work.
>
> Price (2003)

One male author, writing about gay male dancing, also drew on the exploitation discourse to frame his work:

> Central to the virtual self is a constructed sexuality that is not reflective of the desires of the dancer; rather, it reflects the desires of the consumer ... accommodation, rejection, or departure from the occupation may result.
>
> Boden (2002)

A twist on the exploitation frame was to suggest that striptease was a mutual process of exploitation. For example one abstract stated: "[The dancers] do not see themselves as exploited but rather as playing the game of one-upmanship where everyone has the potential to be had" (Salutin 1971).

Liberation

Pro-sex feminists and others drew on the exploitation/liberation frame by claiming that the women who danced for a living were in fact exercising power and freedom when they worked in the sex industry. Examples of this discourse include:

This employment affords women a level of autonomy, flexibility, and economic compensation rarely available to working class women in the labor force.

Bruckert (2001)

Examine[s] the sex industry as a site that encourages women to expand notions of their own sexuality ... invite[s] them to break taboos. Nude dancing represents a form of class opposition to the dominant Neopuritian norms.

Barton (2001)

Contended that strip clubs represent feminist sites because they offer an opportunity to occupy and interpret a space with a freedom of motion not available elsewhere.

Johnson (1999)

Exploited and Liberated

Still others viewed the exploitation/liberation polarization as artificially imposed by the academy, inaccurate, and a potentially harmful construct – a dualism trap that social science researchers fell into. The truth, it was claimed in this version of the exploitation/liberation frame, was that from moment to moment in the lived experience of an exotic dancer, she may experience empowerment *and* oppression. Some studies, typically interactionist studies, sought to explode this arbitrary dichotomy. For example:

"sex wars" have resulted in a polarized debate which perpetuates cultural stereotypes and a failure to let sex workers speak for themselves.

Barton (2001)

The idea of complex personhood explodes victim/agent dichotomies that are typically used to explain relationships between women and their bodies ... Lives and identities are complicated and often contradictory and women move fluidly amidst identities and victim/agent constructions.

Wesley (2001)

The multiplicity of dancers experiences are both exploitative and agentic ... as well as many things in between ... problematizing the binarization of exploited victim and liberated woman as theorized in both radical and pro-sex feminist paradigms.

Egan (2000)

[Makes] the link between strip club pole work & the struggle by feminist theorists against "conceptual poles."

Johnson (1999)

These authors critique the language of exploitation and liberation as applied to the selves and bodies of exotic dancers, but were nonetheless forced to employ the language of exploitation and liberation to make their argument. As they replicated the discursive order imposed by the assumptions inherent in the language of commodification of the body, they further established and reinforced existing power relations between strippers and society. These authors intended to dismiss the polarities, but instead, they reified the poles by using the labels. Two discreet categories became a continuum, marginalization morphed into a different form. Nothing was problematized nor exploded.

Claiming Dancers' Bodies

Overwhelmingly, female striptease dancers were the favourite subject of striptease researchers. It is tempting to conclude that there were fewer abstracts on male dancers than female because the male version of the occupation is a more recent historical development. However, only seven articles were published on female striptease dancing (starting in 1969) before the first male article appeared in 1980. Nonetheless, when female dancers were the subject of analysis, a majority of the abstracts employed deviance/pathology exemplars, exploitation/liberation exemplars, or both. When male dancers were the subject of an abstract, a smaller percentage employed deviance/pathology exemplars and only two referred to the exploitation/liberation exemplar. An exploration of the numbers reveals a great deal.

Out of 87 abstracts, 22 (25 percent) of drew upon both the deviance/pathology exemplars and the exploitation/liberation exemplars. Of these abstracts, 60 (69 percent) used deviance/pathology exemplars in their discussions of exotic dancers. 35 (40 percent) abstracts within the sample used exploitation/liberation exemplars. Of the 35 that used exploitation/liberation exemplars, ten (29 percent) described the activity of exotic dancing as exploitative, three (9 percent) described it as liberating, and 22 (62 percent) described it as both exploitative and liberating. 14 (16 percent) of the 87 abstracts did not employ the language of deviance/pathology or exploitation/ liberation.

Of 87 abstracts, six (7 percent) did not specify the gender of the stripper. Of these, four were abstracts pertaining to the law and one mentioned strippers in a larger discussion of the Australian sex tourist trade. 62 (71 percent) of the abstracts exclusively featured female dancers. Out of those 62 abstracts, 16 (26 percent) drew on both deviance/pathology exemplars and exploitation/liberation exemplars. 45 (73 percent) of the 62 used deviance/pathology exemplars to describe the activity of dancing while 27 (44 percent) used exploitation/liberation exemplars. Of the 27 that used exploitation/liberation exemplars to describe female dancers, eight (30 percent) described the activity of exotic dancing as exploitative, three (11 percent) described it as liberating, and 16 (59 percent) described it as both exploitative and liberating. Six (10 percent) of the 62 abstracts on female strippers did not employ the language of deviance/pathology or exploitation/liberation. Of the six abstracts that did not employ these frames, two focused on male audiences the subject of analysis, one applied Ritzer's (2004) concept of McDonaldization to striptease dancing, and three were stories based on the researcher's personal experience of exotic dancing.

Of 87 abstracts, 14 (16 percent) featured exclusively male dancers. Of the 14 abstracts on male strippers, five (36 percent) used deviance/pathology exemplars to describe the activity of dancing. Only two (14 percent) used exploitation/liberation frames: one characterized it as exploitative only, one characterized it as both exploitative and liberating. Both of these articles were about men who danced for a male audience. Seven (50 percent) of the male striptease abstracts did not employ the language of deviance/pathology or exploitation/liberation. Over all, 14 of the 87 abstract did not employ deviance/pathology exemplars or exploitation/liberation exemplars. Of these, seven (50 percent) were exclusively on male strippers. Of these seven abstracts, five (71 percent) focused on female audiences who watch male strippers the subject of analysis.

Four (5 percent) of the abstracts featured both male and female dancers. Three of these used deviance/pathology exemplars and one specified exotic dance as both exploitation and liberation. The one article focused on transsexuals drew upon deviance/pathology exemplars, specifying identity and stigma as problems for dancers, as well as framing it as both exploitative and liberating.

In 34 (39 percent) of the abstracts, customers were mentioned. In ten (29 percent) customers, not dancers, was the subject of analysis. Five (50 percent) of these abstracts focused on female and five (50 percent) male audience members. 23 (67%) of the 34 refer to male customers and ten (29 percent) to female customers. Of the ten abstracts which mentioned female customers, all of the studies took place in male strip clubs. One was on male striptease and did not specify the gender of the audience. We emphasize here that of the 14 abstracts mentioned earlier that did not employ deviance/pathology exemplars or exploitation/liberation exemplars, ten (71 percent) of these were focused primarily on the customers.

The Uses of Dancers' Bodies: Gender and Politics

In our review, academic discussions of exotic dancers were a gendered and politicized expression and reflection of power. In summary, 71 percent of the female striptease articles used deviance/pathology exemplars as compared to 36 percent of the male striptease abstracts. 44 percent of the female striptease abstracts used exploitation/liberation exemplars as compared to 14 percent of the male striptease abstracts. Females were clearly characterized as pathologized and exploited by the occupation. Males were pathologized to a much lesser degree and only characterized as exploited when they danced for other men, not when they danced for women. However, in five male strip abstracts, where neither exemplar was applied, the focus of the articles was the female patrons. This was a large portion (35 percent) of the abstracts on male striptease. If we were to throw out those cases, the number of male strip articles would fall to nine. Five abstracts out of nine applying the deviance/pathology exemplar would yield a higher ratio of 55 percent, which is still be below the 73 percent we reported for female dancers. Two abstracts out of nine applying the exploitation/liberation exemplar would yield a higher ratio of 22 percent, which is still be half of the 44 percent we reported for female dancers.

In the six cases where female dancers were not characterized by either deviance/ pathology exemplars or exploitation/liberation exemplars, two made male audiences the topic of discussion, one applied Ritzer's concept of McDonaldization to striptease dancing, and three were stories based on the researcher's personal experience of exotic dancing. If we throw out the two cases where the male customers were the topic, there are 60 abstracts on female dancers. 45 of 60, a full 75 percent of the abstracts, applied deviance/pathology exemplars to the case of female exotic dancers. 27 of 60 of the abstracts (45 percent) applied exploitation/liberation exemplars to the case of female exotic dancers. We are now quibbling over numbers – the case has been made; female dancers are constituted by researchers as deviant and exploited significantly more frequently than male dancers.

Gendered Selves and Bodies

In 1986, Chafetz and Dworkin noted that gender bias was a general trend in deviance research. Likewise, Millman (1975:251) noted that "sociological stereotypes of deviance closely resemble those that appear in popular culture." Decades later, little has changed. After a review of Sociological Abstracts, it appears that scholars constitute and disseminate more "knowledge" in general about female dancers than males.

In Foucaultian terms, scholars have regulated, disciplined, and controlled female bodies and selves through the discourse of commodification. When women put their bodies in the sexual marketplace, the language system, which is localized and diffused throughout the culture, specifies that it is either pathological or exploitative. This discourse serves as discursive constraint (Cordell and Rambo Ronai 1999; Rambo Ronai 1997, 1994; Rambo Ronai and Cross, 1998) on both the bodies and the identities of dancers. Through the gendered discourses of the commodified body, the narrative possibilities of the dancer are limited. If she persists in this behaviour, scholars will label her as defective. She is not permitted to define herself. Discursive constraint attempts to limit "who" the dancer is allowed to be and, through negative labels, encourages her to select a different occupation, one in which her body is not for sale.

The commodified male body is subjected to a different scholarly gaze – not so much in need of regulation, discipline, and control as the female body. When males are the strippers, scholars are often more interested in their female audiences as research subjects. A man dancing for women is considered an interesting occupation – a curiosity. Scholars are not as interested in changing his behaviour or constraining the discourses he is permitted to define himself by. Only when men danced for men did scholars constitute them as victims. Homosexual male bodies are frequently targets for discursive constraint, more so if they are commodified homosexual male bodies.

However, commodified bodies are not passive; commodified selves are not passive. Female dancers are painfully aware of how those who research them perceive them and they resist. More on that later.

Politicized Selves and Bodies

When we think in terms of pathology, exploitation, and liberation, we have stumbled into the arena of morality. Researching exotic dancers becomes a sociopolitical act. Exotic dance becomes a sign-vehicle where researchers project their morals. One explanation for the bifurcated research positions under consideration can be found in George Lakoff's (2004) latest book *Don't Think of an Elephant* in which he argues that there is a tendency for political arguments to polarize into a strict father model and a nurturing parent worldview (for instance Republicans and Democrats in American politics). The strict father model is a conservative frame which posits:

> the world is a dangerous place, and it always will be, because there is evil out there in the world ... there is an absolute right and an absolute wrong. Children are born bad, in the sense that they just want to do what feels good, not what is right.
>
> Lakoff (2004:7)

When this metaphor is applied to politics, society must punish harshly to teach the internal discipline necessary to act morally. Applied to stripping, a strict father model would gaze at exotic dancers and see "deviants" in need of discipline and "fixing."

The nurturing parent model assumes "that children are born good and can be made better. The world can be made a better place and it is our job to work on that" (Lakoff 2004:12). Nurturance means empathy and responsibility and that we must take care of our children. When this metaphor is applied to politics, society must provide protection and help its citizens become fulfilled in life. Applied to stripping, the nurturant parent model is empathetic and views strippers as in need of protection and rescue, thus the exploitation/liberation discourse regarding them from feminists.

By labelling their bodies as deviant, exploited, liberated, or both exploited and liberated, well meaning scholars adopt paternalistic tones toward participants in their research, as if arguing with the correctness of their world views and failing to maintain heuristic distance. Regarding what dancers say, Garfinkel and Sacks (1970:339) would call for a "methodological indifference" by "abstaining from all judgements of their adequacy, value, importance, necessity, practicality, success, or consequentiality." When we fail to maintain heuristic distance, we fail to listen to the ways in which dancers make meaning of their experiences. We as scholars are both consumers of localized discourses and agents at local sites, disseminating a gendered discourse of commodification of the body that is paternalistic, moralistic, and sexist.

Dancers Talk Back

Sara Renée Presley, the second author on this chapter, has conducted 14 taped interviews with female dancers for the purpose of categorizing the types of discourses that dancers generate when verbally constructing accounts of the identities of male and female customers. The dancers interviewed have some preconceived notions regarding how the academy perceives them. Sara made no statements to evince the impression she thought negatively of them. Nevertheless, they narratively resisted discursive constraint from the academy.

One exotic dancer, Angie, invokes the idea that dancers are thought to be mentally ill, but resists it: "I would just say I admit, no wait, I am aware of how I use my body. I don't need someone in here counselling me. That's what I hate." Sara, in no way, suggested that Angie "was in need of counselling." What Angie makes very clear is that if she is a research participant, she expects to be perceived as mentally ill – in other words in deviance/pathology terms. Their conversation continues:

Sara: What do you mean "aware of how you use your body"?
Angie: Girls all do it, most of them. I know you probably have, girl. I just pay attention.
Sara: Most women do what?
Angie: You know what I mean girl.
Sara: Yeah I do, I think, but maybe explain if you can.
Angie: It can be anything. Giving your boss head to get a promotion. Or here's one... batting your eyes at some ugly dude in a bar so he'll buy you drinks all night. Most girls have done that. And you *know* that mother-fucker ain't getting any pussy at the end of the night. You know that. I've seen you do it girl. [laughter]
Sara: [laughter] Yeah I have.
Angie: He wasn't really ugly girl, just too old.
Sara: So you're saying I wasn't aware of what I was doing?
Angie: [laughter] No, You probably were. I'm saying most girls aren't. Those are the ones I don't need in there.

Angie resists imputations of mental illness or deviance by suggesting, "Girls all do it," thus she is no different from other women. The ones who are "aware" are narratively positioned at one end of a continuum while those who are "not aware" (most girls) are positioned at the other end and labelled people "I don't need in here." Angie does not need counselling because she is "aware of how she uses her body." This might imply that those women who are "not aware" need counselling. Angie narratively resists (Rambo Ronai and Cross 1998) the discursive constraint handed to her by society regarding her occupation.

Framing Angie's response to Sara as narrative resistance to discursive constraint is a very different perspective relative to the ones offered by more traditional deviance/ pathology theories. One might be tempted, for instance, to see Angie's response as a technique of neutralization (Sykes and Matza 1957) whereby she condemns her condemners (researchers and/or all girls) as hypocrites. What this and other deviance theories imply is that deviance has an obdurate quality that must be neutralized, justified, excused, or somehow worked around. It implies the research participant "knows they are bad" and tries to manipulate the listener into making an exception for them.

Body/Embodiment

The narrative resistance/discursive constraint frame illuminates a process whereby the dancer firmly asserts an identity claim for herself in the face of efforts made by others to constrain her identity and behaviour practices. In no way is she neutralizing or justifying. She actively resists, at the level of her narrated identity, efforts made to control her body and her sense of self. Narrative resistance makes use of existing negative discourses and transforms them into more positive identity possibilities which can be disseminated back into the mainstream discourses regarding exotic dancers.

This next excerpt reveals the perspective of a dancer who attends college:

Lisa: I'm in college now. I think I said that already. Sorry. I know how it goes. I'm oppressing all of womankind. [laughter.]
Sara: [laughter] No, no, no. What do you think about it [exotic dancing as an occupation]?
Lisa: I'm making it. I waitressed before, made like no money. Had no time whatsoever. And that was so many hours with school and everything.

While Lisa does not spell it out that she is talking about feminism, she reveals a perspective she picked up in school where she expects to be labelled as "oppressing all of woman kind" by being a dancer.

In a different example Becky tells Sara directly about stripping and feminism:

Becky: I liked it when women came in. Better tippers. Well, while I was on stage anyways. You know most of your money comes from private dances and stuff and that was almost always a man but as far as tipping while I was out there, women were good for that.
Sara: Any good stories?
Becky: Not really. But you know they were always the same. Sexual girls.
Sara: Really?
Becky: They liked to be around it.
Sara: The sex?
Becky: Yeah. The whole thing. They liked it all. And I liked them, it was fun to have women in there. Strippers are not anti-woman. They don't need a preaching to about feminism. We got it, they don't.
Sara: Got?
Becky: The idea. We own ourselves, no one else does. And girls who are out there with us you know, sexual, open to life, girls. They got it. Get it too. It's a mindset.

And with this mindset, other narrative possibilities for identity emerge:

Becky: I didn't just do it for money.
Sara: What else then?
Becky: The feeling.
Sara: What feeling?
Becky: The attention. The power of it. I could be a dominatrix or a catholic school girl. Whatever I wanted. I liked that they wanted me to just look at them or talk to them. And

I could give it to them, or not. The sex. I mean I never had sex with any of them but I felt like sex.
Sara: Sexy?
Becky: No like pure Sex . . .I felt like sex, I was sex, you know?
Sara: Not exactly no. Explain it to me.
Becky: What they were paying for. They go home and don't have boring housewife sex that night. He fucks her, really good. A sexy passionate fuck and he is thinking about me while he's doing it. Or in the bathroom at my bar, he can't even get to his car he has to jack off right there. Because of me. It's a powerful feeling. They were paying to fantasize about me. Think about it.

Becky's identity work, to claim that she "was sex" resembles pro-sex feminist discourse. However, to argue that Becky is "mentally ill" or "really liberated" because she is free to enact these roles, or a victim of "false consciousness" who replicates the wishful discourse of her oppressor, is to miss the point.

When sex is in the marketplace, it is often stigmatized and problematized – particularly for women. As a culture we paternalistically tell dancers that what they do is illegitimate and immoral. Whether it is due to their flawed character or false consciousness, *we* create the discourses, logics, and situations that *they* exist within. Feminists and other researchers (of which, all three authors claim to be) are agents of social control and purveyors of discursive constraint.

The Reflexive Identity of the Researcher

When Becky tells Sara that she "felt like sex," and "I was sex," Sara, as a researcher, is partially constrained in her interpretation of Becky's words by the existing research literature and research culture. The pre-existing literature guides Sara's thinking about what Becky said. Sara is free to think outside the box, but not necessarily encouraged by the literature to do so. Rewards come to those who come up with variations on what already exists.

Research on sexuality is stigmatized, even while it enjoys enormous popularity. Amy Flowers (1998:13) in her ethnography on phone sex work comments, "To have researched working at phone sex has only slightly less stigma than having been a phone sex worker. Any association with sex work seems to sully the reputation, leaving the researcher vulnerable to prurient interest, paternalistic censure, and general trivialization." Just as scholars constrain the identity possibilities for dancers, they also constrain the identity possibilities for those who research them. With stigma comes questions such as, "Who will risk mentoring those who research sexuality" (the first author was told by some of her professors that her choices of research topics made her difficult to work with and close to unemployable), and "Where will they submit their article(s) for publication?" Carol, Sara, and Don, are all dependant on a system which supports sexuality research which draws upon deviance/pathology exemplars and exploitation/liberation exemplars. Unless you are characterizing commodified sex, or any sex, as something deviant, dysfunctional, or exploitative, what you have to say about sexuality is often not considered "legitimate." These are the normative frames of comfort.

A social semiotic interpretation of exotic dancers' embodied practices does not have as its goal the reification of deep, dualistic, ontological and moral structures which institutionalize theory. In this chapter we did not *use* exotic dancers as accidental evidence to advance our theoretical or moral agenda. Instead we reflected on how researchers like us constitute knowledge and the processes that such discourses generate in terms of practice. Along a similar vein, Saukko (2003:13) criticizes early cultural studies and its structural semiotic foundations for:

> running into contradictions, [by] bring[ing] together a phenomenological or hermeneutic desire to "understand" the creative lived world of another person or group of people, and the distanced, critical structuralist interest in "analyzing" linguistic tropes, which guide people's perceptions and understanding.

Saukko (2003:13) adds that:

> Furthermore, neither the interest in lived realities or the cultures and languages that mediate our perception of reality bode well with the tendency to make statements about the social and political situation, which is always, to an extent, wedded to a realist quest to find out how the world or reality simply "is."

Or, we might add, a moralist quest to establish how the world or reality ought to be.

In conclusion Saukko (2003:14) notes that:

> since the 1960s, women, blacks, and various postcolonial people, and their movements, have accused institutions, including the state, education, media and so on, of institutionalized discrimination. They have also accused that research, which has always had a particular interest in underprivileged groups, has not depicted the realities of women, ethnic minorities, or postcolonial people but used them to back up the scholar's theoretical and political projects, ranging from colonialism to Marxism and liberal humanist feminism.

A reflexive social semiotic perspective on the sociology of the body revealed how we as researchers were engaged in a contest to define the gendered, commodified, bodies and selves of exotic dancers. Some of us saw dancers as deviant/pathologized bodies and selves, others wanted to determine if those bodies and selves were exploited, liberated, or both and still others see them as both deviant and exploited/liberated. A socio-semiotic perspective on the sociology of the body can reveal other research sites where other contests are in process. Most topics in this book could be examined in this manner. Perhaps a symbolic interactionist focused sociology of the body, as it is explored in this book, will illuminate new ways and new specialized technical vocabularies which are not loaded with judgement regarding their research participants.

References

Barton, Bernadette. 2001. "Inside the Lives of Exotic Dancers." *Dissertation Abstracts International, A: The Humanities and Social Sciences*, 61, 9, Mar, 3775–A.

Boden, David Michael. 2002. "A Wink and a Smile: Titillation and the Alienation of Sexuality within the Occupation of Male Erotic Dancing." *Dissertation Abstracts International, A: The Humanities and Social Sciences*, 62, 11, May, 3951–A.

Boles, Jacqueline & Albeno P. Garbin. 1974. "The Strip Club and StripperCustomer Patterns of Interaction." *Sociology and Social Research*, 58: 36–144.

Bruckert, Christine M. 2001. "Stigmatized Labour: An Ethnographic Study of Strip Clubs in the 1990s." *Dissertation Abstracts International, A: The Humanities and Social Sciences*, 61, 8, Feb, 3378–A.

Chaftez, Janet S. and Anthony G. Dworkin. 1986. *Female Revolt: Women's Movements in World and Historical Perspective*. New York: Rowman & Allanheld.

Cordell, Gina. and Rambo Ronai, Carol. 1999. "Narrative Resistance in the Discourse of Overweight Women," in Sobal, J and Maurer, M. (Eds), *Interpreting Weight: The Social Management of Fatness and Thinness*. New York: Aldine de Gryuter.

Egan, R. Danielle. 2000. "The Phallus Palace: Stripping Spaces, Desiring Subjects and the Fantasy of Objects." *Dissertation Abstracts International, A: The Humanities and Social Sciences*, 61, Nov, 2066–A.

Enck, Graves E. and James D. Preston. 1988. "Counterfeit Intimacy: A Dramaturgical Analysis of an Erotic Performance." *Deviant Behavior*, 9, 4:369–381.

Fowers, Amy. 1998. *The Fantasy Factory: An Insider's View of the Phone Sex Industry*. Philadelphia: University of Pennsylvania Press.

Foucault, Michel. 1977. *The History of Sexuality, Volume I: An Introduction*. New York: Pantheon.

Garfinkel, Harold and Harvey Sacks. 1970. "On Formal Structures of Practical Actions," in John C. McKinney and Edward Tiryakian (Eds), *Theoretical Sociology: Perspectives and Developments*. New York: Appleton-Century-Crofts. pp. 337–366.

Hochschild, Arlie R. 1983. *The Managed Heart: Commercialization of Human Feeling*. Berkeley: University of California Press.

Johnson, Merri L. 1999. "Pole Work: Autoethnography of a Strip Club," In Barry M. Dank and Roberto Refinetti (Eds), *Sexwork & Sex Workers: Sexuality & Culture Vol. I*. New Brunswick: Transaction Publishers. pp. 149–157.

Kitinger, Celia. 1994. "Problematizing Pleasure: Radical Feminist Deconstruction of Sexuality and Power." *Power and Gender*, 9:104–209.

Lakoff, George. 2004. *Don't Think of an Elephant: Know Your Values and Frame the Debate – The Essential Guide for Progressives*. Vermont: Chelsea Green Publishing Company.

Millman, Marcia. 1975. "She Did it All for Love: A Feminist View of the Sociology of Deviance," in M. Millman and R. M. Kanter (Eds), *Another Voice: Feminist Perspectives on Social Life and Social Sciences*. New York: Anchor Books.

Price, Kimberly B. 2003. "Context, Ritual, and Gender: An Ethnography of Stripping." *Dissertation Abstracts International, A: The Humanities and Social Sciences*, 64, 1, July, 303–A.

Rambo Ronai, Carol. 1992a. "The Reflexive Self Through Narrative: A Night in the Life of an Exotic Dancer/Researcher," in Carolyn Ellis and Michael Flaherty (Eds), *Investigating Subjectivity: Research on Lived Experience*. Newbury CA: SAGE.

_____. 1992b. "Separating Aging from Old Age: The Aging Table Dancer." *Journal of Aging Studies*. 6 (4):307–317.

_____. 1994. "Narrative Resistance to Deviance: Identity Management Among Strip-tease Dancers." *Perspectives on Social Problems*, (6).

_____. 1997. "Discursive Constraint in the Narrated Identities of Childhood Sex Abuse Survivors," in Rambo Ronai, C., Zsembik, B. and Feagin, J.R. (Eds), *Everyday Sexism in the Third Millennium*. New York: Routledge.

_____. 1998. "Sketching with Derrida: An Ethnography of a Researcher/Dancer." *Qualitative Inquiry*. 4 (3):405–420.

_____. 1999. "Wrestling with Derrida's Mimesis: The Next Night Sous Rature." *Qualitative Inquiry*. 5 (1):114–129.

Rambo Ronai, Carol and Rabecca. Cross. 1998. "Dancing with Identity: Narrative Resistance in the Discourse of Male and Female Striptease Dancers." *Deviant Behavior*, 18 (2):99–119.

Ronai, Carol R. and Carolyn, Ellis. 1989. "Turn-Ons for Money: Interactional Strategies of the Table Dancer." *Journal of Contemporary Ethnography*, 8:271–298.

Ritzer, George. 2004. *The McDonaldization of Society: Revised New Century Edition*. California: Pine Forge Press.

Salutin, Marilyn. 1971. "Stripper Morality." *Trans-Action*, 8, 8, Jun:12–22.

Saukko, Paula. 2003. *Doing Research in Cultural Studies*. Newbury CA: Sage.

Sijuwade, Philip O. 1995. "Counterfeit Intimacy: A Dramaturgical Analysis of an Erotic Performance." *Social Behavior and Personality*, 23, 4:369–376.

_____. 1996. "Counterfeit Intimacy: A Dramaturgical Analysis of an Erotic Performance." *International Journal of Sociology of the Family*, 26, 2, autumn:29–41.

Sykes, Gresham, and Matza, David. 1957. "Techniques of Neutralization." *American Sociological Review*, 22:664–70.

Thompson, William E., Jack L. Harred and Barbara E. Burks. 2003. "Managing the Stigma of Topless Dancing: A Decade Later." *Deviant Behavior*, 24, 6, Nov-Dec:551–570.

Wesely, Jennifer K. 2001. "Lived Experiences and Negotiated Gender: Female Exotic Dancing, Body Technologies and Violence." *Dissertation Abstracts International, A: The Humanities and Social Sciences*, 62, 2, Aug, 782–A.

_____. 2003. "Where Am I Going to Stop?: Exotic Dancing, Fluid Body Boundaries, and Effects on Identity." *Deviant Behavior*, 24, 5, Sept–Oct:483–503.

PART 5
The Narrative Body:
Body as Story

Chapter 16

The Fit and Healthy Body: Consumer Narratives and the Management of Postmodern Corporeity

Charles Edgley

Charles Edgley's chapter is the first of three dedicated to narrative aspects of embodiment. Edgley's chapter is itself a captivating story; the story of a people who – much like the Greek mythological figure Narcissus – have become so obsessed with their own image that they are at risk of becoming engulfed by it. Edgley's story is one of fast slimming diet wizards, obese monsters, and "magic" beautifying technologies. In the mystical world of the commercialized healthy and fit body, saints and sinners are sorted, the sinful are rendered ugly and then, by offering a quick and easy fitness, diet, and plastic surgery plan, are offered a path for redemption – the means to live happily ever after. Edgley's provocative analysis of the discourses common in our beauty culture imply that the American dream itself has now seemingly changed to a vision of our children and grandchildren as thinner and in "better" shape than we.

At the turn of the new millennium, Americans are pursuing the fit and healthy body with an enthusiasm that people living in other times and places would have found startling, if not bizarre.[1] Faced with a deteriorating environment, an uncertain economy, and daily news of intractable and terrifying political events, Americans seem to turn inward toward a preoccupation with themselves; a passion which, for large numbers of them, meant doing something about their bodies. Fighting fat and getting in shape became a national obsession with a torrent of print, film, ether, and omnipresent everyday conversation devoted to advice, products and testimonials about weight loss and exercise. No one, at least officially, had a kind word for corpulence. Fat even became a political crusade where politicians weighed in on the benefits of the svelte life, and citizens were routinely hectored about their general health and levels of fitness.

No matter how dubious these claims were, how economically biased or insensitive they were to questions of race, class, access to resources, gender and genetics, increasingly the message was the same: fit bodies are healthy bodies, the

---

1   This is not the same as saying that preoccupations with health and fitness are anything new in American culture. See Carson 1957; Whorton 1982.

standards of fitness are largely settled, medicine and nutritional science have given institutional imprimatur to a foreordained conclusion, and those who do not measure up are not only courting a self-induced disaster, but are socially irresponsible as well. As waistlines increased, fitness expectations expanded along with them. Ignoring contradictory evidence[2] pouring in from all sides about what constitutes fitness in the first place, what the standards for a healthy body are, and how they might best be achieved, narratives of the public culture of health continued to crank out the conventional mantra of diet and exercise, differing only on the details (Edgley and Brissett 1991, 1999).

These narrative accounts of why Americans were still out of shape flooded both the media and everyday forms of talk. They constitute what Holstein and Gubrium (2000) term "discourses in practice" – those situated narratives available at a given time and place for self construction. These authors distinguish between what they call "discursive practice" – the communicative *means* by which the self is constructed, and "discourses in practice," which I discuss here in terms of narrative stories commonly found in the postmodern world of body consumerism. We take for granted the former[3] – discursive practices such as ethnomethodology, symbolic interaction, and semiotics – in favour of their outcomes and use. In doing so, we develop a critical and interpretive analysis of the practiced discourses of public health and fitness.

Even as Americans grew larger, the popular discourse on fitness and health explained away the contradictions. When increased exercise did not bring about the desired levels of fitness, numerous remedies were sought in the presumed conspiracies of the food industry. Many believed that television and especially the remote control device was to blame. Some believed that fast food outlets were responsible for the obesity epidemic and filed lawsuits against the major chains alleging that eating their food had made the plaintiffs fat. Others opined that it was mass media and automobiles that made Americans lazy and therefore fat. Narrative tales of weight battles consumed obese victims, fuelled by popular television figures such as Oprah Winfrey who shared their personal struggles with corpulent viewers. Winfrey herself lost, regained, and lost again the same 100 lbs – her ratings waxing and waning with every cycle of despair to redemption and back. The diet industry mirrored her plight. As low calorie diets failed, low fat diets became popular. As low fat diets floundered, low-carb diets became fashionable. As weight increased even in the face of Atkins™ and Southbeach™, a host of competitors joined the marketplace trying to cash in on the billions of dollars Americans were willing to spend annually in the battle against corpulence. The mainstream was joined by the bizarre. Blood type diets, rotation diets, negative calorie diets, and diets that promised the eater that certain "miracle foods" – cabbage soup, grapefruit, cranberries, garlic, or vegetable sprouts – would turn the tide in their favour. But like sex, exercise, and other corporeal

---

2   Atrens (2005) reports that while obesity among Americans seems to be increasing; both caloric and fat intake has actually been declining. An examination of cross-cultural data only adds to the diet and exercise contradictions.

3   More technically, we analytically "bracket them" as Holstein and Gubrium suggest.

consummations devoutly wished, more people seemed interested in talking about diets than actually following them.[4]

As the popular discourse sought exculpation from external sources, a blaring profusion of media catering to this appetite for fitness and its associated concerns about health endorsed a different source as an explanation for the problem. Specialty magazines, websites, newsletters, health and fitness columns, books, video tapes, and DVDs, all delivered a message of personal agency: fitness is an individual responsibility and the deteriorating body is evidence not of disease or genetics, but of *moral* failing as the following narrative from a web-based company attests:

> To take control of your health and fitness is to take *full responsibility for what you're doing or not doing.* Its no one else's fault if you don't exercise ... Blaming everyone else for your health is a sure way to stay right where you are – [fat] and hating every minute of it.
>
> Waehner (2005)

Such moral exhortations to personal responsibility are rarely presented without suggestions for improvement. Rather, they are accompanied by an offer of the entire world of exercise and dietary consumer goods as a panacea for corporeal dilemmas:

> The wrinkles, sagging flesh, tendency towards middle age spread, hair loss, etc., which accompany aging should be combated by energetic body maintenance on the part of the individual – with help from the cosmetic, beauty, fitness, and leisure industries.
>
> Hepworth and Featherstone (1982:84)

Somatic salvation and moral rectitude are only a credit-card transaction away. This message of individual responsibility resonated not only with venerable self-denial and abstinence themes in American culture,[5] but also with a burgeoning consumer marketplace that was prepared to meet the needs of Americans anxious to take control of their bodies. The fact that this control is largely illusionary and driven by vanity in no way deterred the fitness enthusiast in search of the perfect body:

> For all their talk of health, what fitness participants achieve on their Nautilus machines and fat-free diets is an *image of healthiness.* They reshape their bodies to exhibit the visual indicators of health demanded by the photographs in the glossy magazines and by the numbers in the Metropolitan Life weight tables.
>
> Glassner (1993:227)

As a result of the emergence of the ethic of health through personal achievement, a cornucopia of consumer products promising to deliver a perfect body to the

---

4 Specialty fitness magazines such as *Runner's World* report that most of their readers do not themselves run. Given the failure rate for dieting, it appears likewise that losing weight is a form of vicarious experience – more interesting to talk about than to accomplish.

5 Gillick traces the moral ethic of individual responsibility for health through clean and upright living to the religious tradition of physical hygiene first enunciated in the work of John Wesley, who's *Primitive Physick*, published in 1764, regarded sickness as punishment for earthly sins (Gillick 1984).

devout flooded the marketplace. Exercise equipment such as treadmills, stationary bicycles, Nordic-track® and Bowflex®, machines, free weights, and power-lifting equipment target every part of the body. Even the brand names themselves suggest different machines for different somatic needs, and the consumer accustomed to the latest technology is required to invest thousands of dollars to cover one's fitness requirements. Butt Buster®, Thighmaster®, and Buns of Steel® assure the user that the machine is tailored to their exact bodily anxieties and fitness requirements.

In addition, workout clubs – sorted by price and class cache – (Nautilus®, Bally®, Dolphin®); "day spas" (Ona®, Wolf Mountain®); and resort "stay spas" (Casa Playa®, Montage®) join with a pharmucopia of drugs, emoluments, herbs, and "nutritional supplements" to create a climate in which health and fitness are consumer commodities to be purchased. Health stores and "Nutrition Centres" dot the landscape. Free-standing businesses such as GNC™ compete with a host of internet operations like Great Earth Vitamins™ and Herbalife™ to hawk the message of vigour and salubriousness. Nutrical™, an internet based operation, even assures that the pets of affluent health enthusiasts have the same opportunities to a fit and health body as their owners.

Formerly mainstream physicians, frustrated with conventional medicine's failures, trumpet the message of health through alternative discourses-in-practice. The success of these crusades has pushed yearly sales of complementary and alternative medicine to more than 27 billion dollars a year (National Academies Report 2005). Chat rooms where devotees can share their health and fitness stories abound. For the more solitary or embarrassed consumer working on fleshly anxieties, there is also the ubiquitous exercise video where a virtual relationship can be enacted with friendly, smiling and proportionately perfect cheerleaders for fitness. Thousands of these video and DVD products are now available and are marketed to every age group, lifestyle and personal taste. From the ubiquitous Richard Simmons to the politically divisive Jane Fonda, there are fitness guides for every taste using these media to promote their own fitness ideal. Finally, we have seen the emergence of "personal trainers," experts on the buff body who are willing to serve as certified fitness nannies: leading cheers, dispensing advice, and, when necessary, badgering clients into the Spartan life of discipline and control.

The Historical Body and the Postmodern Condition

For most of the world's history, human beings have been forced by immutable circumstances to create a self around whatever corporeal circumstances nature and society had dealt them. Many things could be and obviously were done to bodies[6] in an effort to fit whatever cultural insignias and looking-glasses of beauty, power, status and wealth reigned at the time, but the range of possibilities was constrained

---

6 The archeological record is replete with instances of body modification among even the most ancient of cultures. The question is one of current technologies that expand considerably the efficacy of such desires.

by certain obdurate physical realities. It was effectively impossible in the pre-modern world to increase one's height, shorten oneself, or alter one's appearance in any kind of fundamental way. But in the postmodern marriage of consumer culture and medical technology, all of this has changed. Now there appears no aspect of one's body that cannot be modified to suit the self its possessor aspires to be.

Moreover, the growing source of these inspirations – the discursive arena in which these narratives are formed and distributed, is advertising and the consumer marketplace. The postmodern "lifestyle shopper" (Shields 1992) with sufficient resources can surgically enhance, reshape, swell, reduce, or even add to or improve almost any part of the body.[7] In high modernity the body is expected to be a carefully crafted work in progress, open to change, always on the lookout for the most recent trends, and attuned to the demands of image-makers who set the standards. The message is both classist and sexist since the penalties are severe for those who choose to opt out of this game or whose resources are inadequate to the proper playing of it (Wolf 2002).

Technologies of image-making have altered the semiotics of western society in ways that have profound implications for the sociology of both selves and bodies (Gergen 2000; Lyotard 1979; Waskul 2001, 2002). Waskul's work in particular shows that the possibilities afforded by the cybernetic revolution have created a circumstance in which we not only can "embody the self" but also "enself the body." Bodies no longer force or constrain the creation of any particular self around them. The self and the body are now fully and transparently linked, open to manipulation in ways more effective and elemental than ever before, as well as being inseparable from the dramaturgy of politics, advertising, power, imagery, and, above all, consumer markets.

Postmodernity and the Discontented Body

The pastiche of images, contested territories of value, the crisis of representation in which the "real" can no longer be authenticated apart from its representation (Baudrillard 1983), the decline of culture and tradition as a source of stability and direction (Clausen 2000), and the tyrannical demands of what Jameson calls the "perpetual present," (Jameson 1983:125) create conditions which foment discontent in almost every sphere of postmodern life. But the body is particularly vulnerable because it appears at the outset to be the one aspect of a life that can be most easily changed. It seems that virtually no one is happy with the direction in which either society or their own life is headed (Hughes 1994), but if one cannot change society

---

7   While breast implants, face lifts, tummy tucks, rhinoplasty, and liposuction are the most common, virtually anything is now possible in the postmodern world of bodies as medical achievements. Even normally unexposed parts of the body are subject to medical enhancement. In labiaplasty the inner lips of the vagina are surgically reconstructed to give a more pleasing appearance. Hymenoplasty reconstructs the hymen so that a woman can, in a physical sense, regain at least the sign of her virginity. Sullivan (2000) offers a compelling analysis of elective cosmetic surgery.

and if altering the self is difficult because of its inherent connection to existing social arrangements (Mead 1967), at least the construction of a new body might render its occupant immune from the resident frustrations of existence. Pamela Moore's (1997:2) observation about body builders seems to apply to physical alterations in general:

> In one sense, built bodies are the ultimate expression of the postmodern belief in corporeal malleability.... Built bodies are almost absurdly controlled, to the point where flesh no longer is flesh, but metal machines, as when builders describe their arms as guns or their legs as pistons.

Aberrant Flesh

The idea that virtually anyone *can* achieve standards of health and fitness through a proper regimen of diet and exercise quickly translated itself into an ideology that everyone *ought* to. Aligning itself firmly to the therapeutic culture, fitness is no longer simply a succession of positive homilies people offer up to one another and which they can take or leave. The message is intensely moral and negative. Those who do not measure up are variously labelled "couch potatoes", "slackers," "slugs," "thicks," or "chunky/funkys." Aberrant flesh[8] evokes an array of moral opprobrium and interpersonal stigmata that enforce the lesson that fitness is an unalloyed good. Its icons are the unrepentant smoker and the morbidly obese. Like all ideologies, fitness is constituted as a moral framework.[9] Its adherents do not just want to be healthy, they want to be *good*. Those who are not are regarded as representing a danger to those who are.

In this new postmodern world of rapidly developing possibilities, aberrant flesh is no longer tolerated because the view that everything can be altered to fit the societal ideal is now firmly entrenched. Baudrillard's (1993:45) words on this subject, subtitled "Essays on Extreme Phenomenon," no longer seem so extreme:

> We are under the sway of a surgical compulsion that seeks to excise negative characteristics and remodel things synthetically into ideal forms. Cosmetic surgery: a face's chance configuration, its beauty or ugliness, its distinctive traits, its negative traits – all these things have to be corrected, so as to produce something more beautiful than beautiful: an ideal face, a *surgical* face.

But in spite of this consumption-driven view of the body as wholly malleable, in spite of all efforts to stigmatize and to ban those practices and those persons who fail to shape up, aberrant flesh still resists. Shilling's widely-cited and influential view

---

8   I borrow the term from Pamela Moore (1997).

9   Numerous scholars (Gillick 1986; Pronger 2003; Edgley and Brissett 1999) have deconstructed health and fitness movements and shown them to be, at base, moral crusades with both Puritanical and Fascist roots directed toward "the desire to order, organize, control, repress, direct, impose limits – to interrupt the free flow of *puissance* and subordinate it to *pouvoir*" (Pronger 2002:110).

that the body is something of an "absent presence" (Shilling 1993) seems no longer the case, at least from the standpoint of scholarly efforts to render it understandable. But the body still remains in many ways unaccounted for, its fits and spurts strangely resistant to a definitive analysis. The contrast point for fit and healthy bodies remains unfit and sick ones. Diminishing physical capacities and a host of corporal ailments continue to remind us of the triumph flesh exacts over soaring minds.[10]

Moreover, no matter how healthy and fit, bodies still possess repugnant qualities. They leak and smell and the odours they give off must be regulated from birth to death. Shakespeare's "mewling and puking" infant eventually submits to the regulated controls that can be seen in the array of scent depressants resident in bath and body rooms everywhere. But the tamed and socialized body, no matter how meticulously it is attended to, awakens each day to yet another round of renewed suppressions. Bodily orifices that can be rendered hidden are disguised beneath layers of clothing and those that can't be are either discreetly ignored or treated according to implicit aesthetic codes. When it finally dies, typically in a hospital similarly filled with disinfectants designed to erase its presence as a body, it is transported to a funeral home where, as Goffman reports, it is "drained, stuffed, and painted for its final performance" (Goffman 1959:114). The dramaturgical body, carefully staged for proper presentation is, in this sense, an effort to deny that it is a body at all.

Selling and Celebrating the Fit and Healthy Body: Consumer Narratives from Tragedy to Triumph

The electronic revolution that fuelled postmodernity assured a market for visual content separate from the kind of immediate face-to-face narratives that previous generations produced themselves. As Waskul and Vannini point out in the introduction to this volume, symbolic interactionists conceptualize the body as a site of "struggle between institutional discourses and counter-narratives," as well as "struggles between the realm of the symbolic (i.e. the self) and the … corporeal." Nowhere is this struggle more evident than those that rage over the fit and healthy body. Foucault's "docile" bodies that submit to regulation have given way to strident bodies that either enthusiastically celebrate and promote fitness – or actively resist the current definitions of it. Far from being sharply divided in a Cartesian binary, here the body and self are joined in the concept of "embodiment." The embodied self is inherently political, historical, institutional, disciplined (or *un*disciplined), and dramaturgical. It joins at the interstices of recondite flesh and society in ways reminiscent of Moore's discussion of "built bodies" which she describes as "a dynamic, politicized *and* biological site" (Moore 1997:2). The public narratives that promise fit and healthy bodies through the institutionalized vehicle of consumer goods are regularly verified in Cynthian celebrations of those same bodies. Marathons, fitness fairs, wellness centres, cholesterol screenings, and blood pressure checks

---

10 The lament of the aged that "the spirit is willing, but the flesh is weak" strikes to this point.

in shopping malls simultaneously celebrate and monitor bodies. But still more is required to sell health and fitness. The selves that populate bodies, being made out of nothing more than symbols in the first place, are in steady need of narrative stories for support. As Holstein and Gubrium (2000:116) put it, "stories take shape on the occasions of their use, as parts of the very identity projects for which they serve as resources." Consumerism, nutrition and technology unite with willing subjects to generate chronicles of health and fitness sins accompanied by a plethora of consumer products offered up as redemption for flaccid flesh in need of change. The essential message of all these stories is that the perfect body can be purchased and the new media of the postmodern era promote this conventional wisdom.

Following the aforementioned distinctions made by Holstein and Gubrium's discussion of the narrative sources of postmodern identity, this section explores common health and fitness narratives as "discourses in practice" – those stories which form, constitute, and constrain the lived experiences of the self. What is of interest is what these narratives provide: conceived possibilities and resources for the construction of a self around a body, or – in the more postmodern sense we suggest – a body around an idyllic self.

Videos and DVDs

Exercise videos and DVDs provide this narrative support and the range and variety of portable fitness media underscores a pastiche that is inclusive of anyone affluent enough to join the parade. Every lifestyle and taste preference is indulged. There are videos for belly dancers, Yoga aficionados, crunch and abdominal devotees, kick boxers, Hula Dancers, Pilate's followers, Taebo and Tai Chi advocates, as well as those who wish to mix dancing with workouts such as the Salsa™ series and Aerobicise™ enthusiasts. There are exercise videos for persons at every stage of the lifecycle, and even ones for those who wish to combine their appetite for the stimulations of pornography with the stimulations of a workout. Fitness guru and adult film star "Lori Lust" produces a line of adult-oriented sexual exercise DVDs. Her line of Sexercise™, Eroticise™ and Exersex™ videos marry seemingly incompatible decadent flesh with healthy exercise and fitness.

From the pleasures of sex to the results of it, even the nascent foetus is not to be relieved of exercise burdens or be allowed a sedentary lifestyle *in uteri*. "Buns of Steel"'s series of pregnancy and post-pregnancy videos and "Crunch: Yoga Mama Prenatal" hype their products by implying the unverified proposition that the foetus benefits from a "fitness lifestyle." The "Fit Mama" video takes the program to new post-partum heights by assuring that the little tyke gets off to a good fitness start while mom enjoys guilt-free exercise:

> Exercising after pregnancy doesn't have to mean time away from your baby… That's why Leisa Hart created the "FitMama & Me" Exercise Video so that you can include your baby! You'll tone your tummy, hips and thighs while giving your baby a little activity too…
>
> Bellybeats.com (2005)

In the all-promotional advertising environment characteristic of postmodernity, these videos feature jogging strollers with names like "Iron Baby" that assure the post-partum mother that she can get her baby off to a good start by resuming her own fitness program. The sedentary office worker isn't ignored either. Stretchworks™ videos offer a series of exercise regimes designed to be performed at one's desk. Billy's Boot Camp™ Series of Tae Bo videos promise to take the struggling, out-of-shape fitness reprobate and convert him or her into a rock-hard fitness paragon in only a week. Before-and-after success stories are effusive in their praise of the program: over the heading "I've got a flat stomach I'm not ashamed to show anymore" the familiar inspirational narrative characteristic of these products unfolds:

> Jamie is a changed girl. She had always been on the heavy side growing up and vowed that she would never weigh more than 200 lbs. When she got on the scale and saw that she weighed 210 lbs she was completely disgusted. Then she started with Billy, and lost 15 lbs in the first month. Jamie has now lost a total of 85 lbs! So, for her 25th birthday, she got her belly button pierced and wore a bikini to the beach!
>
> http://www.billyblanks.com/Success.asp

The themes in these advertising narratives follow the traditional cycle of despair, hope, reinforcement and, ultimately, triumph. The final exclamation point in Jamie's tale is characteristic of all such before-and-after narratives; the ability to display a part of the body heretofore hidden behind a curtain of shame: the navel, now proudly pierced and displayed in a bikini – the semiotic logo proving the triumph of discipline over aberrant flesh.

Fitness and the Therapeutic Ethic

> Therapeutics need no doctrines, only opportunities.
>
> Philip Rieff (1966:18)

Narrative tales of fitness might never have reached their position as dominant discourses-in-practice about the body or be in a position to create such massive consumer markets had it not been for opportunities afforded by the merger of fitness and therapy. What Philip Rieff (1966) called "The Triumph of the Therapeutic" saw to it that insufficiencies of flesh were translated into discontents that could be revolved by the expedient of medicalization. Every social change requires a convincing rationale and a change in its vocabulary of motives (Mills 1946; Scott and Lyman 1977) was necessary to give fitness and health legitimate imprimatur.[11] Its iconography tied itself to the rising therapeutic enthusiasm that embraced Americans in almost every segment of life (Polsky 1991). Fitness was not just good

---

11 Economic factors alone are insufficient to explain the lure of consumer culture in general or the fitness revolution in particular. What is required is a vocabulary of symbolic motives that gives a storied rationale to the act of buying. The therapeutic provides such purpose and meaning through narrative tales of transformation and redemption.

for the body; it was said, but good for the mind and the soul as well. The rhetoric employed by the founders of the running movement is replete with examples of this marriage of body and soul. George Sheehan (1998), whose book *Running and Being* fuelled much of the enthusiasm for marathoning, devotes as much space to spiritual matters as somatic ones. The subtitles to his many books are indicative of the therapeutic claims which have become standard fitness fare. *How to Achieve the Physical, Mental & Spiritual Victories of Running* and *The Total Experience* let it be known that running was not just a matter of moving one's feet, but that a kind of therapeutic nirvana awaited those who run. James Fixx (1978:28), whose life of devotion to health and fitness was cut short when he collapsed and died of a massive coronary while running, laced his books with quotations and stories from devotees who found "unification of body and mind" and "Alpha" states that protect them from sickness and injury. Originally a movement begun around the simple story of improved cardiac health, running narratives have now expanded to promise an integrated paradise of mind, body, and soul.

God and the Fit Body

Because of the quasi-spiritual nature of these fitness tales, they lend themselves easily to sectarian religiosity. Recondite flesh is open to a host of meaning ascriptions and the symbols produced by the diet industry make it clear that body and soul go together just as bodies and minds do in running. Among the more striking examples is diet workshop guru Gwen Shamblin whose "Weigh-Down Workshops" tie God directly to bodies in ways fully consistent with Wesley's Primitive Physick 200 years before. Like Wesley, the goal is to be "Slim for Him." The principal which underlies her workshops, books, and television appearances is the simple idea that "God is watching everything we eat, and he is not pleased." All-you-can-eat buffets, fat emporiums, and drive-up windows dispensing dietary excess leads directly to the rolls of fat and mounds of flesh that are testimony to how far Americans have strayed from the Godly ideal. Somewhere along the line, she says, "Americans forgot to behave" (Mead 2001:48). They also forgot Wesley, for American Christians have trivialized the sin of gluttony – so much so that churches have traditionally used food as a way of luring people to God. Church suppers, soup kitchens, and, in the case of the rapidly developing urban mega-churches characteristic of the postmodern era, food courts featuring pizza and burgers bring in the faithful. These evangelical tactics have proven to be so successful that two national studies now show that Christians are significantly fatter than American Jews, Muslims or Buddhists (Ferraro 1998).

The sin of gluttony is not to be trivialized any longer and Shamblin and her followers are determined to return the nation to the kind of fit bodies that come from submitting oneself to God. In this sense they are echoing 19th century Christian thinkers such as Sylvester Graham who encouraged a vegetarian diet of whole grains and fruit and the avoidance of meat on the grounds that the latter inflamed animal passions. John Harvey Kellogg, intellectual heir to Graham's writings, developed cold cereal at his Battle Creek sanitarium as a moral food designed to dampen masturbatory ardour thought to be brought on by the consumption of "warm and sensuous" breakfast foods such as eggs and oatmeal. In the virulent anti-masturbatory climate of the time, cold cereals were to be the dietary equivalent of cold showers – an extinguisher of sexual desire (Edgley and Brissett 1990).

No longer satisfied with the charge to save the world, the Christian weight loss movement believes that slimming the self is a more urgent priority. Mead (2001) charts a list of books going back to 1957 which echo this theme and include such titles as: "Pray your Weight Away," "Help Lord – The Devil Wants Me Fat!", "Slim for Him," and "More of Jesus, Less of Me." They find their mandate in the fact that gluttony is one of the oldest of the Seven Deadly Sins, having made the list because it was one of the resident temptations of cloistered monks and, like lust, was believed to take their minds away from God (Lyman 1989). These Christian narratives reframe fat as enemies of God in ways reminiscent of early Christian thinkers' contempt for lust, their concern for which masked a general anxiety for all earthly pleasures. Augustine's Confessions report his anguish over efforts to reconcile his own sexual desires with his monastic commitment to God. The language of the Confessions is replete with references to desire as corrupt and diseased, and sexual interest as leading to perdition. Following the implications of this narrative tale, another early Christian, Tertullian proclaimed that heaven is open to eunuchs, and Eusebius praised those who had made themselves eunuchs, for the kingdom of Heaven's sake" (Matt 19:12). Numerous early Christian fathers accepted this view and castrated themselves (Lyman 1989:61). While hardly requiring such an extreme level of religious devotion, Shamblin and her followers demonstrate how ancient narratives of God and the body can be resurrected in new forms that story the lives of their tellers and rationalize somatic change.

Discordant Narratives: Managing the 'Unfit' Body

Those whose bodies do not measure up to the new symbolism of fitness and health have neither remained silent nor accepted the conventional mainstream narrative. Alternative discourses, honed and practiced in organized opposition to the official version, emerged from those who see themselves as victims of the conventional tale. As Martin (2002) has shown in his study of three organizations, Weight Watchers, Overeaters Anonymous (OA) and the National Association to Advance Fat Acceptance (NAAFA), there are widely differing strategies available to those who see themselves as stigmatized by conventional stories of fitness sins and enforced redemption. While Weight Watchers accepts the official definition of fat bodies as unhealthy and uses societal definitions of appearance as motivation for losing weight, OA and NAAFA reframe fat in ways consistent with their differing views. OA defines obesity in much the same way as its eponymous counterpart Alcoholics Anonymous frames liquor. The overeater, they claim, is sick, a victim of a "disease" the symptom of which is eating too much, a circularity characteristic of the medical model applied to conduct. The solution, they say, is a twelve-step program that combines meetings, support and spiritual strength, all framed within a context of redemption. While these two organizations help their members fight fat, NAAFA helps theirs revel in it. Fat, they say, is a civil rights issue and no one has the right to tell them how much they ought to weigh. Framing the issue in terms of oppression, they organize to oppose "size discrimination" through legal and political remedies.[12]

Martin's work is significant to an understanding of the postmodern body because it demonstrates the pastiche of narrative possibilities for reframing fat in a society where standards of fitness and the vocabulary of motives one articulates about them serve to negotiate and constitute their identity. Each of them makes an effort to story the self; a story that others insist must include an account of fat. For Weight Watchers, calorie control is a way of life. Supplying their members with a vocabulary of motives for weight loss through trimming calories is as crucial to their narrative as cutting calories itself. For participants in Overeaters Anonymous the medical frame transforms participation from dieting to recovery. Similarly, the invocation of the disease model offers an account for the troubles their members suffer. Here we can see that the organizations which attract corpulent consumers sell a framed narrative as opposed to merely a diet program – or in the case of NAAFA, avoidance of diets altogether since pride in one's weight render them unnecessary. Lee Monaghan's recent work on newly developing tales of masculine fat – "Big Handsome Men" and "Cuddly Bears" (fat hairy men) similarly shows entrenched resistance against the dominant narrative. By restoring large bodies in positive ways and infusing them with sexual attractiveness and desire, their members seek to escape what they consider to be the oppressive and negative narratives of obesity and overweight (Monaghan 2005).

Afterword

The societal aftermath of modernity – what in this chapter we called, following Lyotard and others, the postmodern condition – fuelled a variety of social, economic, and especially, semiotic changes in which the self and the body are progressively joined, framed, and evaluated as individual achievements and/or works in progress. The availability of a wide range of health and fitness products generates an expectation that aberrant flesh no longer needs to be tolerated, as well as the social demand that it will not be tolerated. In this arrangement, the status of the body is altered. The self is no longer simply housed within bodies but emerges in a fully interactive process in which the container and the contained have an inseparable, invariant relationship; not simply as residences for selves, but as alterable signs of the self.

---

12 Another discordant voice may be found in "pro ana" websites that give support to anorexics and bulimics looking for narrative rationales for what others term their "eating-disorder." These discordant voices are so at variance with the health and fitness mainstream that there are regular calls for silencing them through internet censorship.

Central to this process is the selling and celebrating of the fit and health body through consumer narratives which chronicle the struggles of the health or fitness offender as they move through predictable cycles of tragedy and triumph. Whether they are narratives that affirm the svelte and exercised ideal or discordant ones which promote alternative views of the body, these stories engage corporeal anxieties as retrospective acts in which the meaning of one's past life is transformed by the present narrative tale. These reinterpretations of the past in the light of the acting present may take the form of tragedies avoided, years wasted, or opportunities lost, no matter whether the narrative is conventional or discordant. This ongoing process of interpretation and reinterpretation offers seductive and powerful rationales for pervasive but ever-changing conceptions of the fit and healthy body.

References

American Sports Data Reports. 2000. http://www.americansportsdata.com/pr-fitnessrevolution.asp.

Atrens, D.M. 2005. "Run for your life." http://www.sirc.org/articles/run_for_your_life.shtml.

Baudrillard, Jean. 1983. *Simulations*. New York: Semiotext(e).

_____. 1993. *The Transparency of Evil*. London: Verso.

Becker, Howard S. and Michael McCall. 1993. *Symbolic Interaction and Cultural Studies*. Chicago: University of Chicago Press.

Berger, Peter L. and Thomas Luckmann. 1967. *The Social Construction of Reality*. New York: Anchor.

Carson, Gerald. 1957. *Cornflake Crusade*. New York: Rinehart.

Clausen, Christopher. 2000. *Faded Mosaic: The Emergency of Post-Cultural America*. New York: Ivan Dee.

Edgley, Charles and Dennis Brissett. 1991. "Health Nazis and the Cult of the Perfect Body: Some Polemical Observations." *Symbolic Interaction*, 25 (2):257–279.

_____. 1999. *A Nation of Meddlers*. Boulder, CO: Westview Press.

Featherstone, Michael, Mike Hepworth and Bryan S. Turner (eds) 1991. *The Body: Social Process and Cultural Theory*. London: Sage Publications.

Ferraro, Kenneth. 1998. "Firm Believers? Religion, Body Weight and Well-Being." *Review of Religious Research*, 39:224–244.

Fixx, James. 1977. *The Complete Book of Running*. New York: Random House.

Gergen, Kenneth. 2000. *The Saturated Self*. New York: Basic Books.

Gillick, Muriel R. 1984. "Health Promotion, Jogging, and the Pursuit of the Moral Life." *Journal of Health Politics, Policy and Law*, 9 (3):369–387.

Glassner, Barry. 1990. "Fit for Postmodern Selfhood." In Howard S. Becker and Michael McCall (eds), *Symbolic Interaction and Cultural Studies*. Chicago: The University of Chicago Press. pp. 215–243.

Goffman, Erving. 1959. *The Presentation of Self in Everyday Life*. New York: Anchor.

Holstein, James A. and Jaber F. Gubrium. 2000. *The Self We Live By: Narrative Identity in a Postmodern World*. New York: Oxford University Press.

Hughes, Robert. 1994. *Culture of Complaint: The Fraying of America*. New York: Warner Books.

Jameson, Fredric. 1994. *Postmodernism, or the Cultural Logic of Late Capitalism*. Durham, NC: Duke University Press.

Lyman, Stanford M. 1989. *The Seven Deadly Sins: Society and Evil*. Dix Hills, NY: General Hall.

Lyotard, Jean-Francois. 1984. *The Postmodern Condition: A Report on Knowledge*. Minneapolis: University of Minnesota Press.

Martin, Dan. 2002. "From Appearance Tales to Oppression Tales: Frame Analysis and Organizational Identity." *Journal of Contemporary Ethnography*, 31 (2):158–206.

Mead, George Herbert. 1967. *Mind, Self and Society*. Chicago: University of Chicago Press.

Mead, Rebecca. 2001. "Slim for Him." *New Yorker*, Jan. 16:48–56.

Miller, W.C. 1999. "How Effective are Traditional Dietary and Exercise Interventions for Weight Loss?" *Medicine and Science in Sports and Exercise*, 31 (8):1129–1134.

Mills, C. Wright. 1940. "Situated Actions and Vocabularies of Motive." *American Sociological Review*, 5(6):904–913.

Monaghan, Lee F. 2005. "Big Handsome Men, Bears and Others: Virtual Constructions of 'Fat Male Embodiment'. *Body and Society*, 11, 2:81–111.

Moore, Pamela. 1997. *Building Bodies*. New Brunswick: Rutgers University Press.

National Academies Report. 2005. *Complementary and Alternative Medicine in the United States*. http://www.nap.edu/books/0309092701/html/1.html.

Polsky, Andrew. 1991. *The Rise of the Therapeutic State*. Princeton: Princeton University Press.

Rieff, Phillip. 1966. *The Triumph of the Therapeutic*. Chicago: University of Chicago Press.

Scott, Marvin and Stanford Lyman. 1968. "Accounts." *American Sociological Review*, 33:46–62.

Sheehan, George. 1998. *Running and Being*. Mission, BC: Second Wind Books.

Shields, Rob. 1992. *Lifestyle Shopping: The Subject of Consumption*. International Library of Sociology. New York: Routledge.

Shilling, Chris. 1993. *The Body and Social Theory*. London: Sage Publications.

Sullivan, Deborah. 2000. *Cosmetic Surgery: The Cutting Edge of Commercial Medicine in America*. New Brunswick: Rutgers University Press.

Waehner, Paige. 2005. "If You're Fat, Whose Fault is it?" http://exercise.about.com/cs/weightloss/a/fatresponsibili_htm.

Waskul, Dennis. 2002. "The Naked Self: Being a Body in Televideo Cybersex." *Symbolic Interaction*, 25, 2:199–227.

Waskul, Dennis, Mark Douglass, and Charles Edgley. 2000. "Cybersex: Outercourse and the Enselfment of the Body." *Symbolic Interaction*, 23, 4:375–397.

Whorton, J. 1982. *Crusade for Fitness: A History of American Health*. Princeton, NJ: Princeton University Press.
Wolf, Naomi. 2002. *The Beauty Myth*. New York: Harper.

Chapter 17

Masks of Masculinity: (Sur)passing Narratives and Cosmetic Surgery

Michael Atkinson

Much like some of the narratives examined by Edgley in Chapter Sixteen, the stories collected by Michael Atkinson in interviews with male customers of the plastic surgery industry show how the alliance between technology, capitalism, and the culture of beauty works: by providing the promise of a technologically advanced "cure" for feelings of body dissatisfaction, plastic surgery can turn lives around by transforming the gender identity of its patrons. From a narrative perspective such an event is a classic turning point distinguishing a life story with the traits of the "before and after" genre. In a cultural universe where it is women who seem to be the exclusive protagonists of stories of beauties and beasts, the value of Atkinson's research resides in its potential to tell the untold stories of men struggling with their own bodies and with the value of plastic surgery. Far from seeking hyper-masculinity, as the stories reported in this chapter illustrate, these men are actively seeking ways of re-writing the story of their embodied self.

Goffman's (1963) description of "passing" points to the body as a key site of self management, as problematic bodies become texts of spoiled identity and interpreted as "stigma signs." From time to time, the structure or natural appearance of one's body is identified as socially problematic; as in the case of stigmas of height, hair, skin, or size of body part(s). By modifying the body's structure as a passing technique, sometimes in invasive and radical ways, people strive to permanently remedy a physical attribute that is deeply discrediting across a spectrum of social circles.

Cosmetic surgery has become, for a wide range of Canadian men, both a passing and covering technique intended to address culturally identified "deficiencies" in contemporary masculinities. Once almost exclusively associated with the pursuit of femininity, cosmetic surgery is now inserted into the body modification practices of a panorama of men, and intersubjectively constructed by them as a tool for fixing aged, overweight, or unattractive masculine bodies. Indeed, cosmetic surgery allows for the literal "re-drawing" of the body into a more culturally recognized, and in some cases hyperbolic, masculine form. Surgery allows men to "(sur)pass" the natural body that is limited or deficient along preferred gender lines. An inspection of the most common invasive and non-invasive cosmetic procedures received by Canadian males highlights how men modify their bodies to fashion veritable aesthetic "masks of established masculinity" in social settings replete with gender doubt, contestation, anxiety, and normative flux. In analyzing narratives collected with male cosmetic surgery patients, and drawing on Goffman's dramaturgical analysis of passing processes, this chapter attends to the contemporary "crisis in masculinity" and reads the cosmetically altered male body as a "fugitive sign" (Goffman 1963) within the symbolic/institutional gender order.

The Crisis in Masculinity

Estimates suggest that nearly 10,000 Canadian men have received some form of elective cosmetic procedure in the past decade, with rates rising sharply in the past five years – a 20 percent increase in participation from 2003–2004 alone (Medicard 2004). In reviewing the most popular forms of elective surgery one immediately gains a sense that men are actively seeking medical-aesthetic solutions to problems of public face work. The embodied performance of masculinity through body modification rituals illustrates the primacy of scripted display in "doing" public identity. The collective willingness of increasing numbers of men to pursue surgery in the pursuit of a more youthful, vibrant, attractive, and healthy-looking body perhaps, at least on the surface, signifies how men's collective sensibilities, or "habituses" (Elias 2002) are shifting; stated differently, it may suggest that men are reframing the parameters of "established" (Elias and Scotson 1965) constructions of masculine body performance to include cosmetic bodywork. In Goffman's (1959) terms, these new codes of "body idiom" among men suggest that social constructions of masculinity may be in flux. However, if social/physical presentation tactics closely jibe with the performance of gender roles in everyday life, we must ask precisely what new forms of masculine bodywork represent.

Sociologists have linked the performance of non-traditional male bodywork with a "crisis in masculinity." Horrocks (1994) and Whitehead (2002) contend that with the gendered fracturing of family, economic, political, educational, sport-leisure, technological-scientific and media power bases, masculinity narratives have been challenged across most social institutions. As such, men no longer possess exclusive ownership over the social roles once held as bastions for establishing and performing masculine hegemony. Hise (2004) and Tiger (2000) suggest that with an increased presence of femininity in most social institutions, a resulting "masculine anxiety" has developed. Couple such masculine anxiety with the proliferation of gender equity movements, ideologies of political correctness, and the spread of misandry in popular media (Nathanson and Young 2000), and realize why some men perceive the existence of a cultural war against men/masculinity in countries like Canada. In the midst of "the crisis," men tend not to acknowledge or embrace new masculinities – despite discourses regarding metrosexual or ubersexual masculinities – but rather retrench themselves into traditional, essentialized and hegemonic masculine images and embodied performances. Increasingly, men are discovering innovative ways to re-write and re-perform their embodied selves as socially powerful.

For the most part, masculinity tends to be framed by gender researchers along very narrow conceptual lines, especially by symbolic interactionists (see Grogan and Richards 2002), who have long been criticized for downplaying the "structuring" aspects of gender in embodied public performances. Very few have studied, for instance, how "everyday" men engage bodywork in order to appear as a "regular guy," or have connected such body ritual to broader cultural critiques of masculine hegemony (see Monaghan 2002). Here, we might consider how re-writing the body through cosmetic surgery produces a body narrative outlining conformity to preferred codes of masculinity. This body narrative, according to Frank (1995) is a "mirroring" body narrative. Or, we might analyze how bodies, through cosmetic narratives, come to articulate a sense of ennui or malaise with hegemonic masculinity; producing what Frank (1995) calls a "communicative" body narrative.

Passing and Covering in the Crisis

In *Stigma* (1963), Goffman highlights how socially discreditable individuals may go to great lengths to conceal outward physical trappings of their "deviant" identities and thereby pass as normal. Since the mid-1990s, there has been a resurgence of passing studies in sociology, with particular emphasis on how passing is not only a routine component of everyday life, but how it is, in some social circles, part of expected body idiom (see Renfrow 2004).

Sociological literatures on these instances of passing uncover how people with speech impediments and other physical challenges (Acton and Hird 2004), homeless statuses (Roschelle and Kaufman 2004), racial/ethic backgrounds (Alexander 2004), sexual preferences (Weitz 1990) or marginalized subculture affiliations (Atkinson 2003) attempt to control information regarding deviant identities/selves in everyday life. Typically couched within the analysis of impression management, extant studies generally construct passers as those who *proactively* manage their bodies/selves in order to frame their identities as compliant with social role and status expectations. Renfrow's (2004) recent "cartography" of passing broadens the theoretical range of passing techniques and purposes enacted in everyday life, via an analysis of passers as increasingly creative, reflexive, and reactive in the identity/information management process. Inasmuch, passers not only attempt to manage discrediting stigma signs they have internalized as "accurate" reflections of the self, but also implied stigmata that are misapplied to them.

In this chapter, cosmetic surgery is analyzed as a reactive passing technique used among Canadian men to confront a perceived masculinity crisis. For a portion of Canadian male cosmetic surgery patients, conceptions and uses of aesthetic body intervention are dialogical with a common fear or anxiety about being potentially targeted as a gender deficient man. These men use cosmetic surgery as a mask of masculinity; as a tool for looking like the hegemonically youthful, intelligent, authoritarian, virile, and strong male even though they experience doubt about their masculine hegemony. Through surgery, men embody and tell narratives about the everyday performance of "threatened" masculinity in Canada. Renfrow (2004:4) comments, "Masking discreditable identities with more socially acceptable ones through passing offers individuals the potential to escape the expectations others impose on them because of their group membership and related stigma." The singularity of the preferred male body image crafted through cosmetic procedures masks many of the plural constructions of masculinity embodied by Canadian men. Cosmetic "masking" procedures allow men to "(sur)pass" the crisis, at least corporeally and socially, by creating a deeply scripted self-presentation of gender confidence. In the process, narratives crafted through cosmetic surgery speak volumes about the active embodiment of the masculine self.

Meeting Patients, Understanding Men

My involvement with cosmetically altered men commenced when I first encountered a surgery patient, Les, in southern Ontario. Les exercises in a local health club I attend, and had learned about my previous research on tattooing (Atkinson 2003). Following a brief conversation, he disclosed his experiences with three cosmetic procedures: Botox injections, liposuction, and an eye lift procedure. Over the course of time, I considered the viability of a study of men and cosmetic surgery and eventually designed a field project on the subject. By the autumn of 2004, I sought out additional patients in the southern Ontario area (e.g. Toronto, Hamilton, Mississauga, London and Burlington) for interviews.

With Les's aid and sponsor, I encountered 44 cosmetic surgery patients in southern Ontario. All of the patients agreed to be interviewed for the study. Subsequently, each patient provided the names of, on average, 2–4 other male patients, and the sample expanded progressively.

Within Ontario patients typically range in age from 19 to 65, a slight majority are single, are largely middle-class, with a mean income of approximately CDN$120,000, and predominantly of Anglo-Saxon heritage (Medicard 2004). Experience with cosmetic surgery varies considerably, as evidenced by the men with whom I have interacted and interviewed. Most male patients in Ontario have undergone one or two treatments, while a minority have received extensive bodywork. The most common procedures Canadian men request includes rhinoplasty, Botox, microdermabrasion and liposuction (lipectomy). However, other men experience hair replacements, breast reductions or reshapings (gynecomastia or mastopexy), eye lifts (blepharoplasty), skin or reductions and "tummy tucks" (abdominoplasty), face lifts (rhytidectomy) and in rare cases, muscular implantations in the chest, biceps, or calves.

Most discussions with men about their cosmetic surgery started with a basic request: "So, tell me about your cosmetic surgery." I wanted the men to craft narratives from the interpretive standpoints they wished, and from starting points they deemed sensible. Over the course of time, I tactically discussed my own personal doubts, interpretations, and scepticisms about cosmetic surgery as a means of encouraging participants to share more intimate details of their personal narratives. As a "bad cop" technique of narrative elicitation (see Hathaway and Atkinson 2003), I challenged the basis of cosmetic surgery as "appropriate" masculine bodywork. Here, I wanted to inspect how practitioners justify and tell stories about cosmetic surgery to outsiders. By engaging such interactive techniques with respondents I wanted our conversations to probe motivations for cosmetic surgery, emotional accounts of its performance, and elements of patients' social biographies.

In the sections that follow, I offer a preliminary introduction to narratives of public passing and covering via cosmetic surgery. Building on Goffman's dramaturgical model, I present one reading of how men socially present and interpret cosmetic "masks of masculinity."

Men, Anxiety, and Cosmetic Passing

> I looked at my neck droop for so long before I mustered up enough courage to have it fixed ... I look like I'm twenty again; well, at least around my neck!! At least no one calls me 'turkey neck' anymore ... you have no idea how many times I wore a turtleneck sweater to avoid derision. I can't buy enough low collar shirts to show off my work.
>
> Tom, age 46, face lift patient

Tom is a 46 year-old advertisement executive living in Toronto. Although one may never glance at him and be suspicious of his "work," he is proud of his body and exudes comfort in his "new skin." Tom's narrative of cosmetic surgery is typical; he tells a story about cosmetic surgery as a pathway toward body liberation, as a vehicle for fitting in, and a technique for building self-esteem; for him, it is a technique of covering his learned fears, doubts, and anxieties about his "frail" masculinity. In Frank's (1995) terms cosmetic surgery becomes a narrative vehicle for telling a story about masculinity in remission. As part of his narrative Tom recounts his intervention in a very plain understanding of his interest in cosmetic surgery; he wanted to be "unrecognized" by others and passed over as normal.

For many men, transforming the body into something socially "invisible" motivates their projects. Stated differently, the act of cosmetic surgery becomes a process of gaining power over others' perceived stares as it tactically contours the image given to others in the social "looking glass" (Cooley 1902). As such, it represents a deliberate narrative rupture in one's life-story of masculinity, and is a designed contingency and turning point in a man's evolving sense of body and social self. As Goffman (1963) suggests, covering work is designed to minimize public condemnation of identity. Cosmetic surgery is not sought out egomaniacally, nor intended to draw social gaze to the surgically enhanced flesh. To the contrary, the intervention is intended to achieve the opposite, to allow the individual to pass into an unrecognizable crowd of "normals." A liposuction patient named Patrick (age 37) described:

There's a comfort every day in walking out of your house and knowing that people won't be looking at your gut when you pass by ... when people ignore you, it's because you are the average person, the non-descript regular guy. I was a fat kid, and then a fat man, and all I ever wanted was to look regular. Yeah, when people ignore you, wow, what a great feeling.

Like many of the men I interviewed, Patrick's cosmetic surgery stories are replete with the idea of passing as "average," of looking "regular," and not standing out. The ability to do so, these storytellers articulate, is a symbolic act of power; a power to control a portion of their public image through surgically-induced embodied work and related narratives. As discussed below, however, the "average" to which these men aspire deeply resonates with images and hegemonic discourses of masculinity. Specifically, I examine the links between looking average, fitting in, and meeting an established masculine body form. Here, three major sites of "crisis" for masculinity are linked to men's uses of cosmetic surgery and the interpretive frameworks men adopt to underpin their bodywork with cultural meaning.

Physicality, Violence, and Masculine Bodies

In a poignant analysis of the gendering of power in Western figurations, Brinkgreve (2004) comments that men's social control has been challenged along a number of lines, especially men's ability to wield violence as cultural practice. In adopting a figurational sociological perspective, she argues that men's agency for expressing aggressive affect has been curtailed seriously over the course of long-term civilizing processes. Indeed, as Maguire (1999) comments, while men have, in no way, been uniformly restricted as aggressive agents, the internal compulsion toward and external control of violence and aggression has both qualitatively and quantitatively increased in the West. This turn represents the end, to a degree, of a long-standing cultural narrative linking masculinity, unproblematically, with overt aggression.

Yet as Godenzi (1999) contends, some men interpret the cultural "attack" on violence as an explicit challenge to masculinity. Labre (2002) examines how selected groups of men perceive the restraint of the male body as a critical condemnation of and control effort on the very basis of the masculine psyche. In feeling that the masculine body is threatened, some Canadian men may be encouraged to reflectively engage in forms of bodywork to physically shore up their public masculinity, power, and stature. Here, the connotation is that men have become socially weak, and must, if only symbolically, appear physically dominant and brimming with masculinity. In Goffman's (1963) analysis, passing through cosmetic surgery is orchestrated to illustrate *what the individual is not*; it is a response to a perceived status problem among men, and a covering technique intended to produce appearances of a traditionally "in control" male. Allan (age 41) explains:

I'd never looked like a handsome guy until I underwent the hair transplantation, you know ... I'm like every other man who's lived with teasing about being bald so young. I feel almost effeminate sometimes, because baldness is positioned as weak in our culture. Women find the look totally unsexy, but all the while like to attack me as a chauvinist just because I am male. I could never win then, and [in our culture] now the only way people leave you alone and accept you, even men, is if you look good, or at least your best.

As Allan and his like-minded peers explain, men may locate substantial social power by "reclaiming" their socially challenged (male) bodies and repackaging them as desirable. Allan's narrative calls us to hear a new masculine narrative that underscores how the performance of masculinity is deeply tied to popular aesthetics. It is, in many ways a narrative adjustment to contemporary challenges to masculine identity. By drawing on long-standing cultural, or established, preferences for the fit, toned, groomed, and slender/muscular body, the men, at least from their interpretive standpoints, contest the contemporary war on masculinity.

For other men, exploring one or another form of surgery displays a peculiar sense of docility and willingness to submit the body to others. Viewed from such a perspective, the masculine man "gives" his body to a professional to be re-worked, proactively acknowledging and admitting a deficiency. It is, in some ways both a self-recognition of weakness (i.e. the failure to physically live up to a set of cultural expectations) and yet a moralistic gesture of the desire for self-improvement. It finds grounding in a middle-class aesthetic (see White, Young and Gillett 1995) that targets bodies as sites of ongoing monitoring, disciplining and identity management. Byron (age 28) comments:

I haven't spoken to a lot of people about the face peeling, because I'm so young and the reaction would probably be seriously negative. But the women I've told react in a similar way; they congratulate me for my body care. Some say it makes me sound more gentle and sensitive, and into looking beautiful ... I should have done this years ago!

At this point, men's stories about cosmetic surgery resonate with the bulk of the literature on women's experiences with the practice (see Davis 2002). When adopted to illustrate reverence toward established gender codes, cosmetic surgery for men and women is an act of (sur)passing. It is, for all intents and purposes, a hyper-real pursuit of a culturally created masculinity standard. The project of cosmetic surgery is not simply designed to "correct" a fractured masculinity, it pushes what constitutes masculinity to new boundaries of embodiment. Bodies are literally manufactured through cosmetic surgery in the desire to attain manufactured cultural constructs of masculinity. In this case, surgery makes the physically unattainable body possible and thus reifies the cultural body standard of masculinity as legitimate. Veritably, a man is able to surpass the constraining organic body and technologically craft his masculine self.

At the same time, men's involvement in cosmetic surgery, especially invasive and painful forms, might be configured as an ironically self-aggressive response to cultural associations between masculinity and violence. As sociologists of the body have commented through the study of tattooing and piercing involvement in painful forms of body modification may be interpreted as a solution to problems of emotional or psychological pain (see Atkinson 2003). Neil (age 39) suggests:

> When the doctor stripped away the layers of fat from around my waist, he removed thirty years of pain from my soul. I'd always been the fat outsider, the little boy who never quite made the cut for anything. Being inside a body that is a gelatinous prison kills a tiny piece of you every moment of your life ... when I woke up after the surgery and looked down, I felt liberated. I could, never in my life, speak to anyone about how much being heavy hurt me emotionally, and now I don't have to ... surgery is the best psychotherapy offered on the market.

Neil's perspective teaches us that the current boom in men's cosmetic surgery might be viewed as an indicator of the cultural imperative for men to not only meet emotional turmoil with self-aggression, but also as a measure of how established constructions of masculinity continue to include emotional withdrawal – indeed, a (sur)passing technique in and of itself as men symbolically manage emotionality through "internal" body work.

For men who respond to ongoing public discourses that connect men, masculinity, and violence through cosmetic surgery, the act of passing involves a degree of public emotion work. The cosmetic procedures are intentionally encoded with reframed images of the non-violent male, but simultaneously illustrate the individual's sense of masculine strength and resolve. Viewed differently, critiques about men's use of violence as a tool of social control (and thus its explicit connection to masculinity) are internalized and indirectly responded to creatively via cosmetic surgery. The cosmetically altered male body appears powerful and in-control within a cultural milieu that has "weakened" masculinity.

Institutional Control and Masculine Bodies

Although marked gaps continue to exist between the genders in relation to established-outsider power balances across most institutional settings, the men interviewed in this study believe their position as established authority figures has been dislodged by women's participation in economic and political spheres. When telling narratives about motivations underpinning cosmetic procedures, approximately three quarters (74 percent) of the men interviewed talked about feeling threatened at work by younger, smarter, and healthier looking women – especially in image-oriented business environments that equate outward appeal with intellectual competency and moral worth. Young, virile, and non-cosmetically altered women become antagonists in these men's narratives. It seems as women have secured preliminary in-roads to power sources in Western cultures like Canada, some men become fear-oriented in their disposition. Again, in Frank's (1995) terms, women's empowerment is a key "narrative disruption" in stories about embodied masculine performance in Canada, and indeed in masculine metanarratives. Resultantly, changes to body regimen among men have followed. Peter (age 54) comments:

Our company hired three new managers last year, and two of them didn't look any older than 25. What makes it worse is that they are well-spoken, bright, charming women who are also gorgeous. So there is me, an aging guy in a changing business environment who appears as if he's missed more nights of sleep than he should have. The superficiality of that realization kind of makes you sick ... but these people won't want me around unless I adapt, unless I change.

Important is that Peter's fear or "threat-orientation" encourages him to consider radical bodywork as a solution to his incompetence anxieties. Peter's masculinity, partly anchored in his ability to physically appear competent in the workplace, as Sennett (1998) might predict, is reconciled through physical intervention; here, the outward ability to "look good" through cosmetic passing supersedes concerns about his ability to perform intellectually as a business administrator.

For other men, their ascribed social positions as established workers within dense chains of interdependency are threatened by subtle implications that their bodies may appear non-masculine. As Connell and Wood (2005) document through the study of masculine business cultures, one's sense of masculinity is often validated by peers' positive comments regarding one's body image and style while "on the job". Therefore, when a man experiences persistent ridicule about his body as lacking the signs of masculinity (i.e. the fat, unhealthy, powerless body), this may manifest into a fear that others view him as inadequate socially. The image reflected in the looking-glass of social interaction is decoded as deficient in masculine terms (Cooley 1902). A man adopting such an interpretive mindset might associate his peers' lack of public acknowledgement of him as a business "expert" in any context as an indicator of their collective interpretation of his deficient body image – leading him to pass as "normal" through cosmetic surgery. Andrew (age 33) explains:

With my job, I don't have time to work out two or three hours a day, and I have to eat most meals on the run ... and most of it is not healthy. And, it's hard to lose weight, so the liposuction gave a little kick-start to the process. Now I'm not the office fat guy everyone pokes fun at and ignores. People listen to me and consider my opinions on practically everything. No one looks at a fat guy and says, there's a real go-getter ... they say the opposite, he's lazy, unmotivated and someone worth firing.

Andrew's cosmetic surgery narrative is filled with self-effacing accounts of his "bigness" and interpretations of his social inferiority. Andrew often speaks in "before" terms through his cosmetic narrative, constructing his previous body like an illness which needed to be corrected through intervention. For him, cosmetic surgery is an act of (sur)passing his "masculine" illness, and social threat management. For these men, it is a more rational and healthy response to body problems then the styles of self-starvation among young men described by Braun *et al.* (1998). Instead, it is a calculated response to long-term emotional distress. The "after" masculine body produced through and self is narratively constructed as a more real representation of one's true masculine identity.

The men who describe risk or threat at work as a motivator for cosmetic surgery equally employ selected techniques of neutralization (Sykes and Matza 1956) to account for their body projects. When challenged about the source of their concerns at work, and the perceived lack of control experienced in the workplace, men respond by arguing that cosmetic bodywork is neither morally problematic nor physically dangerous. Further still, they highlight how the degree to which they are willing to sacrifice their bodies to look masculine jibes with a sense of worth and personal dedication to succeed. Buttressing these accounts is also a present centred mentality, in that the solution to their lack of work control must be immediate. Derrick, a 52 year-old marketing expert who regularly receives Botox and microdermabrasion treatments says:

> I can't wait another 20 years to take action. I need to be the man who walks into the room and no one says, damn he looks tired. If that continues to happen, I'll be out the door. I could have experimented with herbal remedies, creams or lotions to erase the years from my face, but it might take years, if it even works. Why wait when I can have better results it only one day?

For Derrick, any risk in or potential long-term effects of the procedures is secondary to the immediate gains received from passing as young. The means-end, here-and-now mentality is, of course, directly reflective of the consumerist, commodified, and highly rationalized manner by which people come to approach bodies (and body problems) in "civilized" figurations (Elias 2002). It is only the "after" body that matters; merely the outcome of the flesh journey and not the process figuring into the narrative. The end "reveal" of the new, masculine, commodified body is the climax of the narrative. Any service that publicly "covers" his problems of masculinity is thus justified as worthwhile, particularly when the service may be purchased from a qualified medical professional.

What the above narratives underscore is the process by which men come to write and re-write their masculine bodies/identities through surgical intervention. Actively responding to a perceived control threat through bodywork is interpreted by the men as a very masculine endeavour; that is, confronting a challenge through cosmetic passing is ironically configured as a symbol of masculine power, control, courage and leadership (see Sargent 2000). As White, Young and McTeer (1994) describe in the study of how male athletes reframe the injury process as a testing ground of one's masculinity, cosmetic surgery patients often tell stories about how their willingness to endure painfully invasive surgeries in order to pass actually confirms their ability to meet social threats with masculine resolve.

Knowledge Production and Masculine Bodies

Compounding the threat some men perceive regarding their masculinity in the workplace and across institutional settings, is the type of work men are performing and the lack of spare-time exercise they partake. With more men than ever in service or information processing industries, the current generation of employed men are perhaps the most "stationary" workforce in our cultural history. Furthermore, with decreasing amounts of spare-time, dietary habits revolving around high calorie fast-food choices, and leisure time dominated by consumption and inactivity, the physical tolls on their bodies are evident (Critser 2002). The post-industrial economy and associated lifestyles, it seems, is not easily reconciled with traditional images of the powerful, performing, and dominant male (Faludi 1999).

The men I interviewed express a sense of frustration with the form and content of their work responsibilities. For these men, ritually performing daily "disembodied" or "virtual" work (i.e. computer-facilitated) encourages a mind-body separation and neglect (see Potts 2002). Roger's (age 45) words are emblematic of the disaffection some men experience with their work:

> My whole job, the entire thing, involves flexing my mind but not my muscles. Sitting at a desk for 10 hours a day, then a car for 2, then on your couch for 3 more wears your body down. Not to mention that my skin barely ever sees the light of day. At times, I can feel my face literally sagging because of my posture ... Looking in the mirror when you're forty and having a road map for a face should not be surprising. That's not who I am, that's not the image of my inside I want to project.

Instrumentally, then, men like Roger who possess such an interpretive mindset refuse to link external bodies with inner selves. Roger's body is further objectified and instrumentalized in cosmetic surgery, as he views his physical form as a site of much needed identity management. Such an interpretation of the body only exacerbates existing fears about their bodies as socially non-masculine. Once again, cosmetic surgery provides a fast, efficient, and highly rational way of alleviating these psychological strains and social discomfort:

> From the time I was 15 years old, I gained weight. I watched my diet and tried to work out, but I kept packing on inches. By the time I graduated school and started office work [computer programmer], it only grew worse, literally. Liposuction saved me from the self-hatred and the ridicule I faced from others. It's like having the clock re-set, or like a magic wand being waved and your troubles are gone.
>
> Ray, 43, liposuction patient

Narratives about the role of cosmetic surgery in eliminating the unfortunate side-effects of sedentary lifestyles are equally filled with constructions of the masculine body as "vicitmized" by enduring cultural expectations that men are compelled to labour for long hours. Men often cast work or work-related responsibilities as the enemy of masculine bodies, and their narratives contain a litany of "clues" regarding such antagonistic constructions. For men like Leon (age 37), a graphics designer living in London, Ontario, his "need" for facial surgeries results from the social pressure he experiences to work in support of his extended family:

> It's not like I can quit my job, or be there for less than twelve hours a day if I want to earn a living. No one pays me for sitting on my ass and doing nothing, they pay me for sitting on

my ass and designing! If I choose not to work, I'm choosing not to feed my family.... We come from a very traditional Italian background, and it's not questioned that I am the sole provider.... There's an unspoken rule that a man who cannot provide is not really a man.

For nearly ten years, Leon's work habits have, in his terms, "weathered" his body. The three facial surgeries he has received temporarily remove the unwanted "marks" of weakened masculinity from his appearance. Like other men, Leon configures his surgical preferences as a symbol of his dedication to looking his best, even in the context of incredible social/work pressure. This, for Leon, is a decisively masculine (sur)passing response to the social problems inherent in everyday life.

Still, when confronted about such constructions of cosmetic surgery, the men employ another set of neutralization techniques. For the most part, these include classic "denial of victim" narratives. Steve (age 48) tells us:

Why should anyone else care if I did this (Botox)? I'm not hurting anyone, or even myself, so whose business is it? No one should even try to tell me what to do with my own body!

The aggressive posturing Steve adopts might be described as quintessentially, or at least traditionally, masculine. Steve refuses to have his body choices or passing preferences interrogated, and when this occurs, he responds from an overtly powerful position of control. Others prefer to "condemn the condemners," as Alan (age 50) does, by re-directing criticism about "problematic" passing practices back toward the source of critique:

Everyone who picks on me for having my skin re-surfaced I bet never thinks about the million ways they change their bodies every day by going to the gym or eating low-carb, kill yourself diets.

Ironically, while men like Alan frequently position themselves as victims of work through their cosmetic surgery storytelling, they vehemently deny personal victimization in the cosmetic surgery/passing process. Quite predictably, as Davis (2002) mentions, these men never pathologize invasive body interventions as self-victimizing. Instead, they prefer to reframe surgical intervention as masculine character building; that is, the courage associated with partaking in cosmetic surgery is highlighted as a powerful and self-controlled response to their identity/ body problems.

Conclusions

The men discussed in this chapter provide a conceptual composite of what they consider the ideal or "established" masculine body in a time of cultural crisis. It is a body that is at once firm, fit, flexible, and fat-free. But perhaps most importantly, as Frank (2003) notes, it is a body that exudes a sense of cultural awareness and acceptance; a form articulating a deep awareness of the perceived changing roles, statuses, and identities of the "new male". The male's cosmetically altered body is also one that is economically invested in the established cultural standard of masculinity (Schmitt 2001). And, at the same time, it is a performing body that is validated by social recognition and ongoing kudos from admiring others. In these ways and more, the cosmetically altered body is interdependent with others' constructions of masculinity, and derives social meaning from extended social interaction across a range of contexts.

The men in the study comment on how cosmetic surgery tends to be silently managed and privately experienced. At present, men do not openly discuss their cosmetic body projects with many "outsiders". Men typically express how cosmetic surgery is not mainstream masculine performance in Canada, and how an air of stigma still hovers around the practice. The men perceive themselves as, in Goffman's (1963) terms, discreditable deviants whose predilections for surgical enhancement might jeopardize their statuses as "real" masculine men. In response, the men refrain from expressing emotion about the cosmetic surgery process, and instead prefer to suffer the physical pains of surgery in silence. Almost contradictory to the previous point, the widening use of cosmetic surgery among men may be a clever technique of masculine power attainment via collective image work. In a beauty/image saturated and obsessed culture, these men glean significant attention and social accolade for their "improved" physical forms. The "beautification" of men's bodies through cosmetic surgery might be considered the poaching of a traditionally feminine technique of power attainment through the body; inasmuch, men may be colonizing a site of social control traditionally dominated by women. As Sarwer and Crerand (2004) suggest, the movement of men into cosmetic surgery could be an extension of the male gaze in Western cultures like Canada.

The analysis of men's cosmetic surgery illustrates how social constructions of gender are enacted through and inscribed on body practices. While cultural theorists have been reticent to empirically scrutinize how men actively use body modification to wrestle with masculine identity and pass as the "normal" male, the study of cosmetic surgery outlines how cultural contests involving the struggle for "gender power" are embedded corporeal performance. Rather than reaffirming a crisis of masculinity, men's narratives about cosmetic surgery may allude to how established masculinity is being reframed in innovative ways to produce traditional results: social power and distinction for men across a host of social contexts. In this way, the proverbial "song remains the same" for men, masculinity and social control.

References

Acton, Ciaran. and Myra Hird. 2004. "Toward a Sociology of Stammering". *Sociology*, 38(3):495–513.

Alexander, Bryant. 2004. "Passing, Cultural Performance and Individual Agency: Performative Reflections on Black Masculinity." *Cultural Studies – Critical Methodologies*, 4(3):377–404.

Atkinson, Michael. 2003. *Tattooed: The Sociogenesis of a Body Art.* Toronto: University of Toronto Press.

Brinkgreve, Christiaen. 2004. "Elias in Gender Relations: The Changing Balance of Power Between the Sexes." In S. Loyal and S. Quilley, *The Sociology of Norbert Elias.* Cambridge: Cambridge University Press.

Connell, Robert. 2002. *Gender.* Cambridge: Polity Press.

Connell, Robert and Julian Wood. 2005. "Globalization and Business Masculinities." *Men and Masculinities*, 7(4):347–364.

Cooley, Charles Horton. 1902. *Human Nature and Social Order.* New York: Scribner's.

Critser, Greg. 2002. *Fat Land: How Americans Became the Fattest People in the World.* New York: Houghton Mifflin.

Davis, Kathy. 2002. *Dubious Equalities and Embodied Differences: Cultural Studies and Cosmetic Surgery.* New York: Rowma and Littlefield.

Elias, Norbert. 2002. *The Civilizing Process.* Oxford: Blackwell.

Elias, Norbert and John. Scotson. 1965. *The Established and the Outsiders.* London: Sage.

Faludi, Susan. 1999. *Stiffed: The Betrayal of the American Man.* New York: William Morrow & Company.

Frank, Arthur. 1995. *The Wounded Storyteller: Body, Illness and Ethics.* Chicago: The University of Chicago Press.

_____. 2003. "Emily's Scars: Surgical Shapings, Technoluxe, and Bioethics." *The Hastings Center Report*, 34(2):18–29.

Godenzi, Anne. 1999. "Style or Substance: Men's Response to Feminist Challenge." *Men and Masculinities*, 1(4):385–392.

Goffman, Erving. 1959. *The Presentation of Self in Everyday Life.* New York: Anchor.

_____. 1963. *Stigma.* New York: Prentice-Hall.

Grogan, Sarah and Helen Richards. 2002. "Body Image: Focus Groups with Boys and Men." *Men and Masculinities*, 4(3):219–232.

Hathaway, Andrew and Michael Atkinson. 2003. "Active Interview Tactics in Research on Public Deviance: Exploring the Two Cop Personas." *Field Methods*, 15(2):161–185.

Hise, Richard. 2004. *The War Against Men.* Oakland: Elderberry Press.

Horrocks, Roger. 1994. *Masculinity in Crisis: Myths, Fantasies and Realities.* Basingstoke: St Martin's Press.

Labre, Magdala. 2002. "Adolescent Boys and the Muscular Male Body Ideal." *Journal of Adolescent Health*, 30(4):233-242.

Maguire, Joseph. 1999. *Sport Worlds.* Champaign: Human Kinetics.

Medicard. 2004. *Report on Cosmetic Surgery in Canada.* Toronto.

Monaghan, Lee. 2002. "Hard Men, Shop Boys and Others: Embodying Competence in a Masculinist Profession." *The Sociological Review*, 50(3):334–355.

Nathanson, Paul and Katharine Young. 2000. *Spreading Misandry.* Montreal: McGill-Queen's University Press.

Niva, Steve. 1998. "Tough and Tender: New World Order Masculinity and the Gulf War." In M. Zalewski and J. Parpart (eds). *The "Man" Question in International Relations*. Boulder, CO: Westview Press. pp. 109–128.

Potts, Annie. 2002. "The Essence of the Hard-on: Hegemonic Masculinity and the Cultural Construction of 'Erectile Dysfunction'". *Men and Masculinities*, 3(1):85–103.

Renfrow, Daniel. 2004. "A Cartography of Passing in Everyday Life." *Symbolic Interaction*, 27(4):485–506.

Roschelle Anne and Peter Kaufman. 2004. "Fitting in and Fighting Back: Stigma Management Strategies Among Homeless Kids." *Symbolic Interaction*, 27(1):23–46.

Sargent, Paul. 2000. "Real Men or Real Teachers? Contradictions in the Lives of Men Elementary Teachers." *Men and Masculinities*, 2(4):410–433.

Sarwer, David and Charles Crerand. 2004. "Body Image and Cosmetic Medical Treatments." *Body Image: An International Journal of Research*, 1:99–111.

Schmitt, Richard. 2001. "Proud to be a Man?" *Men and Masculinities*, 3(3):393–404.

Sennett, Richard. 1998. *The Corrosion of Character*. New York: WW. Norton & Company.

Sykes, Gresham and David Matza. 1956. "Techniques of Neutralization." *American Sociological Review*, 22:664–670.

Tiger, Lionel. 2000. *The Decline of Males: The First Look at an Unexpected New World for Men and Women*. New York: Griffin Trade Paperback.

Weitz, Rose. 1990. "Living With the Stigma of Aids." *Qualitative Sociology*, 13(1):23–28.

White, Phil, Kevin Young and James Gillett. 1995. "Bodywork as a Moral Imperative: Some Critical Notes on Health and Fitness." *Loisir et Société*, 18(1):159–182.

White, Phil, Kevin Young and William McTeer. 1994. "Body Talk: Male Athletes Reflect on Sport, Injury, and Pain." *Sociology of Sport Journal*, 11 (2):175–195.

Whitehead, Stephen. 2002. *Men and Masculinities: Key Themes and New Directions*. Cambridge: Polity Press.

Chapter 18

The Pregnant/Birthing Body: Negotiations of Personal Autonomy

Rachel Westfall

Pregnancy has clear physiological beginning and end. Yet, the protagonists and antagonists of pregnancy stories are less determined by biology; their stories are framed by social organization. Rachel Westfall's chapter reports in detail the complex process of interaction whereby a pregnant woman and the medical establishment claim ownership over both the pregnant women and the unborn. Through her stories we learn how health care in the modern welfare state is the result of intersecting practices of individual care of the self and institutionally mandated care of medicalized subjects' bodies.

Sociological perspectives on the body can contribute to our understanding of the impact of medical management on the experience of illness, birth, death, sexuality, and other life events (Turner 1992). Medical narratives have subordinated personal, lay, and other alternative narratives of health and illness in modern times (Frank 1995). Regarding illness, Frank (1995:6) described the "obligation of seeking medical care as a *narrative surrender*". Yet, a narrative approach has rarely been used in critiques of medicalized childbirth.

This chapter considers the narrative construction of one woman's experience of childbearing in Canada. I consider the ways in which women negotiate their personal autonomy, choosing to give health professional access to some (but not all) aspects of their private lives, including information which is pertinent to accurate medical diagnosis. Drawing and redrawing the line between the public and private self, women actively shape their experiences of childbearing. Their narratives represent their experience, but also serve to shape that experience (Miller 2000). While built in part out of a locally available stock of narrative resources and embedded in societal institutions (Holstein and Gubrium 2000), these narratives nonetheless present an avenue for self-construction and personal agency.

I begin by examining the literature on the dominant discourses of medicine and public health, considering how these discourses impact the subjective experience of childbearing. I then turn to one woman's childbearing narratives to illustrate how these discourses enter her stories, and how she attempts to resist the subjugation of her own narratives.

The Body in Pregnancy and Childbirth

The process of medicalization is said to limit personal choice and agency, while encouraging dependency on the health care system (Lupton 1997). The medicalization critique of childbearing has taken various forms. Feminist scholars have critiqued medicalization on the grounds that it affects the lives of women more profoundly than those of men (Riessman 1983). Medicalized childbearing can be seen as an interruption in women's accustomed bodily autonomy, as it entitles health professionals access to the body and its intimate history. Some classical feminist writings point to the failings of medicine, while suggesting alternative approaches to maternity care such as midwifery care and home birth (i.e. Oakley 1984; Romalis 1981). Others have described how dominant public perspectives on childbearing impact the experience of pregnant embodiment (Duden 1992; Martin 2001; Young 1990).

Young (1990) and Mackenzie (1995) described the unique phenomenological experience of childbearing as one in which the woman's bodily boundaries shift, on account of her changing physique and the fact that she now contains an additional living being. Longhurst (2001a,b) saw the shifting bodily boundaries of pregnant women as a threat to themselves and society, particularly as they have the potential to leak tears, vomit, and "show". Like cancer patients whose "coherent bodily boundaries erode" (Waskul and van der Reit 2002:487), Longhurst's pregnant respondents experienced abject embodiment. Like the obese or disabled person, in the late stages of pregnancy, a woman may experience her body as a "spectacle – a visible object within the field of social space" (Moss 1992:182). The inability of women to conceal pregnancy in its later stages, the potential for fluid leakage, and the uncertain nature of the timing and outcome of delivery, are all reflected in the dominant societal discourse regarding the fragility and unpredictability of the pregnant body. This discourse, in turn, reinforces the medicalization process.

Martin (2001) and Young (1990) both portray medicine as an interruption in the self's narrative of the body, alienating women from their experiences of pregnancy and birth. Others have noted that prenatal monitoring can have specific implications for women's embodied experiences of childbearing. In a historical analysis, Duden (1992) showed how internal signs of pregnancy, such as quickening (the first movements of the foetus to be felt by the expectant mother), have been replaced by more efficient diagnostic tools such as urine tests, blood tests and ultrasound imaging.

Medical technology has granted women the earlier detection of pregnancy and the reassurance that their unborn children are healthy, but these changes have come with accompanying costs. First, this technology renders public information which was once knowable only to the woman herself. Young (1990) suggested that medical knowledge directly competes with women's embodied knowledge of pregnancy. Additionally, Duden (1992:336) argued that a woman's experience of childbearing is shaped by medicine in a manner which is highly politicized: "science uncovers and professionals mediate her womb as a public space. Her flesh becomes the stage whose proceedings are of immediate interest to the state and the body politic, to public hygiene and the church, and also to the husband."

For some women, a second cost associated with the use of prenatal diagnostic technology has been their peace of mind and enjoyment of pregnancy (Rothman 2001). Related to this, a third problem is technology's use in the expansion of surveillance and the discourse of risk which overshadows everyday life.

Risk Discourse

Foucauldian scholars have explored the concept of surveillance medicine, which monitors not only the health of individuals, but that of populations. Surveillance medicine involves the identification of risk factors which point to the possibility of future illness (Armstrong 1995). It uses epidemiological statistics (Woodward 2003) and moral arguments (Howson 1999; McKie 1991) to locate individuals within a framework of relative risk compared to the rest of the population (Lupton 1999).

In the realm of surveillance medicine, individuals have a personal and social obligation to stay healthy: a "duty to be well" (Howson 1999:402). This is particularly true for pregnant mothers, who are held responsible not only for their own health, but also for the health of their unborn children (Lupton 1999). In lay and clinical settings, pregnant women are given extensive self-care advice, aimed at the avoidance or minimization of risk. Women are held responsible if they reject this advice or fail to seek regular prenatal care, and they may be found criminally as well as morally negligent if their infants are not born healthy (Lupton 1999; Pollitt 2003; Tsing 1990). This form of "victim-blaming" (Ryan 1976) was problematized by Lupton (1993), as it passes the responsibility for illness onto the individual, while de-emphasizing the structural factors which have contributed to the likelihood of illness. In pregnancy, this discourse may lead to critical self-examination as well as stigmatization, two processes which can contribute to the dissociation of the self from the body (Moss 1992).

Risk discourse is pervasive in both lay and medical literature for pregnant women and their care providers. Below, I will illustrate how it is also found throughout the childbearing narratives of one woman.

Risk Management and Negotiations of Personal Autonomy

The remainder of this chapter draws upon the narratives of a woman whom I will call Sally. I interviewed Sally twice in 2002, towards the end of her first pregnancy, and again postpartum. These interviews were part of a larger study of 27 women's experiences of childbearing in British Columbia, Canada (Westfall 2003; Westfall and Benoit 2004). The interviews were tape recorded, transcribed, and thematically analyzed. For this chapter, I returned to the transcripts of a single respondent and examined it in greater detail.

I relied upon several key works on illness narratives to guide my analysis (Bury 2001; Frank 1995; Hyden 1997; Riessman 2003). Following Charmaz (1991), individuals may experience pregnancy, like illness, as an interruption or intrusion in their lives, or they may immerse themselves in the process. While a chronic illness narrative model is not a perfect fit for pregnancy and childbirth, a preferred framework is, at present, unavailable. In popular, medical and scientific discourse, childbearing is a natural occurrence; it is not a disease. Nonetheless, the process of medicalization has placed childbearing conceptually within an illness framework, and its chronology resembles that of acute illness.

In the study region, women have a choice between physician or certified midwifery care, both of which are funded through the public health care system. The research sample included women from both of these styles of midwifery care, as well as some women who, like Sally, had hired a lay (non-certified) midwife, or who were planning an unassisted birth. Sally's pregnancy and birthing narratives were chosen for this chapter due to their richness regarding medical surveillance, risk management, and negotiations of personal autonomy. While each woman's childbearing experience was unique in many ways, parts of Sally's narratives reflect the voices of the other research participants.

Narratives of Pregnancy and Birth

At the time of our first interview, Sally was a massage therapist living in an urban centre. She was pregnant with her first child, and she saw childbearing as an aesthetically pleasing experience in herself and friends:

> I've had a couple of friends who've really inspired me. One of them is just a natural mum. I was always in awe, and just amazed. She had so much confidence, you know, and I remember seeing black and white photos of her after her first one was born, and just thinking, this woman is so brave, and so strong, and just knowing that it's the right thing, and just beaming and beautiful, and sexy and all those things. And I just thought, that's just the way to go. You know? Like, none of this, oh I'm pregnant, and I'm sick, I hurt all the time. So I feel like I've had some really positive, positive influences. So I feel that's affected my pregnancy. I've been able to work full time, you know, be really active, I still go out at night and dance with friends, and go for long walks.

While Sally said she believed that a positive attitude towards pregnancy had helped shape her experience, she chose to avoid extensive contact with people who would view her pregnancy in a different light. She had interviewed several potential maternity care providers, including an obstetrician and a lay midwife, before deciding to opt for the lay midwifery care. Meanwhile, for most of her pregnancy she had seen her family physician for standard prenatal testing.

> I saw my personal MD up until 24 weeks. She tends not to see women after that, she refers out. So, up until that point, you know all the blood tests and what not were done by her. We had a fairly good rapport. She was a little bit concerned about my choice to do a water

birth, particularly with this individual. But, she was, she was fine, you know. She went through all the medical procedures, just as an MD would. And though she recommended that I'd probably want to have medical backup, she also suggested that no obstetrician in their right mind would back me up knowing full well what I was deciding to do. So that was a bit of a difficult conflict. So since then I have not sought out any medical doctor for prenatal care.

Sally's choice to avoid contact with doctors in the latter part of her pregnancy was not unique among the participants in this study. Indeed, several other women talked about avoiding contact with their family doctors, as well as avoiding other people who might question or condemn the choices they had made. Meanwhile, they filtered the information they did receive through those channels, choosing what they wished to comply with, and rejecting the rest. This often took place within a framework of risk discourse, and in some cases the women felt better qualified than their doctors in making decisions about self-care.

The blood tests and everything seemed fine. She considered me low risk. Quote, unquote. But she was very quick to say, well here are the pamphlets for [the local hospital] that you'll want to look through, because that's where you're going to deliver, and these are the prenatal vitamins that you should take and there's a drug store just around the corner there. So I walked out of the first session going okay, well, you know she's doing her job, but I don't want to take prenatal vitamins that are stuffed with fillers. I want to go out there and research what my body should really truly be getting. I don't want to go to the drug store and down these pink pills that, I don't know what's in them. So thankfully for me, my partner's mother is very well informed, and she knows of natural, very high quality vitamins that you cannot even buy in a store, you have to order them. And as soon as his mum found out that I was pregnant, she was sending me information through doctors' journals. So I mean, doctors who have done research on this product, who are in the know, were very happy to bring this to the attention of their clients and patients.

Sally indicated her scepticism of risk discourse by inserting "quote, unquote" after her reference to being "low risk". Meanwhile, she rejected her doctor's advice regarding prenatal vitamins, opting to listen to someone who she considered a more authoritative source of information (her mother-in-law). This sort of lay health advice was commonly reported by the research participants, and like the advice given to Longhurst's (2001b) pregnant respondents, it was not always received favourably. Nonetheless, Sally saw her mother-in-law as a tremendous resource, and she trusted her advice over that of her physician.

[Sally]: So, when I went around to my second appointment [with my family physician], she said, how are the prenatal vitamins, I said great! She said, what kind, and I said, oh you know, the kind you get at the drug store. So, I kind of felt like I didn't want to tell her.
[Rachel]: Why was that?
[Sally]: Because she was telling me what to do, she was advising me. And although, I mean I'm sure she would have accepted it, I'm sure I could have just told her. I just didn't want to stir the pot with that relationship. I know where she stands, and I knew that

what I was doing was right, so at that point I thought well, I know what I'm doing. She knows what she's doing, and I know that I'm taking responsibility and I'm happy with this choice. As long as she knows that I'm taking a prenatal vitamin, she'll probably be happy just to do her little check mark in her box, and move onto the next question.

Sally seemed to think that taking someone else's advice would be a direct challenge to her doctor's authority, so she gave the doctor the impression that she had followed her advice. She described her physician as someone who was merely doing a mechanical job, whereas she believed that her mother-in-law saw her and responded to her as a unique individual. Nonetheless, she had given her doctor some other information which would follow her and impact her future encounters with the health care system.

I did go and see this other obstetrician, because I knew my doctor was only going to see me until 24 weeks. The first four minutes of my obstetrician's visit was absolutely wonderful. She greeted me with very warm energy. And I guess that was because I didn't tell her straight out that my plan was to do a water birth, but because the files from my personal MD were forwarded to her, she saw that in the files, five minutes into the visit. And she obviously had something up with that and some issues around that, and was very vocal about that. And it really stems from her own take on what's safe and who should be doing what.

While the obstetrician framed Sally's birthing plan within a discourse of risk, Sally rejected that discourse, pointing to the physician's training as the reason behind her objection to a home water birth.

I appreciate that because when you go through the training, and you believe in what you do, and you're good at what you do, and you've established your reputation, then it's something that you want to protect. So, although I have respect for that profession a hundred percent, I felt that the way in which she took to my choice was quite harsh and negative. So I thought, oh okay, well, everybody has a right to their opinion. As I have a right to choose which way I want to give birth. But I could just tell that it's the system that creates those walls and boundaries, which is unfortunate. Anyways I could see that that was a struggle for her. Even though she wanted to be a part of my process, she had to protect herself.

Here, Sally described medical knowledge as opinion; she saw it as one narrative among many possible narratives. This reflects the postmodern experience of medicine described by Frank (1995:6) in which the individual tries to hold onto her own narratives, resisting "narrative surrender," but Sally has gone a step further than Frank's ill respondents. She has chosen not to view her pregnancy as an illness requiring medical management, but rather as a holistic "process." Her narratives hinted at the powerful tension that lies between these competing discourses. Not only did she refuse narrative surrender; she also refused to surrender her *body* to medicine. And yet, paradoxically, much of her prenatal narrative centred on issues of risk and health maintenance. She spoke at length of the herbs she was using to support her health in pregnancy, with specific reference to "the uterus" with a disembodied voice that is more commonly associated with medical practice (Young 1997).

> I'm using Blossoming Belly tea, and it says it's a nourishing and tonic tea blend, safe throughout pregnancy. Nettles, which help increase levels of iron I believe, or maintain levels of iron in the body, which is really important. Raspberry leaf, which helps prepare the uterus, strengthen the uterus. And I'm not too sure about these other ones, what their properties are, but also safe in pregnancy. I guess I started taking it in the third month, and I'll use it till the end of the pregnancy. But then I'll also start taking something with blue or black cohosh in it, a month from now. And that really helps prepare the uterus.

Sally's earlier reference to her mother-in-law's high quality vitamins, along with her incomplete understanding of the medicinal properties of the herbs she was using, suggested that the narrative she chose was not entirely of her own making. This is not a novel reflection. Holstein and Gubrium (2000) noted the importance of local cultures and sub-cultures in framing narratives and thereby shaping self-construction. Sally chose to construct her narrative around popular holistic health discourse, an example of what Somers (1994: 631) called "counter narratives," as they contradict dominant belief systems. Meanwhile, Sally drew upon risks discourse when talking about drugstore multi-vitamins and other pharmaceutical products.

> I told my dentist that I was pregnant and I didn't feel comfortable doing a two week course of this bleach product, his eyebrows kind of went together and he said, well why not? You know, it's only a small amount and only a little bit leaches into your system. And I'm thinking, okay, fine for me, I'm a grown 28 year old adult that's developed my nervous system. I know enough about the neural tube and how it develops and how early gestation is such a critical time. I said to him, I'm not comfortable doing this. And he said, there are no studies that prove that this has had damaging effects. Well, okay how long has this particular product been out on the market? And, I mean nobody is going to know the effects that this is going to have. Even if you did do a study. I mean it's ridiculous to play that card.

While Sally was eager to embrace scientific evidence for the efficacy of her chosen brand of vitamins, she was equally prepared to reject scientific evidence supporting the use of the tooth whitening product in pregnancy. She made use of medical and scientific narratives to validate her choices in both cases, alternately accepting or rejecting the outcomes of "studies."

Sally's experience of pregnancy involved a tapestry of narratives, some competing, and others complementing one another. As we have seen, a narrative of risk was one of these, and Sally was actively engaged in risk management throughout her pregnancy. And yet, risk did not enter into her vision of giving birth, from this prenatal vantage point. Her anticipation of her birthing narrative was full of excitement and wonder; she anticipated it as a spiritual quest (Frank 1995) and a potential learning experience.

My vision for the birth is to have a water birth at home, hopefully with the birth attendant of my choice, if all goes well, with my partner. And to just go with the waves of whatever happens when we birth. This is a new experience for me. Yeah, I feel really curious and excited. And there's an element of fear, but I don't feel that, at this point anyway, that it's going to be crippling; I'm more excited. I really see it as a journey and a real spiritual part of a woman's life. It's so exciting. I've got shivers all over my body right now just looking at you with your little one right here, just going, it's just a phenomenon.

Nonetheless, when the time came for Sally to give birth, risk discourse crept back into her narrative, despite her efforts to keep the medical world at bay. Her labour was much longer than she had expected, over three days altogether, and her amniotic membranes had ruptured at the beginning of the process. Both of these circumstances factored into her evaluation of risk, and were compounded by the fact that she developed a fever.

Three days, it was actually longer than three days, it was three and a half days. My water broke, right here, and I went into the washroom so I wouldn't get it all over the carpet. And so we jumped into bed, and then an hour later, contractions started. And I don't have the exact length of the contractions, but I wrote it all down for the first twelve hours. I want to see how this goes, right? Yeah, and it just, it just ended up being 24 hours of the same thing, which wasn't too intense, like I wasn't in a lot of pain. And I thought, hey, this is going to be okay. Because our midwife wasn't available, we decided we were going to try and do an unassisted birth. And unfortunately, because it was dragging out for so long, I just knew that this was longer than I ever anticipated. And I started to feel that I needed that support of whoever was in the area at the time.

At this point, it became apparent that Sally's idealized narrative of childbirth was in need of adjustment. What she had envisioned for the birth was proving to be fictional. Her birthing narrative entered a phase of "chaos" (Frank 1995:97) wherein a sequence of strangers entered her home, each attempting to discern why her delivery was taking longer than expected.

So I think it was the second day that two women came. I think one was a training doula, and the other was a midwife from the States. They were coming from all around. Over the course of the three days, six women came. No, sorry, five, five. Yeah. So I felt like I had lots of, lots of different types of support throughout the three days. Two days later, oh, a new set of helpers. But it seemed that, like I said the 24 hours, was like the same thing, for 24 hours, not really progressing into stronger, or, yeah, and into the second day, it's all kind of a blur. They got me doing some different breathing techniques, and I tried, and that seemed to help. By the third day, I was so fatigued. And my partner was saying, maybe we should think about going to the hospital. You know, just in case. And so before any of that happened, one of the midwives who'd ended up there on the last day, she took my temperature, and I had a fever. So that was sort of an indicator that, hmm, maybe it's time now to have some extra support, because three days is a long time to have your water broken. And I think, in the medical world anyway, if your water's been broken for 18 hours, you're considered high risk. Well at this point, it was into the third day, so it was well beyond the 18 hours. So we figured, okay, we've done well, we've done as much as we can here, and sort of just read what everybody else was feeling, and what I was feeling, and what my partner was feeling, and felt it was time to go to the hospital.

With the progressive shift from a private to a public arena, Sally's birthing experience evolved from one which she constructed herself, in private with her partner, to one which was shaped in part by a number of support people. Her narrative chaos was apparent in the temporal discontinuity of her narrative and her confusion about who had visited her home. This chaos was resolved by her decision to transfer to hospital, at which point her narrative became temporally ordered again.

Though Sally had conducted her own risk assessment, she did not want to be received as an emergency case. Like several other research participants (Westfall and Benoit 2004), in order to avoid a high-risk label, Sally carefully edited the information she gave to health care professionals.

> Actually we didn't end up telling [the hospital staff] it was the third day of labour, but it was 18 hours ago my water broke. We didn't want them to go all crazy on us. But they did anyways. They got really crazy on us, because they were like, well who was your prenatal support, who was your obstetrician? You wanted to do a what, an unassisted birth? So one doctor in particular actually approached my partner and gave him a mouthful about how irresponsible, and how dare you come in here without knowing that this is very serious what you've done.

While this doctor viewed Sally's choice to attempt a home birth as highly risky, she dismissed his objections, pointing to his youthful inexperience as the reason for his strong opinions. Again, this points to her paradoxical use of medical discourse to validate her choices, while rejecting medical discourse when it contradicted her opinions. At any rate, she had no conflicts with the other hospital staff members. Perhaps it was her air of self-assurance that enabled her to negotiate the care she wanted. Whatever the reason, she was quite satisfied with the events that followed.

> Because we were coming from an unassisted birth, supposedly at home, they knew that I was really serious about doing it as naturally as possible. But I'm sure they would have wanted a c-section by that point. Although they didn't appear nervous, they were like, well this is serious. Little did they know that actually it was more serious than we let on.

This last sentence reveals that Sally was aware of the level of risk she was exposed to, yet she still chose to conceal it, actively resisting the assumption of an illness role and rejecting the imperative for narrative surrender (Frank 1995). For Sally, entering the hospital was in itself a transgression, given her plans for a natural home birth. Having gone that far, she wished to retain the right to choose what would happen next, and she believed that the minimization of risk perception (on the part of hospital staff) would help her to achieve this.

> I really didn't want to have any drugs, or a Caesarean, and I was starting to really fatigue. So they suggested that you know, I just wait it out. And they just monitored me, so I was all hooked up to monitors and whatnot. The obstetrician was excellent. She said,

well, these are the options, and then she stepped back and let us make the decision. She didn't say, you should do this or that. I was really impressed. My partner and I finally just weighed out all the options, and because now I was in quite a bit of pain by the end, we decided to get an epidural, because I was so fatigued. And also that would mean that I could go from the 9 centimetre phase at that point and give birth to her vaginally without actually having the pain of the contractions.

For the rest of the delivery, medical measures remained a prevalent part of Sally's birthing narrative. These measures appeared in the birth narratives of all of the research participants who gave birth in hospital, as well as the narratives of those women who gave birth at home with certified midwives. They were the same measures that had begun to creep into Sally's homebirth scenario: measures of cervical dilation, time, and body temperature. How had they entered into the narrative of someone who had intended on giving birth at home without medical monitoring or intervention? Though Sally had originally chosen a non-medicalized birth, she was well versed in the language of medical management. This was true of virtually all of the study respondents, regardless of their personal birth philosophies, and it was not a not surprise, given the predominance of the "grand narratives" of medicine and science in Western societies (Hyden 1997:265).

Though Sally expressed no regrets about her use of the epidural block, she measured her success in terms of other medical interventions that were avoided. The tools and temporal measures of medicine gave her birthing narrative cohesiveness, though they were not the measures she had originally chosen to use. She used the tools offered by the health care system, the epidural pain medication and intravenous fluids, to override her body's messages of pain and fatigue so that she could give birth without other interventions.

Once the epidural was in, I started pushing, and in 5 hours she came out. So even that was long, because they say that they reckon half an hour to three hours is kind of the norm. But you know, they didn't suggest anything else, they didn't suggest oxytocin, or, you know? And I think it's because I had really good support. I mean, my partner was just amazing. And we had his mum in Europe calling us on the phone, a cheering squad. They could see, I think, that there was a really supportive environment, and that I was set on really doing this as naturally as possible. I think I was spent by that point. I wasn't eating, so I was hooked up to an IV as well. I had actually lost quite a bit of weight in the whole process.... And at this point, the epidural was us trying to do it vaginally. And so we did it, finally! And no, no episiotomy, no tearing, which was really great. I think because it took so long, we had lots of time to stretch out the tissue. So that was one good thing. I recovered really quickly, and I was walking around a few minutes after she was born.... It's such a natural process that you just have to trust it as much as possible. And endure. It was a test of endurance, wasn't it?

Unlike chronic illness narratives which may have no clear ending (Hyden 1997), childbirth narratives end with the delivery of the baby and placenta. Sally's narrative was punctuated with the rhetoric of the natural childbirth movement, referring to "trust" and a "natural process", despite all that she has been through. While this may seem incongruous to the reader, for Sally, it was a way of normalizing (Hyden 1997) her experiences. Her closing comments gave her childbearing narratives coherence, fitting them into her personal belief system, and successfully bringing her quest (Frank 1995) to a close.

Conclusions

Narratives are not constructed in social isolation. They reflect the experiences and perspectives of the speaker, while simultaneously drawing from a culture-bound pool of "narrative resources" (Gubrium and Holstein 2001; Holstein and Gubrium 2000). In addition, narratives are told for their listeners; narrators are performers and storytellers (Riessman 2003). Narratives are a form of self-portrayal, in which the individual highlights the personal qualities which they want the listener to perceive. In the telling, the self is engendered (Frank 1995; Holstein and Gubrium 2000; Miller 2000; Somers 1994). In addition, the teller may wish to enlighten the listener through storytelling. "Telling stories in postmodern times, and perhaps in all times, attempts to change one's own life by affecting the lives of others" (Frank 1995:18).

As a narrator, Sally spoke to a researcher who was a mother with a babe-in-arms, and also an advocate of natural home birth. While she did not know the full details of my reproductive history, she could reasonably expect me to be sympathetic to her choice of home birth. Additionally, she may have felt it necessary to rationalize her choice to transfer to hospital and receive an epidural block, given that these things signify a *lack of self-reliance* in the homebirth community. She crafted her story with a purpose, enlightening me about the necessity of the medical interventions she experienced. In order to retain social status in this alternative community, it was essential that she did not appear to have exchanged her personal autonomy for medical help. Indeed, given the context of these narratives, an essential endpoint was her reiteration of her belief in birth as a natural process.

In many ways, Sally's childbearing narratives were like those of the other women who I interviewed. Unlike Longhurst's (2001b) pregnant respondents who experienced pregnancy as a physical disturbance and an abject bodily condition, Sally described pregnancy in a positive light, celebrating the changes she observed in her body. She aspired to be a mother for whom childbearing was a smooth, natural, and aesthetically pleasing process. She worked towards this goal by means of a careful regimen of holistic self-care and a select network of support people. Yet Sally's experiences were, in many ways, shaped by the unique circumstances of her life. As a holistic health practitioner by trade, she had a hands-on, self-directed approach to pregnancy and childbirth. Her body was much like Frank's (1995:41) archetypal disciplined body, using tonic herbs and mail-order vitamins in an effort to assert "*predictability* through therapeutic regimes, which can be orthodox medical compliance or alternative treatment." She sought predictability regarding the inherently unpredictable process of childbirth, for which she worked to prepare her body to "perform well." Her embodied experience of pregnancy was markedly more "active" than that described in other writings, where the body is objectified by medicine (Duden 1992; Martin 2001; Young 1990).

Sally's narratives demonstrate Bury's (1998: 12) theory that a "complicated form of subjectivity" comes to the fore as the lay person acts upon perceived health risks. Prior to giving birth, Sally perceived childbearing as a natural, and even spiritual, process in which medical intervention was viewed as a disruption in the body's narrative. And yet, she viewed the circumstances of her labour within a standard framework of health risk. Her perception of risk led to her decision to open up her body and her private space to an increasingly wider circle of support people, which eventually included hospital staff. Yet, her narrative reflected how she had negotiated with her support people for the care she needed; she acted as an agent of her own health care. She maintained her autonomy by withholding certain information that would cause her to be labelled as high-risk, and by choosing some interventions and refusing others. Accordingly, Sally's narrative clearly represents the "active patient" described in recent sociological work on physician-patient interactions (Bury 2004).

Sally was a maternity patient in postmodern times, resisting "narrative surrender" (Frank 1995:6), interweaving her own subjective experiences with other lines of popular discourse. Only selectively did she allow her body and its birthing narrative to become public, shifting the line between sacred and profane.

References

Armstrong, David. 1995. "The Rise of Surveillance Medicine." *Sociology of Health and Illness*. 17(3):393–404.

Bury, Michael. 1998. "Postmodernity and Health," in Graham Scrambler and Paul Higgs (eds), *Modernity, Medicine and Health*. London: Routledge. pp. 1–28.

_____. 2001. "Illness Narratives: Fact or Fiction?" *Sociology of Health and Illness*. 23(3):263–285.

_____. 2004. "Researching Patient-Professional Interactions." *Journal of Health Services Research and Policy*. 9(Suppl. 1):48–54.

Charmaz, Kathy. 1991. *Good Days, Bad Days: The Self in Chronic Illness and Time*. New Brunswick, NJ: Rutgers University Press.

Duden, Barbara. 1992. "Quick With Child: An Experience That Has Lost its Status." *Technology in Society*. 14:335–344.

Frank, Arthur W. 1995. *The Wounded Storyteller: Body, Illness, and Ethics*. Chicago, London: University of Chicago Press.

Gubrium, Jaber F. and James A. Holstein. 2001. "Introduction: Trying Times, Troubled Selves," in Jaber F. Gubrium and James A. Holstein (eds), *Institutional Selves: Troubled Identities in a Postmodern World*. New York and Oxford: Oxford University Press. pp. 1–20.

Holstein, James A. and Jaber F. Gubrium. 2000. *The Self we Live By: Narrative Identity in a Postmodern World*. New York, Oxford: Oxford University Press.

Howson, Alexandra. 1999. "Cervical Screening, Compliance and Moral Obligation." *Sociology of Health and Illness.* 21(4):401–425.

Hydén, Lars-Christer. 1997. "Illness and Narrative." *Sociology of Health and Illness.* 19(1): 48–69.

Longhurst, Robyn. 2001a. "Breaking Corporeal Boundaries," in Ruth Holliday and John Hassard (eds), *Contested Bodies.* London: Routledge. pp. 81–94.

_____. 2001b. *Bodies: Exploring Fluid Boundaries.* London: Routledge.

Lupton, Deborah. 1993. "Risk as Moral Danger: The Social and Political Functions of Risk Discourse in Public Health." *International Journal of Health Services.* 23(3):425–435.

_____. 1997. "Foucault and the Medicalization Critique," in Alan Petersen and Robin Bunton (eds), *Foucault, Health and Medicine.* London: Routledge. pp. 94–110.

_____. 1999. "Risk and the Ontology of Pregnant Embodiment," in Deborah Lupton (ed.), *Risk and Sociocultural Theory: New Directions and Perspectives.* Cambridge, UK: Cambridge University Press. pp. 59–85.

Mackenzie, Catriona. 1995. "Abortion and Embodiment," in Paul A. Komesaroff (ed.), *Troubled Bodies: Critical Perspectives on Postmodernism, Medical Ethics, and the Body.* Durham and London: Duke University Press. pp. 38–61.

Martin, Emily. 2001. *The Woman in the Body.* Boston, MA: Beacon Press.

McKie, Linda. 1991. "The Art of Surveillance of Reasonable Protection? The Case of Cervical Screening." *Sociology of Health and Illness.* 17(4):441–457.

Miller, Tina. 2000. "Losing the Plot: Narrative Construction and Longitudinal Childbirth Research." *Qualitative Health Research.* 10(3):309–323.

Moss, Donald. 1992. "Obesity, Objectification, and Identity: The Encounter with the Body as an Object in Obesity," in Drew Leder (ed.), *The Body in Medical Thought and Practice.* Dordrecht, Netherlands: Kluwer Academic Publishers. pp. 179–196.

Oakley, Ann. 1984. *The Captured Womb: A History of the Medical Care of Pregnant Women.* Oxford: Basil Blackwell.

Pollitt, Katha. 2003. "'Fetal Rights': A New Assault on Feminism," in Rose Weitz (ed.), *The Politics of Women's Bodies: Sexuality, Appearance, and Behavior,* Second Edition. New York, NY: Oxford University Press. pp. 290–299.

Riessman, Catherine Kohler. 1983. "Women and Medicalization: A New Perspective." *Social Policy.* (summer):3–18.

_____. 2003. "Performing Identities in Illness Narrative: Masculinity and Multiple Sclerosis." *Qualitative Research.* 3(1):5–33.

Romalis, Shelly. 1981. *Childbirth: Alternatives to Medical Control.* Austin: University of Texas Press.

Rothman, Barbara Katz. 2001. "Spoiling the Pregnancy: Prenatal Diagnosis in the Netherlands," in R. DeVries, C. Benoit, E.R. Van Teijlingen and S. Wrede (eds), *Birth By Design: Pregnancy, Maternity Care, and Midwifery in North America and Europe.* New York and London: Routledge. pp. 180–198.

Ryan, William. 1976. *Blaming the Victim.* New York, NY: Vintage Books.

Somers, Margaret R. 1994. "The Narrative Construction of Identity: A Relational and Network Approach." *Theory and Society.* 23(5):605–649.

Tsing, Anna. 1990. "Monster Stories: Women Charged with Perinatal Endangerment," in F. Ginsburg and A. Tsing (eds), *Uncertain Terms: Negotiating Gender in American Culture.* Boston, MA: Beacon Press. pp. 282–299.

Turner, Bryan S. 1992. *Regulating Bodies: Essays in Medical Sociology.* London: Routledge.

Waskul, Dennis D. and Pamela van der Reit. 2002. "The Abject Embodiment of Cancer Patients: Dignity, Selfhood, and the Grotesque Body." *Symbolic Interaction.* 25(4):487–513.

Westfall, Rachel E. 2003. "Herbal Healing in Pregnancy: Women's Experiences." *Journal of Herbal Pharmacotherapy.* 3(4):17–39.

Westfall, Rachel E. and Cecilia Benoit. 2004. "The Rhetoric of 'Natural' in Natural Childbirth: Childbearing Women's Perspectives on Prolonged Pregnancy and Induction of Labour." *Social Science and Medicine.* 59(7):1397–1408.

Woodward, Kathleen. 2003. "The Statistical Body," in Justine Coupland and Richard Gwyn (eds), *Discourse, the Body, and Identity.* Houndmills, Hampshire: Palgrave Macmillan. pp. 225–245.

Young, Iris Marion. 1990. *Throwing Like A Girl and Other Essays in Feminist Philosophy and Social Theory.* Bloomington and Indianapolis, IN: Indiana University Press.

Young, Katharine. 1997. *Presence in the Flesh: The Body in Medicine.* Cambridge, MA and London, UK: Harvard University Press.

CONCLUSION

Chapter 19

Viewing the Body: An Overview, Exploration and Extension

Clinton R. Sanders

While, as Waskul and Vannini (in this volume) and others (e.g. Holstein and Gubrium 2000:197; Shilling 2003) have rightly observed, the body has lurked in the background of the sociological landscape until fairly recently, it has not altogether been ignored. Since the work of Herbert Spencer (1820–1903) – or before – the *physical* body has provided the metaphorical foundation for thinking about the *social* body. Social thinkers who describe society as a system composed of various inter-related parts which work together more-or-less harmoniously, typically present the social system as generally healthy (i.e. orderly), evolving in order to adapt to changes in the surrounding environment, and sometimes suffering from "diseases" such as deviance and social problems.[1]

With the rise of biogenic positivism in criminological theory (see Lombroso 1876; Sheldon 1949), the human body became the overt focus of socio-etiological theory. The body was presumed to determine one's movement into a pattern of law-breaking or reveal his or her physiological propensity to misbehave.

Throughout the 1960s and 1970s the body enjoyed continued – though considerably less speculative – attention as an important element of social life. The rise of the investigation of how people communicate through the movement and relative placement of their bodies (called kinesics and proximics respectively – see Birdwhistle 1972; Hall 1969) spawned popular, practical discussions of how "reading" the bodies of co-actors could reveal hidden thoughts and desires and aid the reader in achieving various interactional goals (Julius Fast 1988 [1970]). In the 1980s, impelled by feminist critiques, academic interest in the body turned to cultural definitions of beauty and the impact those definitions have on women's identities and social experiences (see Freedman 1986; Hatfield and Sprecher 1986).

From the rise of sociology as a unique discipline to the present, the human body has also been a central, though often not overtly examined, element as sociologists have explored various occupations that employ the body (e.g. prostitution, erotic

---

1 For a discussion of this historical development see Ross (1991:3–21). For a critical discussion of the society-as-orderly-social-body view see Mills (1943). For a more contemporary use of the body analogy see Douglas (1996).

entertainment, theatrical and musical performance, sports)[2] or involve activities directed at healing or modifying the body.[3] The importation into sociology of post-modernist perspectives derived in part from psychoanalytic and Continental literary theory in the late twentieth century (Sarup 1989) resulted in a flurry of analytic interest in and discussions of the body (see Featherstone, Hepworth, and Turner 1991; O'Neil 1985; Shilling 2003; Turner 1984). Within this perspective, the body was conceived as a "text" to be "read" or, as Holstein and Gubrium (2000:198) put it, "the narrative embodiment of subjectivity." Presumably, the most accomplished readers were those most familiar with post-modernist theory. Exactly *why* the body became central to post-modern analysis is open for debate. My guess is that, given the sometimes radical critique of meaning (Rosenau 1992:25–41) central to the perspective, the body (and its immediate experience) was one of the few things a committed post-modernist could be moderately certain actually enjoyed some modicum of meaningful existence.[4]

No matter whether employed as a metaphor, implicated in the genesis of bad behaviour, of secondary interest in discussions of certain occupations and professions, or the overt focus of attention in post-modern analyses, the body clearly plays a central role in sociological thought. As Monaghan (in this volume) succinctly puts it, "sociology (is) a body relevant discipline." In what follows I want to examine certain themes that stand out in the selections included in this collection. Because creating typologies is, it seems to me, a basic element of doing sociology (see Prus 1996:141–172), I will start with a typology into which these chapters, and other body-oriented sociological discussions, might reasonably be placed. I do not see this list as definitive and there are obvious overlaps between and among categories. Next I will highlight identity, the self, and emotion – three phenomena central to symbolic interactionist thought and which are the focus of attention in a number of the selections. I move then to a brief discussion of the part the body plays in interaction and as a vehicle of communication and follow this with a discussion of a key theme in this volume – the body as an aesthetic object. Finally, and perhaps most importantly, I focus on the issue that may be found in virtually all of the chapters in this collection – the interesting, problematic, and conflictual relationship between the body and social/self control.

Central Issues in a Sociology of the Body

In one way or another, all of the selections in this volume focus on the most elemental feature of an interactionist sociology of the body – the body as a meaningful object and visibly available indicator of an acting subject within an interactional context. They emphasize that the body is the dominant vehicle of social interaction and must

---

2   For relevant, and overtly body-focused, discussions see P. Atkinson; Kotarba and Held; Rambo, Presley and Mynatt in this volume.

3   See M. Atkinson, Cahill, Charmaz and Rosenfeld, Westfall in this volume.

4   For a far more complete and systematic discussion of the place of the body in sociological thought see Waskul and Vannini in this volume.

be taken into account in all analyses of social and personal identity, constructions of the self, emotional experience, the acquisition and display of power, and other issues of special interest to interactionists. As Cooley (1964 [1902]) observed, appearance and our understanding of other's responses to it are central in shaping internal and interpersonal interaction.

The distinction between bodies that are deemed normal and those that are judged different is another issue found in many of the selections and in interactionist discussions of the body more broadly. Here, an important contrast is between works that focus on differences that are ascribed and not (at least, overtly) chosen by the actor and those that are the consequence of some measure of voluntary action. The first subcategory of the "unusual" body designation incorporates discussions of the disabled, ill, deformed, or socially disvalued body.[5] In this volume specific attention to this "dysappearing" body, as Charmaz and Rosenfeld refer to it, is found in Gardner and Gronfein's chapter on the various problems those with multiple sclerosis encounter in public settings, Owens and Beistle's and Huggins' presentations of the "polluted" black body and the "polluted" addict body respectively, and Charmaz and Rosenfeld's chapter on chronic illness.[6]

Bodies that are moved out of the normal confines of conventionality because of a more-or-less voluntary choice made by the "owners" (or "renters" if one takes a longer view) have been of particular interest to social scientists in recent years. While some have focused on more-or-less permanent forms of body alteration (e.g. Atkinson 2003; DeMello 2000; Hewitt 1997; Sanders 1989), other sociologists have attended to the social significance of relatively impermanent means of alteration such as fashion (Crane 2000; Davis 1992; Finkelstein 1991)[7] and hair style (Lawson 2003). The selections in this volume continue this focus on voluntary corporeal modification as Michael Atkinson connects men's anxieties with their decisions to seek cosmetic/aesthetic surgery, Monaghan describes body building and the desire of adherents to transform their bodies into "living art," Westfall discusses the social consequences of having a body modified by pregnancy, and Edgley takes on the commercially driven messages that "sell" fitness and health.

Following upon the work of Erving Goffman (to which all professed interactionists are indebted), the body as the centre of performance is another focus within a sociology of the body. The piece by Cahill spotlights the important distinction between bodily performances that take place in public settings or those that occur in private. Kotarba and Held's discussion of female football players, Paul Atkinson's chapter on opera, Stephens and Delamont's chapter on *capoeira*, and the material on exotic dancers offered by Rambo, Presley and Mynatt all provide insight into

---

5   For a fascinating historical and sociological discussion of ascribed physical deviance see Robert Bogdan's (1988) book on circus freaks.

6   Goffman's *Stigma* (1963) is the foundational discussion of physical "abnormality."

7   See the importance of fashion in demonstrating one's place in the social world surrounding dance/martial art form of capoeria as discussed by Stephens and Delamont (in this volume).

performance situations in which the actors are most "reflexively agentic" (Schrock and Boyd in this volume). The people described in these chapters operate within the context of staged performances and are, therefore, rather more attentive to matters of overt presentation and the supportive dramatic materials than are those who move through the more customary and casual (though no less performative) situations of everyday life.

A fifth key issue used to orient a corporeal sociology deals with the body as a necessary occupational resource or as the focus of certain occupational activities.[8] Again, Atkinson's discussion of opera, Kotarba and Held's chapter on semi-professional football, and Rambo, Presley and Mynatt's discussion of exotic dancing present forms of work centred around the body's appearance and abilities. The chapters by Charmaz and Rosenfeld, Cahill, Michael Atkinson, and Westfall all, at some level, deal with the occupational control exercised by medical doctors. We will return to the issues of who controls the body, in what situations, and the consequences of conflict around control below.

Yet another way of contextualizing the body is to view it as a source of pleasure or, alternatively, as the source of pain. Many of the chapters in this volume present these aligned issues. Crossley discusses pain and embarrassment, Kotarba and Held deal with the joy a football player experiences when "hitting" another player, Stephens and Delamont discuss the social and physical pleasures that come from demonstrating expertise in *capoeira*, Vannini and Waskul focus on the relationship between the body and ecstatic experience, and Edgley touches on pride and vanity in elements of body building.

Finally, the body may be discussed as an instrument of communication. Brandt's chapter deals directly with this issue as she moves Mead's ideas about gestural conversation between humans into a world of physical interaction that involves two very different species. Here she calls into question the exclusive centrality of human language as the vehicle by which meaning is transmitted from communicator to receiver and offers an alternative model of interaction as an intersubjective accomplishment grounded in the contact and movement of physical bodies.

Whether or not we cast bodies as socially contextualized, as disabled/ill/deformed, as voluntarily or involuntarily modified, as central to social performances, as the focus of occupational activity or an occupational resource, as a source of pleasure and pain, or as a vehicle of communication, we must, at some point, attend to three issues of central import to symbolic interactionists. Identity, selfhood, and emotional experience – the topics to which I now turn – are inextricably intertwined with appearance, movement, interpretation, and the other body-focused phenomena that make up social life.

---

8   For discussions of people (and the bodies they inhabit) as resources, see Becker (1982:78–81) and Lyon (1974).

Identity, Self, and Emotion

As Waskul and Vannini and others in this volume have emphasized, the body is most appropriately seen as a process rather than an object; it is constantly becoming something else and is an ongoing social accomplishment as those who inhabit the bodies "do" (present, alter, redefine, and so on) them. Encased in, or accompanying, these bodies are selves and identities[9] and, as William James (1961 [1892]) emphasized, a central feature of selfhood is the experience of emotion.

Some elements of the body related to self concept and identity – gender, height, skin colour, and so forth – are relatively easy to alter while other features are less amenable to change.[10] Involuntary processes such as aging and disease also shape self and social identity.

Since, as Charmaz and Rosenfeld (in this volume) emphasize, the "self and body are not the same but each informs the other" (see also Mead 1962 [1934]:136), changes in the body effect changes in the self (and vice versa). Alterations of this "embodied self identity" (Kotarba and Held in this volume) typically have either positive or negative impact on one's emotional experience. In short, one may feel pride or embarrassment due to corporeal change and related alterations in self definition. Bodily change that one voluntarily chooses holds the potential, understandably, of providing the most positive emotional experience. One of the tattoo wearers I interviewed expressed the joy he felt because of his having gotten a tattoo as being due to the mark's power to symbolically differentiate his body from that of others:

> Having a tattoo changes how you see yourself. It is a way of choosing to change your body. I enjoy that. I enjoy having a tattoo because it makes me different from other people. There is no one in the whole world who has a right arm that looks anything like mine. I've always valued being different from other people. Tattooing is a way of expressing that difference. It is a way of saying, "I am unique."
>
> Sanders (1989:51)

---

9 Dennis Waskul (personal communication) rightly points out that both older technologies (e.g. print) and new communication vehicles (e.g. the internet and cell phones) sever the body from self and its presentation.

10 Clearly, there is considerable flexibility regarding whether one must accept ascribed physical characteristics. Medical technologies and cosmetic interventions, can, if one has the funds and commitment, lead to significant physical change and the change in self definition and social identity that follow (see Schrock and Boyd in this volume). Less drastic alterations such as changing one's diet, level of physical activity, clothing style, make up, and so on, result in changes that alter the identity and self definition one carries based on physiological factors that are (presumably) more under the carrier's voluntary control. See Goode (2005: 325–328) for a discussion of the shifting boundary between voluntarily chosen physical features and those that are not the bearer's "fault."

Of course, decisions to alter one's body may eventually lead to regret and embarrassment if the change is redefined as unwise, based solely on impulse, or, most importantly, as having negative impact on one's social identity and relationships (see Sanders 1989:53–57).

A person's evaluation of his or her body and the emotions related to that self definition are deemed to be of considerable import in the psychologized perspective of contemporary culture. A "negative body-image" is associated with "low self esteem" and together they are routinely presented by various claims-makers as having significant explanatory weight when one attempts to understand the etiology of "bad" behaviour. As Vannini and Waskul (in this volume) observe:

> Psychological research has been pivotal in claims-making efforts aimed at elevating issues of body dissatisfaction – broadly defined – to wide acceptance amongst social scientists and the general public. Psychologists have been particularly adamant about stressing the psychiatric and psychological problems associated with negative body-image...

This negative body-image analysis is most commonly encountered when forms of misbehaviour are related to presumed damage to or misuse of the body. So this etiological perspective is commonly found in both popular and academic discussions of such phenomena as cutting and other types of "self mutilation," anorexia or bulimia, and drug "abuse."[11]

Underlying essentially all of the chapters in this collection is the basic principle that one's perceived appearance has significant impact on his or her social experience. One's location along the identity continuum between attractive and unattractive has much to do with his or her interactions and social chances. Attractive people enjoy higher chances of economic success (Feldman 1975) and are regarded by others as more healthy, competent, and personally appealing than are those who are less attractive (Jones *et al.* 1984:53–56). As established within the conventions of popular cultural products, moral character is reflected in physical appearance. Those who are evil are typically ugly with "bad" teeth and hair, small deep set eyes, pocked and blotchy skin, and other visible signs of their moral failure (Warner 1990).[12]

As Charles Horton Cooley (1964 [1902]) famously observed, one's self concept is constructed out of how one understands certain impressions that are given off by others in the course of face-to-face interaction. Physical appearance is the most

---

11 The current "social problem" surrounding the increasing tendency for Americans to be "overweight" or "obese" (some 60 percent of the population is said to fit into this category of physical deviance; see Stein 2005) is an interesting case in point. Despite the decidedly negative presentation in the mass media of being above a certain Body Mass Index, a recent Gallup poll found that 61 percent of Americans profess to being "happy" with their current weight (*The Week,* January 6, 2006, p. 22).

12 For an overview of bodily characteristics that are defined as attractive cross culturally see Ford and Beach (1951:85–105). There is some evidence that in Western society the relationship between beauty and positive social experiences leading to happiness is not entirely clear cut. See Douglas' (1985) discussion of the social experiences of the beautiful women he labels "goddesses."

immediate source of these impressions and is therefore centrally implicated in the linked processes of self definition and social identity construction. As such, the body is an instrument of communication whether or not the actor employs conventional verbal symbols or intends the meaning of the message received by co-interactants (Goffman 1959). We turn now to look briefly at the body in relationship to communication within face-to-face (or body-to-body) interaction situations.

The Body and Communication

The body is the central resource in the drama of social interaction (Goffman 1959; Waskul and Vannini, Charmaz and Rosenfeld in this volume). Presenting one's self – both to others and to the self (as in being "self-conscious" or "self aware") – is a communicative act. Communication takes place in identifiable situations, moves along lines characterized by specifiable relationships, and is directed to coordinating shared activities ("collective action") and ensuring some measure of social control and situational predictability (see Prus 1996:141–172).

While, at some level, all of the selections in this collection deal with the body as an instrument of communication, the issue is most in the foreground in Brandt's discussion of the cross-species relationship between a horse and his or her rider/caretaker and the communicative process by which human and nonhuman interactants express their wishes within and definitions of the immediate interaction situation. Here is a unique form of social performance in that, while directed at dramatizing the situation and establishing one's place within it, the co-interactants establish these shared understandings primarily through physical, rather than linguistic, means. The intersubjectivity is, as Brandt emphasizes, "embodied." In presenting the communicative act as not being grounded solely upon a shared ability to use linguistic symbols, Brant builds upon and furthers the work of a number of interactionists who are exploring people's relationships with nonhuman animals (see Alger and Alger 2003; Irvine 2004; Sanders 1999) and ostensibly human actors who are unable to manipulate conventional symbols (see, for example, Goode [1994] and Bogdan and Taylor [1989] on interactions with severely disabled humans, Gubrium [1989] on interactions with Alzheimer's sufferers, and Stern [1985] on social exchanges between adults and preverbal infants).

Brandt's discussion is of additional interest to symbolic interactionists because it moves beyond the nonlinguistic communication of demands or desires ("go here," "move that away," etc.) from humans to nonhumans. The interspecies interaction she describes involves the mutual communication of emotion. Clearly, what Mead (1962 [1934]) discounted as mere gesture has far greater import in the communication of fairly complex meanings and subjective experiences than has been, until fairly recently, acknowledged by interactionists. As I observe in a recent article:

> Because of the linguicentric constraints imposed by our Meadian heritage we have emphasized the differences that exist between humans and nonhuman animals.... (W)e have ignored an area of social life that is commonplace, emotionally rich, and of significant

analytic interest. Moving nonhuman animals and people's relationships with them into the realm of "sociological visibility" ... promises to shed light on commonplace worlds of sociological interaction to which conventional interactionism has, until recently, turned a blind eye.

Sanders (2003:420–431)

In her chapter, Brandt reveals the importance of the body in the communication of emotion and meaning even when interactants are separated by differing bodies, mental and physical abilities, and personal interests.

The Body as an Aesthetic Object

The body as an aesthetic construction and an object of defined beauty are also central themes in the chapters included here. Conceptions of physical beauty are important to the typological systems people share, used to give order to reality, and provide the core of culture. While corporeal aesthetics vary from culture to culture, there seem to be some common definitions of human beauty. In general, people with bodies that appear to be strong and healthy (for women in most cultures this translates into being plump and having large breasts) and who have good complexions are deemed to be attractive (Ford and Beach 1951). Body aesthetics vary over time, between racial and ethnic groups, and by locality. In a real sense, concepts of attractive (or, at least, passably appropriate) appearance are best seen as embedded in the linked phenomena of fad and fashion.[13]

Like all fashion (broadly defined) and other shared cultural interests, modes of altering the body for aesthetic purposes (e.g. "aesthetic" surgery, clothing, dieting, body modification) provide the focal centre for what Gans (1999) refers to as "taste publics" (see Crossley in this volume). Groups composed of men who have an avid interest in "overweight" women (see Goode 1996; Monaghan in this volume), or fans and practitioners of tattooing (like the National Tattoo Association), or willing "victims" of anorexia or other eating "disorders" (see Vannini, McMahon and McCright 2004) seek others with similar inclinations, pass on lore, seek status, make evaluations, and otherwise behave in ways common to subcultures (Prus 1997).

Of course, all social worlds (Strauss 1978), whether they have bodies as the central focus or not, develop evaluative principles, ethical prescriptions, and other ideological materials useful in ordering reality and acting as the foundation for action and interaction. Edgley (this volume) offers an excellent example of this as he connects physical "fitness" with moral virtue and the movement of the individual from being out-of-shape to being fit as a moral passage. Similarly, Stephens and Delamont (this volume) in their chapter on *capoeira* emphasize the body type and

---

13 Kunzel (1982) offers an interesting historical account of corseting, tight-lacing and other forms of "body-sculpture." For a discussion of the "tattoo rage" that swept Europe and the United States in the late nineteenth and early twentieth centuries see Sanders (1989:13–18).

fashions considered attractive, the key skills displayed by certain practitioners, and the aesthetic evaluations of these skills as they are acquired and demonstrated.

Because of the central role the body plays in the establishment and presentation of identity, where the "owner" locates his or her body along some aesthetic continuum (from, say, grossly ugly to outstandingly beautiful) is of special importance. Of course, one has some control over corporeal aesthetic definition and the impact of the body's impact on identity. He or she may, among other things, choose not to reveal offending parts of the body in public or private situations, reject a particular system of aesthetic evaluation and employ another, discount the legitimacy or ability of those making the appearance judgements and the validity of their opinions, or take active steps to alter his or her body in order to change its positioning on some attractiveness scale. Mechanisms such as those described in this volume provide not only opportunities to alter the body and its aesthetic evaluation but they also reinforce – for the self and others – the understanding that the body, first and foremost, ultimately belongs to its "owners." As an example, in speculating about what motivates people to acquire tattoos, a tattoo artist with whom I talked presented a view of the body as the ultimate piece of personal property.

> Tattooing is really just a form of personal adornment. Why does someone get a new car and get all of the paint stripped off of it and paint it candy-apple red? Why spend $10,000 on a car and then spend another $20,000 to make it look different from the car you bought? I associate it with ownership. Your body is one of the things you indisputably own. There is a tendency to adorn things that you own to make them especially yours.
>
> Sanders (1989: 51–52)

Viewing the body as a possession leads to an issue that is central to many of the selections in this volume. Is the person an owner of his or her body or simply renting it from the political and legal systems, the medical community, religious institutions, and other networks of power? We turn now to matters of corporeal control – both control exercised by the individual over his or her own body ("self control") or exercised by external forces who present their control of the body as for the owner's individual welfare, the good of the society, or as advancing the interests of the individual or group exercising power.

The Body and Control

At one level, control of the body is control over the self (see Charmaz 1995). At another level, control over the body is an elemental political issue (Foucault 1977). Who exercises what kind of corporeal "mastery" (Waskul and van der Riet 2002), in what situation, for what purpose are questions central to both social and self control. Since, as various social analysts (e.g. Merton 1976; Sanders 2006; Weigert 1991) have stressed, ambivalence is the dominant experience in contemporary society, people have "mixed emotions" regarding bodily control. As with many social phenomena we may see the linked issues of physical ownership and control as involving how individuals interact with themselves and how cultural forces, corporate actors, and institutional structures shape and constrain the appearance, placement, and disposition of bodies.[14] Self control refers to both the ability to personally exert control over bodily actions, as when one does not display or act on anger generated in a social exchange, and to who or what has the legitimate right to exercise control over the individual body. Many of the chapters in this volume deal directly with these matters.

Personal efficacy and relatedly positive views of the self typically are based on physical skills and appearance. Acquiring skills – becoming accomplished at a martial art, sport, or dramatic activity, for example (see Stephens and Delamont; Kotarba and Held; P. Atkinson in this volume) – offers both intrinsic satisfactions and demonstrates to the self and others that the accomplished person is in control of his or her body. Interestingly, as Stephens and Delamont (this volume) show, the process of acquiring this sort of bodily self control typically is contingent upon ceding control of the body to others. Coaches, trainers, directors and similar "experts" with license to exercise control over others' bodies frequently present their controlling actions and instructions – their exercise of power – as leading to individual achievement and the related enhancement of the individual's self-esteem or to the eventual success of the collectivity (team, performance company, and so forth). The controlling expert who appears to revel in his or her role based ability to control the bodies of others is often viewed with distaste by controllees and the public. However, this distaste is commonly tinged with admiration if the autocratic controller's activities lead to success.

Similarly, enhancing one's positive definition of his or her appearance entails offering the body up to experts. When the individual submits his or her body to the cosmetic surgeon (M. Atkinson in this volume; Joanisse 2005), tattoo artist (Sanders 1989), fashion consultant (Crane 2000), or hairdresser (Lawson 2003) he or she is giving up control in order to achieve a more aesthetically pleasing body. Again, achieving self-control entails giving up self-control.

In a carcereal society (Foucault 1975), control over bodies is more commonly taken than given. A number of the pieces in this volume focus on people's attempts to escape, or at least take a furlough from, the control exercised by parents, religious organizations (see Griffith 2004), fashion designers, and, especially, the medical "community." In this case, self control involves wresting control away from those in power. The chapters by Charmaz and Rosenfeld, Cahill, Gardner and Gronfein, and Westfall all present people offering resistance to medical definitions and practices. Basing his discussion in part on the work of Norbert Elias (1978 [1939]), Cahill presents the control of the body by the self or by others as being closely linked to the cultural ascendancy of civility and the related split between public and private arenas of action. Of particular interest are those liminal settings and situations – gyms,

---

14 Like most dichotomies, this is a false one. As Collins (1975) observes, social forces, institutions, and such like do not actually exist. What does exist are people and their relationships and the central issue regarding power – including the power to exercise control over the body – is "who gives orders, and who takes orders."

public restrooms, and medical facilities – that exist on the boundary between public and private.

Cahill focuses on an important element of this public/private cultural split – the control one exercises over excretory activities (also see Weinberg and Williams 2005). Excretion is conventionally regarded as a private activity. Yet, in medical settings (especially hospitals) where "patients reveal their most intimate bodily secrets" (Cahill this volume), excretion is both a matter of concern as an indicator of the patient's health or medical progress and a private activity observed and officiated over by relative strangers. Because they need to have assistance when performing bodily functions or need to be cleaned when they soil themselves, patients are symbolically reduced to the status of infants whose bodies (and excretory activities) are under the total control of adults.

This issue of the connections among excretion, control over one's physical self, privacy, and infantalization came to be of considerable personal concern during the spring of 2005. While on vacation I contracted a serious case of babesiosis – a tick-borne disease – and was required to spend almost two months in a hospital. Once having regained consciousness in the Intensive Care Unit, I was confronted with the helplessness inherent in the patient role. The fieldnotes I wrote toward the end of this ordeal reflect my special interest in the symbolic and practical elements of excretory control.

> The main thing I remember is the humiliation of having to ask a nurse to help me when I needed to move my bowels or urinate. The latter wasn't so bad since I could do it into a urinal-bottle but shitting was, for me, a degrading experience. A nurse would roll a commode on wheels to the bed, I was helped onto it, I eliminated (because I was being fed through a tube I had serious diarrhoea) and was helped back into bed while nurses dealt with the leavings. On occasion I didn't make it and had to be rolled and cleaned by two nurses. It was a helpless, humiliating, child-like experience.... [later after having been transferred to the rehabilitation floor] So far there have been a few high points to this whole thing but the best so far since being let out of ICU was getting my "green card." This was, literally, a green card taped to my door (along with a green band attached to my ankle) that indicated that I now no longer had to ring the buzzer to call the nurse to come and get me out of bed, help me to the bathroom, stand around to make sure everything was working ok, and help me back to bed. Getting the green card allowed me back – at least partially – into the world of adults.

My physical condition during this time made it difficult (but not altogether impossible) for me to wrest bodily control from the hands of those in charge. Medical personnel were also adept at convincing me that doing what they demanded was "for (my) own good" (something those in charge are always eager to have those being controlled believe).

Human beings (at least those in contemporary, Western, low-context cultures) frequently do what they can to resist the physical dictates of authorities. This resistance is seen in many of the selections. The women football players described by Kotarba and Held, for example, resist the cultural conventions related to women's physical abilities and what they should do with their bodies. The mother described by Westfall resists "narrative surrender" (Frank 1995) by rejecting the imposed role of "sick person" and the helplessness attached to that role. Vannini and Waskul present theorists who regard fatness as a revolutionary response to a phallocentric cultural system. Gardner and Gronfein focus on people with disabilities and their attempts to resist and avoid the "uncertainty" and imposed constraints they experience when they encounter "normals" public settings (see also Cahill and Eggleston 1994; Sanders 2000).[15]

A final issue related to the body and control is raised overtly by Huggins in his chapter on the addict's body. Here the author makes the important point that the debilitation and decay thought to characterize the addict's polluted and deviant body are established as elements of contemporary "reality" in the same way much of the rest of social reality is constructed – through mass media messages. Consequently, as Huggins observes, official control over certain bodies – in this case, the "polluted" bodies of heroin addicts[16] – is shaped by, and gains social support because of mass marketed popular cultural images (see Sanders and Lyon 1995). The media offer legitimation of the bodily control exercised by established authorities and institutions, portray appropriate and (presumably) effective models of control, and, somewhat paradoxically, demonstrate the means by which those being controlled can resist this control.

It is a rare issue, phenomenon, or object that relates to so many matters of central interest to symbolic interactionists as does the body. Attention to the body directs us to consider identity, power and control, selfhood, interaction, pride and shame, status, and deviance. But the paramount importance of the body as the focus of serious analytic attention is that it is most closely associated with the lynch-pin of the interactionist perspective – the social construction and communication of meaning. As anthropologist Olivia Vlahos (1979:12) succinctly puts it: "Vessel of life, the body is, as well, the ultimate vessel of meaning. And meaning, after all, is the beginning and the end of being human."

---

15 An issue raised by Gardner and Gronfein and these cited articles (Cahill and Eggleston on wheelchair users and Sanders on guide dogs) that is not explored at any length in this collection is the extension of the body through technical, material, and interpersonal means (see Belk 1988).

16 When I was involved in doing field research with heroin users in Chicago during the late 1960s and early 1970s, addicts and treatment personnel commonly presented the view that heroin "preserved" the bodies of male heroin users but "destroyed" the bodies of women users.

References

Alger, Janet and Steven Alger. 2003. *Cat Culture: The Social World of a Cat Shelter.* Philadelphia: Temple University Press.

Atkinson, Michael. 2003. *Tattooed: The Sociogenesis of a Body Art.* Toronto: University of Toronto Press.

Becker, Howard. 1982. *Art Worlds.* Berkeley: University of California Press.

Belk, Russell (1988), "Possessions and the Extended Self," *Journal of Consumer Research*, 15:139–168.

Birdwhistle, Ray. 1972. *Kinesics and Context.* New York: Ballentine.

Bogdan, Robert. 1988. *Freak Show.* Chicago: University of Chicago Press

Bogdan, Robert and Steven Taylor. 1989. "Relationships with Severely Disabled People: The Social Construction of Humanness," *Social Problems*, 36 (2):135–148.

Cahill, Spencer and Robin Eggleston. 1994. "Managing Emotions in Public: The Case of Wheelchair Users," *Social Psychology Quarterly*, 57 (4):300–312.

Charmaz, Kathy. 1995. "The Body, Identity, and the Self," *The Sociological Quarterly*, 36:657–680.

Collins, Randall. 1975. *Conflict Sociology.* New York: Academic Press.

Cooley, Charles Horton (1964 [1902]). *Human Nature and the Social Order.* New York: Schocken.

Crane, Diana. 2000. *Fashion and Its Social Agendas.* Chicago: University of Chicago Press.

Davis. Fred. 1992. *Fashion, Culture, and Identity.* Chicago: University of Chicago Press.

DeMello, Margo. 2000. *Bodies of Inscription.* Durham, NC: Duke University Press.

Douglas, Jack. 1985. *Creative Interviewing.* Beverly Hills, CA: Sage.

Douglas, Mary. 1966. *Purity and Danger.* New York: Routledge.

Elias, Norbert. 1978 (1939). *The History of Manners.* New York: Pantheon.

Fast, Julius. 1988 (1970). *Body Language.* New York: Simon and Schuster.

Featherstone, Mike, Mike Hepworth, and Bryan Turner. 1991. *The Body: Social Process and Cultural Theory.* London: Sage.

Finkelstein, Joanne. 1991. *The Fashioned Self.* Philadelphia: Temple University Press.

Ford, Clellan and Frank Beach. 1951. *Patterns of Sexual Behavior.* New York: Harper.

Foucault, Michel. 1975. *The Birth of the Clinic: An Archaeology of Medical Perception.* New York: Random House.

———. 1977. *Discipline and Punish: The Birth of the Prison.* New York: Pantheon.

Frank, Arthur. 1995. *The Wounded Storyteller: Body, Illness, and Ethics.* Chicago: University of Chicago Press.

Freedman, Rita. 1986. *Beauty Bound.* Lexington, MA: Heath.

Gans, Herbert. 1999. *Popular Culture and High Culture*. New York: Basic Books.

Goffman, Erving. 1959. *The Presentation of Self in Everyday Life*. Garden City, New York: Doubleday.

_____. 1963. *Stigma*. Englewood Cliffs, NJ: Prentice-Hall.

Goode, David. 1994. *A World Without Words: The Social Construction of Children Born Deaf and Blind*. Philadelphia: Temple University Press.

Goode, Eric. 1996. "The Ethics of Deception in Social Research." *Qualitative Sociology*, 19:11–33.

_____. 2005. *Deviant Behavior* (7th Edition). Upper Saddle River, NJ: Prentice-Hall.

Griffith, M. Marie. 2004. *Born Again Bodies: Flesh and Spirit in American Christianity*. Berkeley: University of California Press.

Gubrium, Jaber. 1986. "The Social Preservation of Mind: The Alzheimer's Disease Experience." *Symbolic Interaction*, 9:37–51.

Hall, Edward. 1969. *The Hidden Dimension*. New York: Doubleday.

Hatfield, Elaine and Susan Sprecher. 1986. *Mirror, Mirror: The Importance of Looks in Everyday Life*. Albany: State University of New York Press.

Hewitt, Kim. 1997. *Mutilating the Body: Identity in Blood and Ink*. Bowling Green, OH: Bowling Green University Popular Press.

Holstein, James and Jaber Gubrium. 2000. *The Self We Live By: Narrative Identity in a Postmodern World*. New York: Oxford.

Irvine, Leslie. 2004. *If You Tame Me: Animal Identity and the Intrinsic Value of Their Lives*. Philadelphia: Temple University Press.

James, William. 1961 (1892). *Psychology: The Briefer Course*. New York: Harper.

Joanisse, Leanne. 2005. "'This is Really Who I am': Obese Women's Conceptions of Self Following Weight Loss Surgery," in Dorothy Pawluch, William Shaffir, and Charlene Miall (eds), *Doing Ethnography*. Toronto: Canadian Scholar's Press. pp. 248–259.

Jones, Edward, Amerigo Farina, Albert Hastorf, Hazel Markus, Dale Miller, and Robert Scott. 1984. *Social Stigma: The Psychology of Marked Relationships*. New York: Freeman.

Kunzle, David. 1982. *Fashion and Fetishism*. Totowa, NJ: Rowman and Littlefield.

Lawson, Helene. 2003. "Working on Hair," in Douglas Harper and Helene M. Lawson (eds), *The Cultural Study of Work*. Lanham, MD: Rowman and Littlefield. pp. 370–396.

Lombroso. Cesare. 1876. *L'uomo Deliquente (Criminal Man)*. Milan: Hoepli.

Lyon, Eleanor. 1974. "Work and Play: Resource Constraints in a Small Theater." *Urban Life*, 3:71–97.

Mead, George Herbert. 1962 (1934). *Mind, Self, and Society*. Chicago: University of Chicago Press.

Merton, Robert. 1976. *Sociological Ambivalence and Other Essays*. New York: Free Press.

Mills, C. Wright. 1943. "The Professional Ideology of Social Pathologists." *American Journal of Sociology*, 49:165–180.

O'Neil, John. 1985. *Five Bodies: The Human Shape of Modern Society*. Ithaca, NY: Cornell University Press.

Prus, Robert. 1996. *Symbolic Interaction and Ethnographic Research*. Albany: State University of New York Press.

_____. 1997. *Subcultural Mosaics and Intersubjective Realities*. Albany: State University of New York Press.

Rosenau, Pauline. 1992. *Post-Modernism and the Social Sciences*. Princeton, NJ: Princeton University Press.

Ross, Dorothy. 1991. *The Origins of American Social Science*. New York: Cambridge University Press.

Sanders, Clinton. 1989. *Customizing the Body: The Art and Culture of Tattooing*. Philadelphia: Temple University Press.

_____. 1999. *Understanding Dogs: Living and Working with Canine Companions*. Philadelphia: Temple University Press.

_____. 2000. "The Impact of Guide Dogs on the Identity of People with Visual Impairments." *Anthrozoos*, 13:131–139.

_____. 2003. "Actions Speak Louder than Words: Close Relationships Between Humans and Nonhuman Animals." *Symbolic Interaction*, 26:405–426.

_____. 2006. "'The Dog You Deserve': Ambivalence in the K-9 Officer/Patrol Dog Relationship." *Journal of Contemporary Ethnography*, 35:1–25.

Sanders, Clinton and Eleanor Lyon. 1995. "Repetitive Retribution: Media Images and the Cultural Construction of Criminal Justice," in Jeff Ferrell and Clinton Sanders (eds), *Cultural Criminology*. Boston: Northeastern University Press. pp. 25–44.

Sarup, Madan. 1989. *An Introductory Guide to Post-Structuralism and Postmodernism*. Athens: University of Georgia Press.

Sheldon, William. 1949. *Varieties of Delinquent Youth*. New York: Harper and Row.

Shilling, Chris. 2003. *The Body and Social Theory* (2nd Edition). Thousand Oaks, CA: Sage.

Stein, Bob. 2005. "Americans Badly Out of Shape, Study Finds." *The Hartford Courant*, December 21, p. A3.

Stern, Daniel. 1985. *The Interpersonal World of the Infant*. New York: Basic Books.

Strauss, Anselm. 1978. "A Social World Perspective." *Studies in Symbolic Interaction*, 1:119–128.

Turner, Bryan. 1984. *The Body and Society*. Oxford: Basil Blackwell.

Vannini, Phillip, Martha McMahon, Aaron McCright. 2004. "Not a Pretty Site: Pro-Anna's Discursive De-Problematization of Easting (Dis)Orders." Paper presented at the Couch-Stone Symposium of the Society for the Study of Symbolic Interaction, March, 2004.

Vlahos, Olivia. 1979. *Body: The Ultimate Symbol*. New York: Lippincott.

Warner, Pricilla. 1990. "Fantastic Outsiders: Villains and Deviants in Animated Cartoons," in Clinton Sanders (ed.), *Marginal Conventions: Popular Culture, Mass Media, and Social Deviance*. Bowling Green, OH: Bowling Green University Popular Press. pp. 117–130.

Waskul, Dennis and Pamela van der Riet. 2002. "The Abject Embodiment of Cancer Patients: Dignity, Selfhood, and the Grotesque Body." *Symbolic Interaction*, 25:487–513.

Weigert, Andrew. 1991. *Mixed Emotions*. Albany: State University of New York Press.

Weinberg, Martin and Colin Williams. 2005. "Fecal Matters: Habitus, Embodiments, and Deviance." *Social Problems*, 52:315–336.

Index

For Product Safety Concerns and Information please contact our EU
representative GPSR@taylorandfrancis.com
Taylor & Francis Verlag GmbH, Kaufingerstraße 24, 80331 München, Germany

www.ingramcontent.com/pod-product-compliance
Ingram Content Group UK Ltd.
Pitfield, Milton Keynes, MK11 3LW, UK
UKHW021014180425
457613UK00020B/943